THE
HEALING CRYSTAL FIRST AID MANUAL

A practical A to Z of common ailments and illnesses and how they can be best treated with crystal therapy

Michael Gienger
author of CRYSTAL POWER, CRYSTAL HEALING

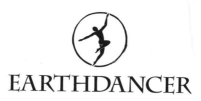

EARTHDANCER

A FINDHORN PRESS IMPRINT

Publisher's note
The information in this volume has been compiled according to the best of our knowledge and belief, and the healing properties of the crystals have been tested many times over. Bearing in mind that different people react in different ways, neither the publisher nor the author can give a guarantee for the effectiveness or safety of use in individual cases. In the case of serious health problems please consult your doctor or naturopath.

1   2   3   4   5   6   7   8   9   10   11   12   11   10   09   08   06

Michael Gienger
The Healing Crystal First Aid Manual

This English edition © 2006 Earthdancer Books
English translation © 2006 Bjorn Mieritz
Editing of the translated text by Astrid Mick, Carol Shaw and Stuart Booth.

Originally published in German as *Die Heilsteine Hausapotheke*

World copyright © Neue Erde GmbH, Saarbruecken, Germany
Original German Text copyright © Michael Gienger 1999

Cover photography: Christopher Cornwell, GB; Ines Blersch
Cover and book design: Dragon Design UK
Typeset in Garamond Condensed
Printed and bound in China

ISBN-10: 1-84409-084-1
ISBN-13: 978-1-84409-084-6

Published by Earthdancer Books, an imprint of:
Findhorn Press, 305a The Park, Forres IV36 3TE, Scotland.
www.earthdancerbooks.com
www.findhornpress.com

Dedication

This book is dedicated to all of those whose contributions
and experience have made possible its publication.

Bernhard Bruder	Elke Lißner
Wolfgang Dei	Ingrid Melcher
Petra Endres	Inge Moser
Erwin Engelhardt	Andrea Müller
Erik Fey	Gabriele Neugebauer
Dagmar Fleck	Walter Panter
Rainer Fromm	Ursula Pantze
Monika Grundmann	Gudrun Peukert
Walter von Holst	Petra Pick
Klaus Hüser	Francoise Schwab
Annette Jakobi	Rainer Strebel
Dieter Jakobi	Birgitta Zerluth
Ulla Lietmeyer	Michelle Zeuner-Mayer

It is also my way of thanking all involved and repaying
all the generous help and support I had from them
during its research and writing.

Contents

Part 3 Home Remedy Kits

Appendices

Preface

The analysis, diagnosis and treatment of patients using crystal healing have developed and advanced very rapidly since the book *Crystal Power, Crystal Healing* was first published in Germany (as *Steinheilkunde*) in 1995.

Crystal healing is a natural therapy that is clearly structured and easy to implement. This book offers mineralogical explanations for the established healing effects shown to exist within certain crystals. As a result it is a therapy, which has been adopted by many alternative practitioners. Against the background of experience that has accumulated since the publication *of Crystal Power, Crystal Healing/ Steinheilkunde*, it is now possible to summarise in a single handbook a wide range of practical applications that have been tried and tested in real, everyday situations.

So, this new handbook contains the essence of all this experience. Furthermore, it is structured in such a way that readers can use it to improve their health and use the treatments described in order to relieve and possibly heal a whole range of complaints without professional help.

However, it must be stressed at the outset that any handbook like this should not be – and indeed cannot be – a substitute for either one's doctor or alternative practitioner. Even a "simple" stomach pain or head ache can have different causes which require professional medical help – unless one can be absolutely certain that the head ache is caused by tension or that the stomach pain is caused by unwise eating (e. g. too much "fast food").

It is, however, extremely important to take responsibility for one's own health. You do not need to visit the doctor every time you have cold. Moreover, hugely increasing expenses in the health sector also make it a priority that we take better care of our own bodies and well-being.

The increasing resistance of diseases to antibiotics and other types of medication is continuing to limit their use to emergencies only – which is another excellent argument for us to treat diseases with alternative methods. In this context, crystals are particularly good for daily use; and it is perfectly valid to say this as we are dealing, to a large extent, with a treatment that has no adverse effects and is non-toxic – provided you apply the crystals in a responsibly correct way. Another advantage of such therapy is that germs and viruses do not become resistant to this alternative method – and this in itself one of the reasons for the great success now being achieved by the use of healing with crystals.

Another important aim of this handbook is to identify those crystals, among the enormous range of those available (some books mention up to 700), which actually make sense for anyone to purchase or acquire for daily use. So, as a good standby, you should always have to hand the following "first aid" crystals: Rhodonite for healing wounds or easing insect bites, Heliotrope for colds and inflammations, Pyrites for most painful conditions.

As with many other treatments, there are certain "classics" among the crystals, whose effectiveness has been proven in thousands of cases. There are also special crystals that only appear to be effective with certain individuals and in specific situations. If no clear distinctions were made here, as a layperson one would often be overwhelmed when trying to find the "right crystal" – but this book offers clarity and safety when choosing that crystal.

I have stressed later – in the final section of Part 1 – the need for a complementary approach combining the information in this book and the involvement of professional medical help. In writing *Crystal*

Healing First Aid, I have no intention of encouraging anybody to do everything "all by oneself". Just as it is harmful to hand over all responsibility to omniscient specialists, so it is also dangerous to let ambition and pride lead to ignorance of symptoms and other physical and emotional warning signs. "It will be O.K...." is sometimes all right, but not always. In addition, sometimes it is important, at certain moments of one's life, to admit to oneself, "I need help". Sometimes, it is this self-knowledge that is the first step towards an improvement of the situation.

Therefore, I would like to make the following request to all doctors and alternative practitioners who read this book: allow your patients, who have also read the book, the opportunity to actively participate in their healing process! This book's explanations in connection with specific illnesses and complaints can contribute to a better understanding of one's own situation, and one will, therefore, be able better to support one's own healing process using crystals.

In the years following publication of *Crystal Power, Crystal Healing,* it has only been possible to compile *Crystal Healing First Aid* through the willing cooperation between many scientists and alternative practitioners. I am particularly grateful to participants from the Cairn Elen Network who, along with myself, collected all the experience contained in this book. Without this cooperation and the exchange of experience within the network this book would never have seen the light of the day. Even though already cited in the dedication, I would once again like to express my heartfelt thanks to all members of the Cairn Elen Network – and in particular, to Rainer Strebel, an alternative practitioner in Schorndorf, for having proof-read this book and for his many brilliant references to alternative treatments; also to Michelle Zeuner-Mayer for having laid out the third part of this book so meticulously!

Likewise, I would like to thank Andreas Lentz of the Neue Erde publishing house for his commitment to the subject. I am pleased that my book is being published by Neue Erde/Earthdancer, where books are published because of their content and where it is natural that an equal relationship exists between the publishing house and the author – a rare phenomenon in today's "media-business" style of the major publishing houses world-wide. I would also like to thank Fred Hageneder of Dragon Design for his extraordinarily positive cooperation over the graphic presentation and the layout, just as I would like to thank Ines Blersch for the photographs that not only make the crystals and their qualities visible, but also appear to allow one almost to "feel" them.

Finally, I would like to extend my thanks to Astrid Mick, Carol Shaw and Stuart Booth for their wonderful work in editing this translation into English for publication thereby ensuring that my intentions and words as the author remain faithful to the original – no easy task when translating.

However, enough of the preliminaries: I present to you *Healing Crystals First Aid,* which, I hope will contribute to the powers of the gems, minerals and the crystals being used to heal and so contribute to the wellbeing of us all.

Michael Gienger
Tübingen

Part 1

An Introduction to Crystal Healing

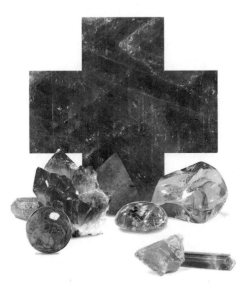

The Art of Crystal Healing

Traditions derived from the ancients and from archaeological discoveries in India, Chaldaea, Mesopotamia, Egypt and ancient Greece indicate that the art of crystal healing has existed within humankind from its very beginnings. For several thousand years, the art of crystal healing has always been seen as a natural part of medicine, a tradition that continued in the West until the Renaissance.

With the beginning of the Age of Enlightenment, which began at the end of the 17th century, however, this method of healing went into a temporary decline. The Age of Enlightenment incorporated a philosophy that emphasised rational thinking and which was highly critical of traditions. Those aspects, along with the newly emerging natural sciences, considered the healing power of the crystals to be simply superstition. In practice even though it was known that there was no lack of success with this "old" method, the real problem for the new thinkers was that it was impossible to explain scientifically the process of crystal healing. Neither the early knowledge of chemistry nor the mechanically-orientated study of physics had any understanding of molecular structure and associated energetic fields.

Things are different today. Following the developments in modern science and associated fields of study, it is clear that all bodies (living beings and inanimate objects) exchange forms of energy with their surroundings. Light, heat, and other kinds of radiated electromagnetic energy are absorbed, transformed and released again in this way. Unfortunately, it is mostly the negative phenomena, such as nuclear radiation damage, atmospheric pollution, electromagnetic/radiation effects and so forth that tend to be the preoccupying concern regarding the connection between energetic interaction and health. Nevertheless, there are certainly also positive and healing effects, including those originating from crystals.

Crystals do also resonate with their own energy signatures. Depending on the mineral, they display a measurable oscillation across the entire range of the electromagnetic spectrum. Even if the energy levels of crystals are of relatively low intensity, they still have a discernably great impact because their magnetic resonance is both harmonic and continuous. By way of comparison, imagine a vibrating guitar string, which might be barely audible if it vibrates freely in space. Nevertheless, it can make the body of the guitar resonate. Correspondingly, the weak electromagnetic vibration from crystals may cause strong reactions in the human organism.

However, other than in the case of radioactive minerals, crystals do not have their own source of such energy. Instead, they transform received light and heat into "radiation". It has been scientifically proven that the nuclei of human body cells emit light impulses that are used for internal communication between cells and for coordinating tissues and organs (see Marco Bischof *Biophotone – Das Licht in unseren Zellen / Biophotons – the Light in Our Cells*, Verlag Zweitausendunseins, Frankfurt, 1995). These so-called biophotons are apparently affected by the electromagnetic resonance of crystals, although the exact mechanism still has to be explored. Spontaneous changes of brain waves that occur when gemstones are applied to the body do at least confirm that some effect is taking place (see also the Appendix).

When the electromagnetic field of a crystal comes into contact with the human organism, it influences the following:

- energy flow through the meridians (energy pathways of the body)
- the activity of the chakras
- the stimulation of electrical nerve impulses
- the activity of the hormonal glands (as a reactin to electromagnetic stimulation)
- metabolism of cells, tissue and the organs (as the exchange of matter through the cell membranes is stimulated electromagnetically)

In principle, the electro-magnetic field of a crystal affects all areas. However, it is only effective where it meets similar frequencies (e. g. because it is the same mineral) or a similar energy structure. This phenomenon is called "resonance" (Latin *resonare*). At the point of contact with the body, an echo is generated, where similar substances, particles or structures of the body can oscillate harmonically with the frequencies entering through the crystals. Not only physical parts of the body are stimulated in this way, but also the corresponding emotional, mental and spiritual planes. The art of crystal healing is therefore a holistic science.

(As another illustration of how the energy levels in crystals can be made to resonate and then enhanced by applying higher levels of electromagnetic energy, consider the phenomenon of lasers, where crystals are used extensively to create high-energy coherent light sources by being stimulated by outside energy sources under controlled conditions.)

The healing effect of a crystal is caused precisely by the constancy and regularity of its energy vibrations. Chaotic, confused frequencies inside our bodies can be harmonised, when they are "tuned" by the crystal. Harmonically attuned oscillations and rhythms within us will also consume less energy than those that are erratic and confused. Just as a whole orchestra can be dominated by a stable flute melody, the entire symphony of one's body can be attuned to a single crystal's oscillation.

Therefore, the natural qualities of a crystal reflect the principles that apply to body, soul and spirit. (See also *Crystal Power, Crystal Healing*, Cassell, London/Sterling, New York, 1968).

Methodology

How can crystals best be used for physical, emotional and mental healing? Modern methods of crystal healing take advantage of four different methodologies, i.e. four approaches which, in practice, complement and enhance each other.

The Intuitive Method

This detects the healing effects and the practical applications of crystals by following what can best be described as an "inner feeling". Using both intuition and trained powers of observation, very subtle changes can be perceived as soon as a healing crystal is touched on, placed on or worn on the body. If you can sense and then follow the positive, strengthening reactions, when performing these actions, you will be able to detect the correct crystal without any theoretical knowledge. Spontaneous personal feelings like, "the crystal speaks to me", or "I suddenly noticed it", "I felt attracted by it", etc. are all expressions relating to the previously described resonance between the body and a crystal. So, refrain from dismissing such reactions as accidental or "coincidence" and, instead, subject them to further investigation.

The Energy Method

This deals precisely with such further explorations. By the means of dowsing measurements, where divining rods or pendulums are used and by the means of kinesiological muscle testing ('kinesiology' – the study of the mechanics and anatomy of human muscles), the subjective feelings described above can then be made more objective – which organ, which energy pathway (meridian), or which other physical, emotional or mental function responds to this crystal can be tested quite accurately. In this way, individual reactions to a specific healing crystal can be very quickly verified.

The Analytical Method

Another method whereby not only the effect of specific healing crystals on the individual is investigated, but, basic principles can also be identified, by the comparison of many individual effects in research groups. It has been stated as fact that both the geological formation of a crystal, its molecular structure, the minerals it contains and its colour each contribute independently to its healing effect (In this context see also *Crystal Power, Crystal Healing* as previously sited).

With the knowledge obtained from these principles, it is possible to identify the exact healing crystal for a specific human being in a particular state of health or life situation.

Using a combination of these first three methods, in which the intuitive type of crystal healing appears to correspond to the emotional aspect, the energy type to the physical aspect (and that of the organism), and the analytical type to the mental (logical-rational), a great deal of knowledge was collected during the nineteen-nineties in this alternative field. Alternative treatment centres, where both doctors and alternative practitioners began to apply crystal therapy, were particularly important for this process. This led to a realization that specific crystals could be applied often, occasionally, or only rarely.

This treasury of practical experience formed the basis of a fourth method of crystal healing.

The Empirical Method

This is built on experience from the other three methods and focuses on those practical applications that have been confirmed repeatedly in treatment practice. Here, no individual method or theory stands alone in its practical effectiveness. In effect, after an interruption of over two to three hundred years, a valuable tradition is being revived and redeveloped – and the circle of people who are contributing their experience is becoming ever larger.

The concept of "crystal healing first aid" was created in this way. The experiences and results that have been repeatedly confirmed in practice have now been brought together in this volume. By using this information, added practical applications are now available for preventive and healing purposes by anyone on an everyday basis.

Using this Book

Healing Crystal First Aid is a first–ever attempt to present a simple and intelligible overview and listing of more than 130 illnesses, ailments, physical and emotional problems, accompanied by a clear description of how they can be treated and cured with crystals. Throughout, ailments, complaints and conditions are arranged alphabetically for quick and easy access and each one is set out in the following uniform manner:

- name of the ailment, etc.
- general description of the illness or the emotional problem
- listing of crystals that are suitable for healing
- methods of use/practical applications of the crystals in therapy

An overall holistic viewpoint is always emphasised. As a result, for physical diseases, reference is also made to any possible psychosomatic causes or emotional roots of the problem, the resolution of which can sometimes be the real cure of the actual disease on a causal level.

The introductory explanations for each illness or complaint make the book very much more than a mere reference work;

they also fulfill the requirements of a practical handbook which provides for the further possibility of a more profound understanding and healing of a specific condition. The better we understand the physical and emotional processes within us, the more we will be able to influence them positively. Because of this wherever it makes sense to do so, the book not only names the healing crystals, but also suggests other complementary home remedies.

In describing the crystals, great care has been taken to emphasise the different characteristics of their effects. It is important to know precisely which crystal has the best effect upon application in any given situation. This precise distinction is often lost when the descriptions of effects are subordinated under the headings of the individual crystal – a common practice in the literature until now. When the arrangement is made according to illnesses and emotional complaints, these differentiations become the essential element. The same goes for the different practical applications. Many options exist, of which those chosen have proved to be the best and most effective practice.

23

Practical Applications

The aim of the different methods of use is to make the crystals work as efficient basis possible.

Sometimes, it is necessary to confine the application to a limited area, so that it becomes preferable to place or wear a crystal on a particular part of the body. If an overall effect on the whole body is desired, it often makes more sense to spend time in a circle of crystals for longer periods, or to take a gem essence. A wide range of practical applications has been developed in the light of all these different requirements.

If a crystal is **placed** or **held on** specific parts of the body, a localised effect is usually obtained. In this way, a specific organ can be stimulated or calmed, while others remain unaffected. The crystals can also be **fixed** with adhesive plaster, **placed** inside a bandage, or even **fixed into** specific articles of clothing (e. g. shoes).

Additional practical applications include crystal **massage** of specific parts of the body using tumbled stones, the application of "**ear olives**" (small crystals that are ground to an oblong, oval shape that can be fixed in the outer ear) and the application of **crystal ointments**. The latter is made by mixing gem essences with an ointment base, which consists of 1 part bee's wax to 4-5 parts of jojoba oil (usually 10 drops of essence are mixed with 10 g of ointment).

A local effect can also be obtained if one **carries** healing crystals in the form of bracelets, necklaces or pendants worn on a very specific area (e. g. over the heart, over the thymus gland, etc). On the other hand, necklaces or bracelets worn uninterruptedly for long periods will, in turn, have a general effect on the whole organism. Their effect is then spread through the blood, nerves and the energy pathways to the whole body.

Crystals held in the **hand** have a similar blanket effect, as there is a connection to the whole body via the reflex zones of the hand. Carrying a crystal in a **trouser pocket** has similar value, as one can hold the crystal in one's hand from time to time. An overall effect is always needed where a physical problem is not limited to a certain part of the body, i. e. where the whole connective tissue, the lymph or the blood system is affected.

Crystals which are **placed in one's surroundings** also have an effect on the whole body. Such an external influence can be obtained when crystals are placed on a work desk or in one's home. The advantage is that only a part of one's life is affected by a specific crystal. Crystals placed under the pillow – or arranged in a circle, for example, around the bed – are good examples of this kind of application, as is the idea of generally spending time sitting or lying, inside a circle of crystals (raw or tumbled stones). As the size of the crystals and the diameter determine the effect, one can adapt these to accommodate personal requirements.

Furthermore, the whole body can be affected by taking gem water or a gem essence. Whereas external application has a rather localised effect (e. g. by rubbing the gem essences into the skin), this can have a much wider effect. Gem water is made by placing crystals in water for a period of time ranging from a few hours to a number of days. Gem essences, on the other hand, are made by placing crystals in water or alcohol for a longer period, or by means of special procedures that differ from one producer to the other.

Hildegard von Bingen's Amethyst Water

The famous abbess and healer known as Hildegard von Bingen lived in 12th century. In her pioneering work on crystal therapy entitled *Lapis Lapidarum*, she wrote about her use of crystals in treatments and healing; and her methods remain just as valid

and applicable today, for they really do work. Most widely used of her tried and tested treatments is her famous Amethyst Water.

This treatment remains important and is described here specifically because of its special preparation and its widely recommended use throughout the book. In order to prepare this healing water, hang up a clean, purified piece of an Amethyst druse over a pot of boiling water, so that the steam can condense on the pointed Amethyst crystals and drip back into the pot. After about half-an-hour, turned off the heat, so that the water slowly cools. Once the water feels just warm to the hand, the Amethyst druse is taken down and placed in the water until the liquid reaches room temperature. This water is very soft, cleansing and good for taking care of the skin in a gentle way. It can be used for personal hygiene without adding soap or any other kind of cosmetic or alcoholic agent.

The simultaneous application of gem water or gem essences, together with locally applied crystals, has a mutually fortifying effect. The double application of water/ essence and crystals also focuses the internal effect of the water/essence on a specific area and so has a very powerful effect.

A slightly weaker effect is obtained when crystals are placed in the mouth (which is also recommended by Hildegard von Bingen). While the crystal has a localised effect on the mouth, teeth, and mucous membranes, etc. via a transfer of information to the saliva, a kind of gem essence with a healing effect on the whole body is produced. Naturally, one must *always* refrain from using toxic crystals and only apply this procedure to the crystals and cases described in these pages (mostly in the form of smooth tumbled stones).

Finally, mention must be made here of special **energy treatments** with crystals. In these examples, the conductive abilities of certain crystals (e. g. Tourmaline and Rock Crystal) are exploited in order to stimulate and guide the flow of energy and liquids within the body, and to further the regeneration and conductive ability of the nerves. When crystals are arranged in specific ways upon the body, pains, complaints in nerves and joints (caused by inadequate circulation or scars) and functional disorders of the large intestine can be treated. The relevant treatments are mentioned under the appropriate ailment.

A method of stroking with pieces of **Amethyst druses** in order to relieve tension and lower the blood pressure also belongs among these treatments. The pieces are not placed on the body, but instead are moved calmly, but firmly over the body along certain paths or lines. In this way, the flow of energy and liquids in the body can be controlled over large areas.

At this point, it must be stressed once more that the practical applications described for the individual conditions, etc. should not be regarded dogmatically as the only treatment, but rather as representing some tried and tested possibilities. If you discover a new, practical application that seems more meaningful than the ones described, or if you have an idea for a new method, then why not go ahead and try it out? However, in so doing, *always remember any restrictions* that are listed or mentioned for specific crystals, especially those that might be toxic under certain circumstances.

It now merely remains to give one more practical warning:

NEVER take pulverised minerals internally!

Many healing crystals are toxic if they are supplied to the body as a physical substance. The effects of the crystals described in this book are not chemical, but come about through a transmission of the crystal's own internal "information". Crystal healing is therefore an information-therapy, rather like homeopathy, Bach flower remedies or aromatherapy. The outer, practical applications of the crystals and the consumption of gem water, gem essences or preparations that do not contain the actual substances, or only in extremely diluted form, are sufficient in themselves to obtain the necessary healing effects.

Cleansing and Recharging Crystals

While applying healing crystals, one occasionally discovers that they either become ineffective, their effect changes, or they actually feel downright unpleasant. The reason for this is that crystals not only transmit energetic information, but also absorb it. In particular, in the case of intense healing processes "disease information" can be absorbed. This, after some time, may then overshadow the crystal's inherent "healing information".

Therefore, prior to beginning, the crystals being applied should be "cleansed" of electrical charges after use. In particular, with direct body contact, many crystals absorb an electrostatic charge. The most extreme case occurs with the use of Amber, which can become quite hot after a couple of minutes application. The best method of discharging the static charge is to hold the crystal under running water for 10-20 seconds.

The absorbed information, however, still remains stored in the crystal after the discharge. Without further cleansing, the information will still be active during the next treatment. In order to delete this information, the crystal can be placed either inside an Amethyst druse or on a piece of an Amethyst druse. Amethyst has a strong, fiery radiation caused by its finely distributed iron atoms and energy concentration; crystals that are energised in this way are freed of the absorbed information. As a rule, this process takes about a day. If the crystal has only been applied for at short time, an hour will be sufficient; however, it will not be harmed if you allow it to remain in the Amethyst druse for a longer time.

As the intensity of a crystal's effectiveness is connected with the absorbed energy, the cleansed crystals can be recharged in one's hand or in sunlight (morning or evening). The absorbed heat energy intensifies the crystal's effect. In many cases, however, such recharging is unnecessary as the crystal has already been warmed up and stimulated by body contact.

Self-treatment – or Professional Help?

The treatment of an illness on one's own and without professional assistance is a controversial issue. On the one hand, our overburdened health services and authorities are demanding that we assume greater responsibility for our own health. On the other hand, reports of complications arising through lack of professional help are a deterrent to acting on one's own.

Sick people find themselves faced with the following dilemma: should they now assume responsibility for their own recovery; or should they leave it to their doctor or alternative practitioner?

The answer is simple: the best way is to assume responsibility *and* also to get professional help. This increases the certainty of a proper diagnosis of any illness (Greek: *diagnose* – to distinguish; to perceive). At the same time, it is always good idea to participate actively in the ensuing healing process.

One has to work on the positive changes of one's own life circumstances, and to exploit all possibilities of healing in accordance with professional advice. However, this process requires an ongoing dialogue.

A dialogue about the practical applications of crystals is most successful when both parties, i.e. the patient and the doctor/alternative practitioner, enjoy practically the same level of knowledge.

Consequently, this book is intended for both these parties. It provides detailed descriptions of different pathological situations and conditions, while, at the same time, having been written in such a way that it can be read and used by the layperson without too much effort.

The use of difficult words or medical jargon has been largely omitted, and where necessarily included, they are immediately explained. In this way it is hoped to revive a genuine dialogue (Greek: *dialogos* – "conversation between two") between the doctor/alternative practitioner, on one side, and the patient, on the other.

This is important as so often such conversations are hampered simply by the use of different terminologies and, in particular, by not having properly defined, understood technical terms. When mutual understanding is achieved, and when you are able to communicate in a common language, confidence can be established. Thus, if one's options and limitations in connection with the treatment of illnesses and emotional suffering have become clearer through the study of this book, then it will have fulfilled its purpose.

Part 2

Practical
Crystal Healing

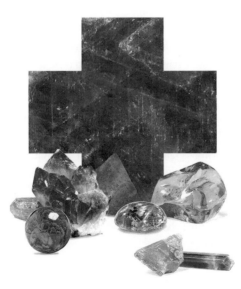

The A to Z of Crystal First Aid

The following pages describe practical applications of healing crystals in connection with a wide range of some 160 specific illnesses, ailments, conditions, emotional problems and maintenance of a healthy body. Each entry is structured in the same way as described earlier in "Using this Book"

It is important to take in **all** the information within an entry before any treatment is begun! This also applies to any examinations by a doctor, an alternative practitioner – and for therapeutic consultations and assistance, in cases of emotional problems.

When looking at the possible emotional causes of physical conditions, it is often very difficult to generalise about such connections in order to make a holistic evaluation. Indeed, it can be extremely difficult – even be impossible, on occasion – as the emergence of a specific pathological picture is unique in every case. There may be many different causes leading to a specific condition. As a result, any suggested causes described in the following pages represent only qualified suggestions, or are presented as an incentive to start thinking about

whether similar situations or experiences exist in the actual case (or vice versa, of course!). So, if you do indeed end up with a better understanding of why you are suffering from a specific illness, or repeatedly suffer from it, then examine this information more closely. Conversely, if you experience a sense of confusion, or feel that something is not right, then ignore it.

The term "emotional" (in this context) refers to unconscious reactions that take place without the awareness of our day-to-day consciousness. The cause of these reactions may be related to specific goals and intentions, to emotional backgrounds (previous experience), or to mental attitudes (convictions, opinions). However, these can all be summed up as being "emotional". After all, as a rule, they are all unconscious, in one way or another, and can only be understood or revealed after serious thought specific self-enquiry about them.

As long as a reaction or a mechanism is not investigated consciously, it cannot be changed! That is also the reason why many things happen to us all the time (they slip pass our conscious awareness) and repeatedly trigger unconscious mechanisms and physical illnesses. Conscious problems, on the other hand, far more rarely lead to illnesses. Exceptions to this are cases where the conscious and the unconscious are combined: Conscious problems involve all of our attention in order that unconscious problems can carry on undisturbed. Yet, generally, consciousness-raising is a process with a curative effect – in particular because we want to change conditions we are conscious about.

Putting all this together, trying to create a simple formula understandable to all, one arrives at the following concept: if we are unable to change something, even though we would like to, then an important factor still remains unconscious. This is where therapeutic help may be necessary. The suggestions given in the individual entries which follow may also be a key to consciousness-raising; but always keep in mind the above recommendation: do not worry too much if a specific reference neither makes sense nor causes a definite "a-ha!" revelatory experience.

There may also be causes other than those mentioned. The best practical application is always the one given in the entry, along with the description of the individual crystals and their effects. The references given are based on practical experience, but should still only to be regarded as suggestions or possibilities. Even then, there are often several ways to arrive at the same conclusion or outcome. Therefore, in order to facilitate an overview of possible symptoms and treatments, cover flaps can be folded out to give "at a glance" all the practical applications mentioned (inside the rear cover flap) and the types of crystal to use (inside back cover flap). Simply allow those two pages to remain opened out, while you are looking up something in Part 2 or in Part 3 of the book.

Overall, It is hoped the next chapters may help you become well or contribute to your staying well. Furthermore, I would be very happy to receive feedback from your experiences with the healing effects of crystals. Please send your questions and descriptions of experiences to Edition Cairn Elen or to Steinheilkunde eV. (addresses as in the Appendix). All such correspondence will be answered in due course.

Abscesses

Abscesses are pus-engorged swellings of the skin. They are the result of the body's natural way of bringing to the surface dead cells and toxic substances. Sometimes, they are accompanied by a raised temperature this is an integral part of the body's healing process.

Since abscesses can be the outer sign of some deep-rooted, inner inflammatory condition, always seek professional medical advice, especially for abscesses that appear along with fever symptoms. Further, in the cases of large abscesses there is also the danger of sepsis (blood poisoning).

If abscesses appear repeatedly, or particularly during in periods of anxiety or severe emotional upset, it may help to think about what it is in your life that you are finding hard to cope with, are having a hard time getting on with or is really bothering you so much that you would prefer to pretend it is not there, i. e. to "reject" it. Any help in solving or coping with such problems can reduce the tendency towards abscesses.

A tried and tested home remedy for an abscess is the application of a cold herbal poultices – in addition to following crystal therapy.

Amethyst helps the body to break down toxic waste from inflammation, so that the abscesses soon shrink and disappear.

Place a tumbled stone, a section/slice, or a whole crystal on the body; apply Hildegard von Bingen's Amethyst Water (page 25) to the affected spot; or take gem essence (3-7 drops, 3 times daily), in order to reduce the tendency towards abscesses.

Heliotrope helps when abscesses suddenly appear and are accompanied by a rapidly developing fever. A crystal with yellow spots (a pus-signature) is especially effective. Place tumbled stones or section/slices on the abscesses or take gem essence (3-9 drops, 3 times daily)

Whilst Heliotrope can be applied as an immediate measure, seek professional help immediately.

Ocean Jasper stimulates the dissipation of abscesses and, in general, reduces any inherent tendency toward their formation. Crystals with many small brown spheres surrounded by a green colour are particularly effective.

In acute cases, place a tumbled stone or a flat section/slice on the affected area. Ocean Jasper can be worn as a bracelet, necklace or pendant for a longer period (up to several months). Alternatively, take as gem water (200–300 ml taken in sips during the course of the day).

Abrasions, Scrapes and Grazes

Abrasions are generally injuries of an area of the skin caused by contact or scraping against rough surfaces. Whilst they may often only bleed a little, more annoyingly they can produce an extremely uncomfortable, burning pain, where the sensitive nerve endings in the skin have been damaged. In addition, and especially with an abrasion where dirt has entered the area, there is real danger of infection and pus formation. The minimal bleeding is insufficient to wash away dirt and germs. As a result abrasions should always be treated rapidly with medical disinfectants before covering the wound – although any large areas of abrasion may require treatment by a professional medical doctor.

See also: Burns; Cuts; Injuries

As with cuts, it is possible to use the 'repeat' process for a faster improvement of the condition and the healing, if one becomes fully conscious and aware of the incident that caused the abrasion.

Repeat the events which led to the abrasion once again – exactly as it took place, at the place of the incident and as quickly as possible after the incident (of course, without hurting oneself again!). Sometimes it is necessary to repeat the whole thing a couple of times, until the pain suddenly increases and then decreases. This is the stage at which to stop. This is a consciousness-raising exercise that focuses the attention of your life energy upon the affected spot and thus furthers the healing process.

Obsidian can be used if the above process is not possible one can take a polished piece in one hand, or place it close to the wound in order to dissolve the state of shock in the cells. One can also rinse the wound with diluted gem essence (10 drops in 100 ml of clean water) or gem water of Obsidian before applying a plaster or a bandage.

Rhodonite or **Mookaite** are useful as a supplement in the form of a tumbled stone or a slice on the skin next to the abrasion, or taken as gem essence (5-9 drops) or gem water (100 ml). Necklaces or pendants of Rhodonite or Mookaite also support the healing process.

Acidification

Although popularly supposed to be principally associated with the stomach, when it is called acidosis, acidification is a more universal process caused by an excess of acid in the body, resulting from an unbalanced diet or some form of metabolic upset. The process of digesting food and metabolic processes within our bodies leads to the formation of acids and alkalis (or bases) in the body fluids. As long as this continues in the normal and natural way, there is an overall chemical balance – in that the alkalis neutralise the acids.

However, if the ratio of acid to alkali veers significantly in either direction, so to speak, there is a chemical imbalance. This when the body employs it natural and automatic buffer mechanisms, usually in the form of various phosphate compounds and other mineral salts, that combine with any superfluous acids and bases to re-harmonise the system. This chemically neutral situation is particularly important for the circulation – though only approximately as blood operates optimally when it is *slightly* alkaline.

If there is a constant surplus of acid, the body starts to use mineral salts from its deposits in the bones and the teeth in order to neutralise this acid. The consequence is that the bones and teeth become damaged in the long term. Also, the resulting compounds of acids and mineral salts are, in effect, toxins and waste products that cannot always be excreted adequately via the kidneys.

Our body's solution is to shift such waste to some part of us where the least damage occurs. This is the connective tissue, the body's "waste dump", in effect (see also Detoxification).

Obviously, this is never a situation or condition that can carry on for long without significant consequences. Whilst only the connective tissue is affected initially by unwanted accumulations of acid and toxins, other parts of us begin to show the signs. The impurities affect the skin as dandruff; eczema and skin diseases; the intestines are affected with resulting diarrhoea; constipation; the airways (which always have a tendency toward infection) become blocked; the blood vessels have deposits and exhibit a dangerous tendency towards bursting and disturbances in blood circulation; and other organs will soon show their own adverse reaction.

Emotional downs and depression can also be made worse by such "acidification" of the body. Indeed, it can be postulated that most common diseases in modern society are associated or connected in some way or another with the condition.

The process of acidification occurs most frequently within those of us living in urban industrialised societies and with nutrition rich or high in animal products (particularly proteins and fats) along with heavy consumption of coffee, alcohol, nicotine and sweets. I would describe these last as "the four sins" associated with the process of acidification).

All of the above is compounded and exacerbated by the enormous pressure "to achieve" in our society. Aspects of living such as hectic activity, a disrupted lifestyle, stress, lack of sleep, irritation and environmental pollution all contribute to acidification – emotionally as well as physically. Leisure time, tranquillity, meditation and relaxation are weapons we can use to counteract the process; each will contribute to a reduced amount of acid in the body. In addition, we should al find more time for such activities.

A de-acidifying diet, sleep and restoration are immediate measures to take in order to fight acidification, for any form of crystal therapy and applying crystals would be meaningless without this support. Further, it is worth adopting a beneficial type of diet, agreed with and under supervision of a doctor or an alternative practitioner, who should also be able to advise on other de-acidifying measures – especially if some action has to be taken rather quickly. The overall regimen ought then to become the rule, with coffee, alcohol, nicotine and confectionary the exception.

Diaspor and **Turquoise** will both encourage de-acidification. Both crystals stimulate a reduction of acid within the blood and body tissue and also promote the cleansing process therein. Emotionally, both have a harmonising effect and reduce stress.

Place or carry a Diaspor crystal on the stomach, or wear Turquoise as a bracelet, necklace or pendant with direct body contact for a lengthy period. As an alternative, take gem essence (5-7 drops, 3 times daily), or gem water (100–200 ml taken in small sips over the course of the day).

Acne

The term covers a number of different skin diseases that accompany accumulations of fatty tissue, inflamed swellings and pus-filled pustules. The most common case is *Acne vulgaris* (also called *Acne juvenilis*, which often starts to appear at puberty and, as a rule, disappears before the age of thirty.

Acne in puberty is triggered by hormonal changes, but is also exacerbated by a fatty diet, sweets, coffee and nicotine. It is often just as harmful to cover acne with cosmetics, as it is to clean the skin excessively with (often commercially promoted) soap or alcoholic solutions. Therefore, if you want to reduce the number of pimples, eat food low in fats and exercise some sense in the number of chocolate bars, etc. you eat and use only skin-care products that are free of soap and alcohol, e. g. Amethyst water as below).

However, crystal therapy only makes sense if accompanied and complemented by the simultaneous implementation of sensible nutrition and gentle skin care

Amethyst cleanses the skin. Hildegard von Bingen's Amethyst Water (see page 25) is particularly recommended

Chrysoprase stimulates detoxification and excretion of toxins and thus relieves skin problems. Place a polished or raw stone regularly on the liver every night

Otherwise, wear it as a bracelet, necklace or pendant for a long period. Alternatively, take it as gem essence (5 drops, 3 times daily), or as gem water (10 ml, 3 times daily).

Moonstone regulates and harmonises hormonal changes during puberty. Wear it as a pendant or – even better – as a necklace or bracelet for several months.

Rhodonite prevents the formation of scars from open spots and pimples, if placed on the affected area in the form of a flat, tumbled stone, or a section/slice.

If you wear it as a bracelet, necklace, or pendant for a longer period, it will also prevent emotional stress that acne can cause.

Allergies

An allergy is an acquired hypersensitivity to specific substances in ones environment and immediate surroundings. An allergy tends to develop as a result of repeated exposure to the irritant and can manifest itself in several ways, as follows:

- skin eruption
- inflammation of the skin (dermatitis, eczema)
- swelling of the mucous membranes and secretions from them (hay fever)
- impairment of respiratory passages (allergic bronchial asthma)
- anaphylactic shock, in extreme cases, with rapidly falling blood pressure, leading to unconsciousness – a truly life-threatening situation.

In addition to the last condition, however, ANY case of severe allergic reaction merits the summoning of an ambulance or emergency medical attention immediately!

A tendency towards allergy develops rapidly as our organism is increasingly loaded with toxic substances that can be neither used nor excreted. Environmental pollution and hypersensitivity toward spe-

cific foods play an important part, of course. Other factors include stress, as well as insufficient rest and sleep, all of these inhibit the body's opportunity for regeneration and it becomes overstressed; and an "allergic" reaction is the result.

Healthy eating, toxin-free living (in so far at this is possible today!), use of only natural medicines and – importantly, I feel – a reduction in direct and indirect exposure to any form or electromagnetic radiation (pollution from such modern technology as TV, computer monitors, microwave ovens, telephone masts, etc.) is helpful.

In particular, diet should be examined professionally and, if necessary, be examined specifically with regard to the personal threshold of tolerance. Furthermore, rest, adequate sleep and detoxification on a regular basis (e. g. intestinal cleansing and fasting under professional medical supervision) may help in the necessary renewal of the body. Finally, focus your attention on what you may be allergic to emotionally.

See also: Asthma; Hay Fever

Self-help treatment strategies for allergies have limited scope. However, in mild cases, such as hay fever, crystals can be a big help. In more problematical cases, seek professional medical advice – and ALWAYS in severe conditions or life-endangering situations such as anaphylactic shock

Aquamarine helps with many allergies, in particular, when they are intensified by psychological or emotional pressures. It can be used in cases of respiratory reactions (anything from hay fever to bronchial asthma) and in cases of violent, acute circulation problems. Emotionally, Aquamarine brings ease and relaxation.

Amber helps with allergies that mainly affect the skin and the mucous membranes. In any case, it should be applied when pronounced aversion to specific contact can be identified.

Blue Lace Agate stimulates lymph flow and ensures a rapid decrease of allergic reactions. It helps cleanse the body and thus heals the starting point of the allergic state. Furthermore, it eases the ability to handle conflict and promotes the correct emotional reactions, so that you no longer react allergically toward specific situations.

Chrysoprase helps with allergies that occur after intoxication (or adverse reactions to certain medication), or those that are the result of an inappropriate diet. It also alleviates any allergy that is a by-product of grief, jealousy, and loss of peace of mind.

Landscape Jasper helps with all allergies as it cleanses the tissues that have been polluted by toxins and waste substances. It relieves nervousness and calms states of excitement. It also helps with stress and, at the same time, strengthens willpower and the ability to "hold your own".

Ocean Jasper, especially with green/white inclusions or transparent areas of pure Chalcedony, helps cleanse the body and regulate the immune system. It reduces allergic reactions quickly and, in the long run, reduces any intrinsic tendency toward allergies.

For all the above crystals, wear as a bracelet, necklace or pendant for a long period. Alternatively, take gem essence as a supplement (3-7 drops, 3 times daily); or gem water (200–300 ml taken in sips during the course of the day) for a longer period.

Ametropia

Ametropia, or defective vision, is caused chiefly by a deformation of the eyeball, which produces a blurred image on the retina (the eye's "screen", where images formed by the lens in the eye are focused and then interpreted by the brain via the optic nerve) at certain distances.

In cases of **short-sightedness** – myopia – the eyeball is too long, and the focal point of the eye's lens is situated "in front" of the physical location of retina, as it were speak. Only objects that are close by can be seen at all sharply.

In cases of **long-sightedness** – hypermetropia – the eyeball is too short and so the eye's lens focus images at a point that is somewhere behind the retina, so to speak. Only relatively distant objects can be seen sharply.

Other causes of ametropia can be changes in the refractive/focusing ability in the eye's lens or in the cornea (e. g. in cases of diabetes or an incipient cataract) or a loss of flexibility of the lens (age-related long-sightedness).

In the most usual and common cases of ametropia, the underlying deformation of the eyeball is often regarded as "hereditary" and consequently as "unchangeable". However, this is a false assumption. Whilst there can be some predisposition, the degree to which it can develop into ametropia can actually be influenced. In this context, it is worth noting that deformation of the normally quite flexible eyeball is often connected with some malfunction of the eye muscles – either being used too little or have become shortened. The tension in the muscles causes or increases the deformation of the eyeball and, in the worst cases, a gradual deterioration. Yet our eye muscles can be relaxed loosened and be trained, so that the deformation is reduced and the ametropia decreases. There is an extensive literature about such eye exercises, seminars and schools, where the person's vision is trained and where training programmes are provided. Positive results can also be obtained by wearing grid glasses, which break our vision habits.

Apart from this, ametropia may also have psychological causes. If we do not want to accept a particular point of view, we will automatically avoid the corresponding physical attitude, e. g. eye positions.

As a consequence, certain eye muscles are not used as much as they should be and become shortened. This lack of "stretching" or exercise can result in ametropia. This applies to everyone; and it can be demonstrated with a simple exercise as described below.

Try rolling your eyes in the maximum possible circle. Can you roll them regularly without stopping or suddenly breaking off and skipping part of the circular motion on? Not usually, in most cases.

Next, identify a specific point where you are looking every time the rolling of the eyes stops or skips on. Turn your eyes in that direction.

Now, in most cases, the angle is uncomfortable to maintain; sometimes, it is even connected with distinct physical discomfort or dizziness.

Normally, this is a way tin which we never use or move our eyes. If there is some reason or need to look into that direction, we always prefer to turn our whole head. The precise nature of discomfort that results in adopting this awkward perspective varies from one individual to the other. Nevertheless, in specific eye therapies and exercises, it can often be that previously uncomfortable eye positions will become easier to adopt and that any associated ametropia may sometimes also be reduced.

Moreover, the connections between eye movement, eye musculature and ametropia show why working at a desk computer or a laptop, with long and concentrated focus on the screen can have an aggravating effect on ametropia. It is even possible that use of incorrect eyeglasses or spectacles can have an effect – and with smaller spectacle lenses, we prefer to turn the head instead of the eye, which shortens the eye muscles even more. All these factors limit the movement of the eye. So, walking (without glasses, if possible), where one consciously changes between looking at objects both nearby or far away (and in as many directions as possible), may provide a good counterbalance.

See also: Cataracts; Eye Problems; Squinting

Crystal therapy can always be combined with eye exercises in cases of ametropia. This results in much faster improvement. The crystals actually make many exercises easier, while first and foremost stabilising the success of these exercises. The effect can be confirmed quite clearly during the pauses between exercises.

Aquamarine and **Emerald** both belong to the Beryl group of minerals and the use of Beryl in cases of ametropia has been known since antiquity. (There is, for example, the story of a cut Emerald being famous for having helped the Roman emperor Nero to improve his sight). The crystals relax the surroundings of the eyes and give the eye musculature the correct tone. Apart from that, they have a positive effect on the associated nerves. Aquamarine and Emerald also have an emotional effect, as they broaden one's inner sight and mental horizon.

Place small crystals or tumbled stones directly on the eyes or wear a necklace or a pendant. Alternatively, you can take gem essence (5-9 drops, 3 to 5 times daily) or gem water (200–300 ml taken in small sips over the course of the day.

Rock Crystal and **Amethyst** can also have a positive effect on ametropia. This goes for Amethyst, in particular. After that, Rock Crystal, Aquamarine and Emerald can be placed (carefully!) directly on the eyes.

Agate may also be used where ametropia is not caused by a deformation of the eyeball, but by a change of the refraction in the lens and the cornea. In particular, Agate slices or thin sections, with Rock Crystal in the centre, often show good results, if they are placed on the eye for a quarter of an hour (preferably in the evening).

Arm and Leg Pains

Pains in the legs and arms are most commonly experienced as the side effects of colds, flu and other feverish illnesses. They are caused by anti-bodies produced by the body's own immune response, as well as by metabolic and waste products of bacteria. In turn, these cause a reduction in the supply of nutrients with a resulting irritation of the tissues nerve endings, disrupted blood circulation and an accumulation of lymph fluid. Usually, such pains are not a severe or dangerous symptom, and, as a rule, will disappear again quite naturally. Nevertheless, they can be quite unpleasant at the time.

See also: Joint Pain; Pain

Banded Chalcedony, Magnesite and **Amber** in combination have proved to be very effective in reducing such pains. Chalcedony encourages lymph flow whilst Magnesite relaxes and soothes the pain. Amber supports the metabolism and promotes the supply of energy to the tissues.

Moss Agate, Ocean Jasper or **Sardonyx** also show good results when worn as ankle and arm bracelets. All three are members of the Chalcedony group of minerals and so help with the overall healing process and the purification and regeneration of the body. They also prevent relapses and their cleansing effect is apparent by the rapid relief they provide from leg and arm pains.

Arteriosclerosis

Arteriosclerosis is a process of thickening of the arterial walls, initially by proteins and coagulated blood and, later by fatty substances (e. g. cholesterol) and calcium deposits. The blood circulation in certain organs, particularly the heart and the brain, is thereby considerably reduced. In addition, there is a danger of spontaneous thromboses, i. e. a total blockage of the ves-

sels, by coagulated blood. In turn, this may cause heart failure or an embolism.

Arteriosclerosis begins slowly and insidiously. Initial symptoms are: calf pains when you walk (indicating poor circulation); cold, colourless and bluish limbs; sudden heart pains; decreased physical capacity, memory and concentration problems; dizziness; headaches; sleep disturbances; irritability; easily recognised emotional problems.

A diet omitting animal protein is an indispensable part of treatment for arteriosclerosis. Furthermore, the diet should also include food rich in vitamins (particularly vitamins C and E), adequate exercise, sleep, and time for overall regeneration. Treatment should always be carried out under professional medical supervision as a wide range of background ailments and conditions can cause arteriosclerosis.

Three crystals in particular have turned out to have a positive effect in its treatment.

Aventurine furthers detoxification and thereby prevents deposits in the walls of the arteries. In addition to that, it prevents inflammatory states and coagulated blood in the blood vessels and thus reduces the danger from deposits, which can cause narrowing of the blood vessels.

Wear it as a bracelet, necklace or pendant for a long period. Also, try taking gem essence (3 drops, 3 times daily), or gem water (200–300 ml taken in small sips during the course of the day).

Diamond breaks down deposits in the blood vessels. Place small, raw diamonds for a day in 200–300 ml of water and drink the water over the course of the following day.

Heliotrope prevents further deposits in the blood vessels. It is particularly effective when blood vessels are inflamed.

Wear it as a bracelet, necklace or pendant for a long period. Also, take it as gem essence (5-7 drops, 3 times daily), or gem water (200–300 ml taken in sips during the course of the day).

Asthma

The term "asthma" (from the Greek *azein:* "to breathe hard"), in its widest sense, covers several types of severe breathing difficulty, ranging from chest tightness to severe breathlessness. Each condition has a different background, such as heart asthma, asthmatic bronchitis, etc.

In its more specific sense, i. e. bronchial asthma, it is considered to be an allergy and can sometimes because by a number of suppressed skin diseases; and it is this type of asthma, which is dealt with here.

Bronchial asthma is characterised by difficulties in exhaling, as the small bronchial muscles becomes tightened when breathing out, the mucous membranes swell and an excess of thick, transparent "goo" is secreted. This causes a severe case of breathlessness. If it persists, it is a definite emergency and an ambulance or emergency medical services should be called!

In this state, air that should be exhaled is held back, and this impedes inhalation. This causes a lack of oxygen, which, in turn, leads to deterioration in basic lung and heart functioning, with immediate impact on the circulation. During the asthma attack, the latter effect shows up in the form of cold hands and feet and bluish lips, with a considerable danger of later complications through damage to the heart.

Bronchial asthma is notable in that it is caused by allergy, but displays clear psychosomatic characteristics. So, an asthmatic attack is not only caused by allergy-provoking phenomena such as pollen, house dust, flour, mould fungi spores, chemicals, but also by cigarette smoke, fog, physical strain, anxiety, fear and other stressful situations.

Consequently, one has to investigate both the physical and the emotional causes of asthmatic attacks. Worry and anxiety can cause chest tightness and impede the natural rhythm of breathing

Because asthmatic attacks may also become life threatening, a professional should supervise any kind of treatment medically. In addition, and as complimentary aids, crystals therapy can relieve attacks and can reduce their occurrence.

Apophyllite is the best crystal to use in cases of acute asthmatic attack. It has a relaxing effect upon bronchial spasm, works as an expectorant and thus soothes breathlessness very quickly. Both Green and Clear variants have this effect. Green Tourmaline, however, has turned out to be the most reliable.

Rutile Quartz is the second best choice of crystal. Strictly speaking, it is better suited to the therapeutic treatment of asthmatic bronchitis – but, as the two diseases are similar, it also shows beneficial effects in cases of bronchial asthma. This holds true in the long term, particularly.

Tiger's Eye and **Turquoise** relieve asthmatic attacks. The form of Tiger's Eye known as Gold Quartz is especially recommended for the treatment of acute attacks.

For all of the crystals mentioned above, particularly in acute cases, press a crystal hard against the chest.

Between the attacks, wear Rutile Quartz in the form of a necklace or pendant on the chest. Apophyllite can be fixed with a plaster or placed in a trouser pocket, as it is usually only available in the form of a crystal cluster.

Athlete's Foot

With cases of athlete's foot, most causes are often thought of as being external, e. g. the danger of fungal infection in public swimming baths or bad footwear. It is true that good foot hygiene and shoes without 'excessive humidity' lessen the risk of suffering from athlete's foot. However, even with this complaint, the internal environment of our bodily fluids is a much more important factor.

Fungal infections in particular can only gain a foothold in skin, mucous membranes or tissues if there are already large amounts of toxic substances in the body. The disinfectants and so forth that are used in swimming pools can, therefore, be downright harmful. A thorough cleansing with skin-friendly remedies is much more sensible as prevention and treatment. (See also: Fungal Infections)

However, a long-term solution can only be ensured through thorough detoxification (see Detoxification). Effective home remedies such as ointment of tea tree oil in a 10% solution, or the crystals cited below, only help relieve annoying symptoms. Their use, of course, remains fully justified; but without a diet and further detoxifying precautions, one cannot obtain a permanent cure.

Chrysoprase and **Smoky Quartz** in combination has turned out to be an effective remedy for relieving athlete's foot as the detoxifying Chrysoprase and the soluble Smoky Quartz complement each other in a significant way.

First, take gem essence of Chrysoprase (5-7 drops, three times daily) or gem water (20–100 ml taken in small sips during the course of the day). At the same time, regularly place a tumbled stone on the affected spot. After two or three days, start wearing a necklace or a pendant of Smoky Quartz. This treatment needs to be carried out for several weeks, but will then show results. Apparently the detoxifying Chrysoprase and the dissolving Smoky Quartz complement each other in a meaningful way.

Back Pain

Back pain can have many different causes. If only temporary, then its cause is usually tension in the back musculature, which, in turn, is caused by strain, poor sitting posture or lack of physical exercise. Apart from that, spinal problems, inflammation, and side effects of other internal ailments or even emotional stress can all lead to back pain.

In connection with the latter, feelings of guilt often can often become transformed into shoulder pains. In addition, pressure to perform in a job and emotional conflict can also emerge as pain in the upper part of the back (around the chest vertebrae). Similar pains in the mid-to-lower back can be caused by financial worries, whilst sexual problems and emotional distress can show up as pains around the sacrum and the coccyx.

However, these are only some of the possible causes. In principle, any kind of stress or concern may result in similar aches and pains, as the back and spine are synonymous with a sense of both physical and psychological "straightness" of attitude.

See also: Lumbago; Joint Pain; Slipped Disc

When treating back problems, the physical and the emotional causes both require equal attention. A treatment that consists solely in dealing with the symptoms – say, through massage or crystal therapy – will only supply relief for a very short time if the real emotional or psychological causes remain untreated. Thus, a professional medical examination is always to be recommended for any form of persistent back pain – along with other forms of therapy if sever emotional strain is involved.

Kunzite is helpful for back pain that is caused by the trapped nerves resulting from a slipped disc or sciatica. It relieves the pain and relaxes the affected area; and it is only when the area is fully relaxed that massage or chiropractic treatment can take place without damaging side effects. Emotionally, Kunzite furthers commitment and humility, and at the same time being true to oneself. That is exactly what the spine stands for, as it must both support and remain flexible.

Place a crystal or a tumbled stone directly upon the aching area – or, as an alternative, take gem essence (5-9 drops, 3 times daily) or gem water (100–200 ml taken in sips over the course of the day).

Magnesite is helpful in relieving tension in the upper part of the back and the neck, especially when the pain results from feelings of being under pressure or where any future confrontations are anticipated. It induces patience and increases the ability to withstand any type of mental or emotional strain.

Wear a bracelet, a necklace or a pendant on the back for the best effect. Alternatively, take gem essence (5-7 drops, 3-5 times daily) or gem water (200–300 ml taken in sips over the course of the day).

Smoky Quartz is helpful with all types of back problems. It relieves tensed muscles and assists with achieving a better posture. Further, it increases greatly the ability to withstand pressures and strains by inducing a sense of calmness, even under great stress. Worn for longer periods, it also reduces any inherent tendency to becoming stressed.

Place a crystal or a tumbled stone on the aching spot; or wear as a necklace or a pendant. As an alternative, take gem essence (5-7 drops, 3-5 times daily) or gem water (200–300 ml taken in small sips over the course of the day).

Ruby is helpful first and foremost with problems in the lower part of the back – the lumber region, sacrum and coccyx. It induces courage and strength when faced with complex worries and has also been show to help many people with sexual problems and anxieties.

Place or fix a crystal, a slice or a tumbled stone on the sacrum – or wear as a necklace or a pendant over the hip.

Emerald is helpful for people with back problems that can occur at those times when there is sense of having 'lost one's bearings' or when suffering some injustice, feelings of disharmony, a sense of failure, or general fatigue and inability to bounce back. It can also be applied when any type of inflammation plays a role, even if the affected area has only an indirect influence on the back (e. g. inflammation in the intestines or other organs).

Place (or fix) a crystal, a section/slice or a tumbled stone on the tender spot. As an alternative, take gem essence (3-7 drops, 3-5 times daily) or gem water (200–300 ml taken in sips over the course of the day)

Black Tourmaline relieves all kinds of back pain and helps with stress and emotional burdens of any kind. Place or fix a crystal on the aching spot – with the point downwards for the most effective outcome. If an actual Tourmaline crystal is not available, then a suitable alternative can be section/slices or tumbled stones.

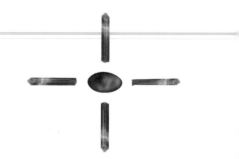

Fig. 1: Pain treatment with Black Tourmaline and Obsidian (Apache's Tear).

Obsidian when used with **Tourmaline** is particularly helpful with pain that radiates from a clearly identifiable point.

Place a small piece of tumbled Obsidian (the so-called "Apache's Tear" form is best) on the aching spot. Place four Tourmaline crystals around it, pointing outwards. The Obsidian helps to relieve the pain, while the Tourmaline crystals drain off excess energy.

Bedsores

Bedsores are painful damage to areas of skin, caused by pressure and disrupted circulation, which, in a progressed state, may also reach deeper seated tissue layers, even as deep as the bones. They are prevalent in patients who have to remain in bed for long periods and who are no longer able to turn around by themselves.

If the condition progresses without treatment ever deeper-lying tissue layers become affected, penetrating even as deep as the bones in truly sever cases. Bedsores are usually classifies by a four-stage progression in which the overall process affects tissue, which is inadequately supplied with nutrients and begins to die The so called first degree involves localised reddening of the skin and tissue; the second degree includes the formation of blisters; then progresses to the deep open wounds of third degree sores and finally, bone marrow inflammation as fourth degree bedsores.

Even the first-degree stage can often be worse than it seems at first glance! Sometimes, a bedsore can extend deep into the surrounding fat and muscle tissue.

Additional, aggravating factors associated with bedsores include being overweight (too much body pressure); underweight (too little natural padding), a tendency towards accumulation of fluid (oedema), moisture, high temperature, lying in the wrong position, anaemia and diabetes.

In order to prevent bedsores, and to treat a first-degree case, consistent pressure relief is necessary; with the position in which the patient lying in is changed at least every two hours and actual physical exercise if at all possible. Depending on which areas of the body are affected, special air-filled rubber rings can be placed in the bed for the patient to lie on, along with the use of special mattresses. Bed sheets should be smooth and wrinkle-free and there should also be thorough skin-care (no creams, which may clog up the pores) (see Skin Care), a balanced diet rich in vitamins and enzymes, and consumption of clean water (gentle detoxification). In cases of incontinence, ensure that the person affected is not lying on soggy bedding for too long. Professional assistance in the form of a doctor, alternative practitioner or nurse should be sought in all cases of incipient bedsores, the sooner the better. If the bedsores have already exceeded the first degree, medical treatment is imperative!

Depending upon on the severity and extent, healing of bedsores can be supported by a number of crystals. This supplementary treatment, however, presupposes accompanying professional medical treatment. An old home remedy, which has proved to be effective, recommends that a bowl of spring water and a raw egg be placed under the bed for prophylaxis and treatment of bedsores. The result is even better, using pure water and organic eggs, instead of tap water and battery-farmed eggs. It may sound odd, and rather quaint; but try it anyway. It cannot do any harm.

Amethyst aids skin care in cases of bedsores, especially when Hildegard von Bingen's Amethyst Water is used (see page 25 and Skin Care) for cleansing the affected areas (only up to first degree cases), or the water may be taken internally (10 ml, up to 3 times a day, but not more!)

Carnelian, **Garnet Pyrope** and **Rose Quartz** improve the blood circulation in the affected area and reduce the risk of bedsores. However, they should not be used in cases of raised temperature or when there is already infection present (as they may have a contradictory effect).

Rhodonite and **Mookaite** are, however, the most important crystals to use in connection with bedsores. As crystals that further the healing of wounds, they also stimulate the healing process of the bedsores. However, please note that any open wounds (as in third degree sores) should be cleaned

regularly and carefully during this process.

Emerald can be applied as a supplement, if the bone is already affected, as it impedes inflammation of the bone marrow and relieves pain.

For all of these, place raw or tumbled crystals around the bed, or place them between the bed frame and the mattress. Also, if necessary, wear as a bracelet or a necklace, as long as this does not increase the risk of creating bedsores, or problems of the lying posture.

One of the simplest measures though is to take gem essence internally (3-7 drops, 3 times daily), or gem water (100–200 ml taken in small sips over the course of the day.

Bed Wetting

As a general rule, bed wetting during the night, particularly in children, has no physical cause. Rather, it tends to be emotional in origin, with the principle underlying reasons being fear, personal loss, jealousy (of younger siblings) or the child's perceived insecurity (e. g. after major changes in family or surroundings). In addition, one ventures to suggest that natural earth radiation fields and electromagnetic pollution may also lead to an emptying of the bladder during sleep. In fact, all of these causes should be investigated and clarified if the problem persists.

50

In contrast, adult incontinence, i. e. involuntary urination, is caused by weakened bladder control. This, in turn, may be caused by bladder infections and illnesses, prolapsed pelvic organs, nervous disturbances, prostate enlargement or a weakness of the pelvic floor muscles. Further causes, though tending to be more obscure in identification, may sometimes be chronic fear, insecurity or the feeling of losing control of your life (or a part of it). Any professional medical examination should therefore include both the latter aspect and physiological causes.

Amazonite helps with bed-wetting that is associated with grief, a sense of failure or strong revulsion. Very restless children, who tend to develop faster intellectually than they do emotionally, also respond positively to Amazonite therapy in this context.

Chrysoprase stops bed-wetting very quickly, particularly with children. It relieves the feeling of jealousy or lack of care and allows the child to rediscover its own security. As Chalcedony mineral, it also strengthens the bladder.

Citrine is particularly helpful with incontinence which is caused by a weak bladder or pelvic floor musculature. In addition, it boosts self-confidence and helps one regain control of one's own life.

Heliotrope helps with incontinence cause by serious worries, a feeling of loss of control over one's own life or in incontinence occurring after bladder infections

and related illnesses.

For all of the above, wear the crystal as a bracelet, necklace or a pendant. Alternatively, or as well, place a crystal directly over the bladder area – taping it in place with sticking plaster. If required,

If none of these have any effect, or because the bed-wetting is caused by a bladder infection – or by a weak bladder – try using crystals described below under Bladder Problems.

Bites

see Insect Bites and Stings

Bladder Problems

Bladder problems can be categorsied in two ways. One is a weak bladder with a tendency to infections, frequent urination and possibly incontinence. The other is a bladder with an infection that withholds of urine.

A weak bladder is often caused by a general lack of basic energy, often in association with fear and difficulties in life. Here, the control of one's own immediate situation, or specific parts of one's life, threaten to slip out of personal control. The result can often be an inflamed bladder with retention of urine. In effect, the latter is a kind of backlash, whereby you try, through exaggerated means, to get things under control.

Of course, an inflamed bladder may also be caused by disease, though any existing weakness will exacerbate the condition.

All bladder infections should be treated professionally. Any advance of an infection, through the urethra to the kidneys, may well cause dangerous complications.

Agate with a bladder signature – and, in particular, with a pink spot in the middle – is particularly good for treating chronic and acute bladder infections. Furthermore, it enhances emotional stability, so that crises and problems can be solved more easily.

Place a polished crystal, section/slice, over the pubic bone – or wear it there as a pendant.

Aquamarine helps with a weak bladder, any frequent need to urinate and with incontinency. It helps both regain control of the bladder function and of any other lifestyle problems.

Wear it as a bracelet, necklace or a pendant for a long period, although it does not have direct body contact. Alternatively, take it as gem essence (3-7 drops, 3 times daily)

Garnet Pyrope, however, is the "number one" crystal for treating a weak bladder and any accompanying tendency to infection. Furthermore, it helps in dealing with difficult life situations.

Place it as a crystal or a polished crystal over the pubic bone.

Heliotrope also helps in treating acute bladder infections, as they usually need to be cured by bed rest. However, do not rely on Heliotrope alone – but if used, place a section/slice or polished crystal over the pubic bone and stay in bed.

Nephrite or **Blue Chalcedony** helps with alleviating urine retention. Both crystals remove the need to retain everything, and also help one remain emotionally "fluid

Place a tumbled stone over the pubic bone. Alternatively, wear it as a bracelet, necklace or pendant for a long period; or take as gem essence (3-7 drops, 3 times daily)

Ocean Jasper helps both with a weak bladder, acute inflammation there and with urine retention. Its effect can best be described as regulating the bladder function. In severe cases, it helps emotionally and assists in the creating of a sense of hope, optimism, *joie de vivre* and renewed power – so that life becomes much easier.

Place a tumbled stone on the upper part of the pubic bone – or wear as a necklace, pendant or gem crystal for a long period.

Bleeding

see Minor Bleeding

Blisters

Blisters manifest as a consequence of mechanical pressure or rubbing (e. g. tight shoes or unaccustomed handling of tools).

Fast healing can be achieved using crystals. Blisters should not be lanced, as there could be a risk of infection. Further known household remedies for blisters are Bach's Rescue Remedy (drops onto the blister) or comfrey leaves placed inside the shoes where they rub.

Agate (containing an appropriate signature), Amethyst, Blue Chalcedony and Ocean Jasper will heal blisters that have not been pricked. The body will reabsorb the fluid in the blisters and the damaged skin layer will be renewed. The Blue Chalcedony and Ocean Jasper can be applied first to help drain the fluid. Then Agate is applied to stimulate the replacement of dead skin layers. Finally, Amethyst is applied in order to alleviate possible tenderness of the affected spot. If you only have one of the above crystals to hand, any of the crystals can also be applied on its own.

Rhodonite is best for open or burst blisters. It relieves any pain and assists faster healing of the open and tender spot.

Blue Tourmaline is particularly good for stimulating re-absorption of water from the blister. It will even prevent the formation of blisters if you place it on spots that have previously been exposed to pressure. Gem essence applied to the spot will have the same effect.

Place (or fix with sticking plaster) a tumbled stone or a flat slice or section of the crystal on the affected spot. Then, apply drops of special gem essence for effective external treatment. When using amethyst, also use Hildegard von Bingen's Amethyst Water (see page 25) on the blister.

Essences containing ethyl alcohol (ethanol) must be diluted (10 drops per 100 ml of water) if they are used for treatment of open blisters.

Bloatedness

A rather colloquial term, "bloatedness" or "feeling bloated", is the name we tend to use for the sensation that we experience as a consequence of increased formation of intestinal gas, This can be caused by certain foods (beans, cabbage, etc.), or because the normal release of the gasses is impeded by constipation. One might feel bloated for longer periods if the intestinal flora is out of balance or if there are other digestive problems.

Occasionally, even "mentally indigestible" situations or problems may also cause bloatedness. Furthermore, a lack of exercise, in particular together with sedentary work, is also a cause. So regular exercise (e. g. visits to the gym and regular walks), stomach massage, a careful combination of certain foods (along with eating such things as fennel and drinking caraway tea) are among proven home remedies.

Agate also relieves bloatedness, as it regulates and harmonises the intestinal flora. Section/slices or tumbled stones, with inclusions of uniform curving bands, can be placed on the stomach for rapid results. In addition, Agate also brings about a vital and necessary emotional stability needed in order to tackle and "digest" any uncomfortable issues. Most effective, however, are Agates worn as a necklace or pendants for long periods.

Emerald relieves any kind of feeling of bloatedness. Take it as gem essence before meals (5-7 drops, 3 times daily). Alternatively, it can be used as crystals or tumbled stones arranged in the shape of a large horseshoe on the stomach, to follow externally the course of the colon. Other wise, wear it as a necklace or a pendant for a longer period

Black Tourmaline is particularly helpful, if bloatedness accompanies constipation. Use it as above for Emerald. When forming a horseshoe of Tourmaline crys-

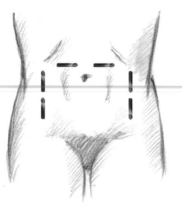

Fig. 2: Tourmaline crystal rods placed on the stomach in the form of a horseshoe.

tals, take care that they point in the same direction as the flow of waste matter through the colon, i. e. upwards on the right side of the stomach, across the stomach and, finally, turning downwards on the left side of the stomach.

Blood Circulation

As a rule, problems with the circulation only arise if the flow of blood is impaired. Usually, the supply of blood to the tissues varies in different parts of the body, depending on the needs of those parts of our organism. Where increased activity is required, the circulation is stepped up; where activity is reduced, blood circulation is slowed down. A really drastic reduction of blood circulation only takes place in emergency conditions, when the body needs to secure the blood supply for the most important of our organs (brain, heart, liver and kidneys) and, as a precaution, restricts the flow to the "less important" organs and parts of the body. Examples of such emergency situations may be loss of blood, a high fever, or dangerous situations. Traditional Chinese Medicine calls this regulating system the "triple-warmer".

If the triple-warmer is impaired or interrupted in any way, the emergency mechanism may kick in, even when it is not required. Among other things, this can result in chronically cold hands and feet.

Apart from this, the circulation of blood may be disturbed by low blood pressure, a weak heart, or by the narrowing and blocking of blood vessels (arteriosclerosis). Malnutrition (too much fat and animal protein), smoking, and certain types of medicines (always read the description and instructions on all drug and medication packaging) can result in such narrowing. Therefore, a regime of detoxification and a change to a healthier diet are some of the most important precautions in dealing with any problems with blood circulation.

Slight disturbances of the blood circulation manifest themselves as a feeling of coldness, limbs that have "fallen asleep" or feel tingly, increasing feelings of great tiredness, pain that appears when one feels anxious, and under certain circumstances, feelings of dizziness. Continuous disturbances of the blood circulation may become dangerous. They can result in damage to the organs and tissues (see Leg Ulcers). Therefore, the crystals, which are mentioned here, are only intended for use in cases of minor disturbances of the blood circulation. In cases of repeated disturbances, or those of longer duration, professional advice should be sought without fail.

Garnet Pyrope is the most important crystal both for cases of general or localised circulation problems. The Garnet fortifies the triple warmer and ensures that energy is spread evenly throughout the body. In this way, it helps with cases of rapid onset of tiredness, feelings of coldness and pains caused by general stress.

Place a crystal or a polished crystal on the affected areas to obtain localised improvement of the circulation. In cases of generally reduced blood circulation, preferably wear necklaces or pendants or take gem essence (3-5 drops, 5 times daily).

Obsidian helps particularly with chronically cold hands and feet, when parts of the body have "fallen asleep", and even in cases of hardening of the arteries in the legs caused by smoking.

Preferably hold a crystal in your hand, place one (cabochon) in your shoe, or place/fix it on areas of the body with bad blood circulation.

Rhodocrosite stimulates the blood circulation. Also, like Garnet, it has a positive effect on the blood circulation. Compared to Garnet, the effect is much faster and Rhodocrosite should never be applied if there is a tendency to high blood pressure.

Wear a necklace or a pendant on the body or take gem essence in small doses (3 drops, 3 times daily are sufficient)

Rose Quartz is well suited in cases of localised disturbances of the blood circulation. For coldness, prickling feelings, or sensations of the affected part "going to sleep", massage the general area with rose quartz balls spheres or polished crystals.

See also Circulation Problems

Blood Pressure

The blood pressure in the arteries is caused by two factors: the quantity of blood pumped out by the heart into the arterial system and the resistance to its flow caused by the elasticity and the condition of the walls of the blood vessels and the blood's own fluidity. Narrowed arteries and "viscous" blood can lead to an increase in blood pressure, while dilated, slack arteries and "easily flowing" blood lead to decreased blood pressure. Normally, blood pressure rises with physical exertion, faster breathing, stress, or dangerous situations. Blood pressure tends to drop when you are calm, relaxed (in particular, when lying down or under the influence of narcotics) or when taking certain medications.

However, blood pressure that is persistently too high or too low can cause problems – some of them quite serious. High blood pressure – called hypertension – manifests as tiredness, headaches, and reduced energy levels Furthermore, under certain conditions, it can result in heart and/or kidney problems, or in nervous illness.

In order to eliminate those instances where such symptoms are caused by a serious disease of the internal organs, and to avoid further serious complications, high blood pressure should only be treated professionally.

So, always consult your doctor if you experience any signs of high blood pressure.

Symptoms of low blood pressure include tiredness, weakness, dizziness, pale or cold skin and a fast but weak pulse. There might also be a tendency to faint or have "black outs", or even become unconsciousness. Like high blood pressure, professional medical help should be sought as soon as possible in order to clarify the causes.

Changes in blood pressure can be a symptom of many different emotional states, which makes it almost impossible to give any real general advice. Indeed, the only help in determining any individual background cause may be by simply observing an apparent connection between high blood pressure and tension, stress or excitement – and any equivalent connection between low blood pressure and lack of energy, unconsciousness and sluggishness. One might have to ask oneself questions about personal or related life issues, or anything at all which might be causing these symptoms to appear?

Many crystals either raise or lower blood pressure. Nevertheless, their practical application only makes sense if physical and emotional root causes are clarified at the same time.

A diet free of animal proteins, regular fasting and other detoxifying measures (see Detoxification) should, in any case, accompany the treatment of any blood pressure condition that is too high or too low.

High Blood Pressure

Here are some crystals that can be used in conjunction with the medical advice and treatment obtained professionally.

Amethyst quickly lowers blood pressure. Using a druse of the crystal the size of a saucer, make gentle stroking movements (as if it were a brush) – without touching the body – from the forehead over the top of the head, the back of the neck, the back, and the legs and arms respectively, towards the floor (see Fig. 3). Should the person's blood pressure fall too rapidly, and symptoms of dizziness or similar are experienced, the pressure can be stabilised with an equalising movement over the body (over the central axis of the body, starting from below in front – over the head and down the back – see Fig. 4). This treatment will provide a comfortable and relaxing effect, both physically and emotionally.

Blue Chalcedony lowers blood pressure in the long term. It is less suited for short-term alleviation, but more so for a long-term stabilisation of "normal" blood pressure.

Lapis lazuli has a very fast lowering effect on blood pressure as long as does not contain traces of Pyrites (Fool's Gold)! Best suited is blue-white spotted Lapis lazuli with Calcite, which is particularly appropriate for lowering acute high blood pressure. It should only be applied for a short while.

Sodalite also has a rapid lowering effect on blood pressure and, contrary to Lapis

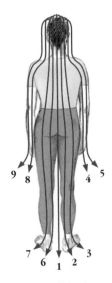

Fig. 3: Lowering of blood pressure with pieces of Amethyst druses.

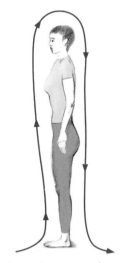

Fig. 4: Equalising trace of crystal for stabilising blood pressure.

57

Lazuli, can be applied for a longer period of time.

Low Blood Pressure

Similarly, and complementing normal medical treatment, the following can prove effective.

Fire Opal provides rapid relief for too low blood pressure and can, therefore, help during sudden attacks of dizziness or unconsciousness, e. g. when "everything goes black" when you stand up.

Hematite stabilises blood pressure during phases of persistently low blood pressure or weakness, e. g. when the body is experiencing rapid growth, or when one is living through a difficult life phase.

Rhodocrosite causes the blood vessels to contract, and raising blood pressure. It should only be applied for a short time for low blood pressure. This is caused, for example, by a lack of sleep.

Ruby generally raises blood pressure and stabilises it within the normal range.

Take a pair of the crystals mentioned above in your hands in order to achieve a rapid change of blood pressure via the circulation meridian (one of the twelve main energy pathways of the body).

Wear bracelets, necklaces or pendants (on the chest), or take gem essence (3-5 drops, 3 times daily) or gem water (100–200 ml taken in sips during the course of the day) for long-term treatment.

Borellia

see Tick Bites

Breast-feeding

The main reason for problems arising during breast-feeding is usually a lack of peace and quiet and/or insufficient rest for the nursing mother. Such conditions or circumstances prevent her from focusing fully upon the feeding baby. Quietness is particularly important at the early stages of breast-feeding phase, when everything still seems new and there is, as yet, no familiar routine. In addition, for the actual process of milk production, peace and quiet and a protective, secure atmosphere should never be underestimated (see also: Lactation).

Once any immediate problems with lactation are overcome – particularly the first flow of milk and any inflammation of the breast – there can still be further problems in breast-feeding. For example, there may still be some feeling of pain when the milk first starts flowing, as the milk ducts leading from the individual milk glands to the nipples are initially still relatively narrow during the early stages, making it difficult for the milk to flow easily. In this case, the application of poultices of quark-type fresh white cheese, firm massaging and use of the crystals mentioned below may help.

Breast inflammation, on the other hand, occurs because bacteria can penetrate the fine cracks and fissures of the nipples. This can be partially prevented in advance by an invigorating massage of the nipples (pulling and pushing) during pregnancy. However, if inflammation does occur whilst nursing, nipple shields can help prevent further aggravation. Quark poultices will also bring relief and the crystals described below have also demonstrated extraordinary results in healing nipple inflammation.

A disturbed emotional relationship between the mother and the baby is something that is often blamed for problems with breast-feeding. However, this has to be rejected most empathically at the outset. Not only is this assumption wrong in nearly every case, it is particularly unhelpful in that it is a concept that, under certain circumstances, can in itself serve to create real feelings of guilt in the mother.

Obviously it is only natural that the baby be breast fed by the mother. In most cases, where there are problems, it is well worth looking at the mother's own "emotional nurturing". For instance, a breast inflammation is more likely to occur where the mother is spending too much time taking care of others and neglecting herself. Furthermore, it is the actual stress and strains caused by childbirth and the often enormous changes of life within the family that are equally responsible for problems with breast-feeding. Undue worries and concerns for others should therefore be avoided by the nursing mother (Chalcedony can help here – see below) and be replaced by a concentration on her own well-being as far as possible.

Chalcedony, particularly the light blue, pink or white one without stripes, is the best crystal for all types of problems during breast-feeding. It relieves inflammation of the breast, stimulates milk production, eases the first flow into the milk ducts and also provides the necessary inner peace that is best for breast-feeding. After all, it is not for nothing that white Chalcedony is commonly called "milk crystal". It has been applied for centuries in order to stimulate milk production and ease breast-feeding.

All the varieties of Chalcedony referred to can be worn as necklaces or pendants on the breast.

Broken Bones

Once broken bones have been set and fixed with a splint, crystals can support the healing process. However, before such application, always ensure that the fracture really has been set properly.

Apatite, in particular, stimulates the healing of broken bones – so effectively, in fact, that if it is used when the bone has not been set properly deformations may occur that, in turn, can lead to long lasting problems. Therefore, use Apatite ONLY when the X-rays have established that the bones are fully in the right position and this has been confirmed medically

Because Apatite furthers the healing of broken bones to such a degree, the parts grow together again almost twice as fast as usual. This is thought to be due to the fact that Apatite is chemically a form of calcium phosphate, and so is very similar to human bone composition, enabling it to trigger the appropriate growth impulse.

Calcite also furthers the healing of broken bones, though not as intensely or effectively as Apatite. It stimulates the calcium metabolism, which, in turn, has a positive influence on bone growth.

For both Apatite and Calcite, place or affix a tumbled stone or a crystal as close to the fracture as possible. Unfortunately, in many cases, a plaster cast is generally in the way, even though this too has a healing chemical make up largely of calcium. Therefore, taking gem essence is recommended as an additional treatment (5-9 drops, 5 times daily) or gem water (200–300 ml taken in small sips over the course of the day).

The same goes for pain relieving crystals and crystals that heal bruising, injured tissues and nerves.

Kunzite, Obsidian or **Sugilite** are additional crystals that encourage the healing process of the bone and which can aid in pain relief

Rhodonite helps heal bruising and contusions.

Tourmaline should be applied if injury to nerves is also suspected with symptoms of numbness or temporary paralysis.

Bruising

Bruises are formed when blood vessels are damaged or torn and blood flows into the connective tissue, muscles or limbs. The causes are usually severe blows, dislocations, sprains, broken bones, or (more rarely) simple pressure points made on the body. The skin covering a bruise appears bluish at first; then, later on, a greenish-yellow, as the red colouring agent of the blood – haemoglobin – is broken down. Bruises generally disappear after a couple of weeks – but the time can be reduced with a suitable treatment. Standard household remedies for this include the application of a cold poultices and arnica cream to the skin, along with taking homeopathic arnica preparations orally. (See also: Contusions)

Rhodonite and **Obsidian** crystals, in particular, expedite fast recovery from bruising and they provide pain relief and so help overcome the shock experienced from painful injuries.

Place or fix (with sticking plaster) a flat, tumbled mineral or a slice/section onto the affected spot. If necessary, place it inside any existing bandaging there.

Gem essence taken internally (5-9 drops, as required), or gem water (100–200 ml taken in sips during the course of the day) may also be helpful.

Bronchitis

Bronchitis is an infectious disease of the bronchia, often developing as a complication from the common cold. It affects the two main branches of the trachea and their ancillary branches leading to the lungs. The complication of the original illness is often caused by clogging of the tissues with toxic substances, e. g. those from dairy products. Nowadays, many cows are raised for mass production of milk and dairy products. As a result, their the milk, now lacking enzymes but with a high content of antibiotic residues and other harmful substances, can only be humanly digested only with some considerable difficulty. This, in turn, leads to a clogging of our tissues. Such "pollution" curbs the activities of the natural immune system and so increases our susceptibility to infection.

A simple, common cold can develop relatively easily into bronchitis. It manifests itself first as a cough, producing phlegm (particularly in the morning), a raised temperature, and general weakness and, occasionally, chest pains or breathlessness. Although an attack of bronchitis will normally resolve itself naturally during the course of several days, professional medical advice should always be sought to prevent the disease from spreading unnoticed and – finally – affecting the lungs. Many household remedies have proved to be very effective when it comes to supporting the healing process. Hot poultices of potato, goose grease, or onion, in particular, are tried and tested folk-style remedies for fast relief.

Bronchitis should be treated with great care, as it may become chronic if you have had recurrent bouts. The emotional background of the illness should also be taken into account. As with other illnesses of the common cold variety, personal interaction with other people and one's environment also play a part. Furthermore, especially in the case of bronchitis, there may be issues of sadness and grieving involved for some sufferers – along with a deeper effect of any hidden fears that one may be harbouring. The crystals described below are also effective in alleviating these effects

Apophyllite may rapidly relieve acute bronchitis, aid with complete recovery from the illness and stimulate regeneration of the mucous membranes. It also helps with shyness, anxiety, feelings of apprehension, tightness in the chest and insecurity.

Ocean Jasper helps with both acute and chronic bronchitis. It relieves coughs and breathlessness, regulates raised temperatures and prevents dangerously high temperatures. It also strengthens the will to recover and lends hope and an optimistic outlook.

Rutile Quartz helps equally with acute

and chronic bronchitis. Opaque crystals containing many Rutile threads are most effective. Emotionally, Rutile Quartz has a mood-lightening and anti-depressant effect. It dissolves hidden [unconscious] fears and helps sustain hope and the will to recovery in the case of stubborn diseases.

Emerald helps with acute bronchitis, in particular where it has developed very rapidly from a cold. It slows down an accelerated course of an illness, in this way, preventing further complications. Furthermore, Emerald supports a fast and total recovery. You can generally apply Emerald when an attack of bronchitis is declining, so that it can be completely cured and not become chronic.

With Apophyllite, place or tape a crystal, or small group of crystals, directly onto the bronchial area.

For Ocean Jasper, Rutile Quartz and Emerald, place, or tape if necessary, a polished crystal on the bronchial area, and wear a necklace, or a pendant for a longer period. Gem essence can also be taken internally (5-7 drops, 3-5 times daily) or gem water (100–300 ml taken in sips during the course of the day).

Burns

Burns are what we call the painful damage to the tissue caused by a localised exposure to temperatures of more than 50 degrees centigrade (about 120 degrees Fahrenheit). Naked flames, hot gasses, steam, heated fluids and objects can lead to burns or scalding – as can also exposure to electrical power and radiation (ultraviolet, X-ray, microwaves and radioactivity).

Burns are categorised under four degrees, depending on the depth and the scope of the damage.

A first-degree burn is characterised by painful skin that is reddish and swollen for a couple of days.

A second-degree burn causes blisters and can, if extensive, lead to the formation of scars. Under no circumstances should such blisters be damaged, burst or opened, as the danger of infections and the formation of scars are greatly increased.

With third-degree burns, entire areas of skin are destroyed. Ironically, these areas are often more or less painless, as the nerve endings themselves have also been destroyed. Such burns only heal very slowly, from the periphery toward the centre, and leave distinctive scars. Skin transplants are usually required in order to support the healing process.

In cases of fourth degree burns, the underlying tissue is damaged, too. Full recovery is impossible, in most cases, implying permanent damage.

All serious burns or scalds require the **immediate** attendance and treatment of a doctor or emergency medical services.

In other cases of burns, first aid always

involves placing and keeping the affected area under cold, running water until the initial severe pain is reduced or ceases. In cases where hot liquids cause scalding, the wet clothes should be removed at once. After that, cover the burned or scalded area with a sterile burn bandage or pad and ensure the wound is seen by a doctor. Treatment of large-area burns ought also to involve drinking lots of fluid (about 1 litre of water mixed up with 3 g salt), in order to offset the loss of liquid from the wound and to prevent shock from the burn.

In cases of first-degree burns, or small second-degree burns but with no blisters, many home remedies, such as irradiation with orange light application, treating with juice from the Aloe Vera plant, oil from St. John's Wort, or etheric oil from wild mountain lavender (only for closed blisters!) may speed up the healing process.

Blue Tourmaline can be applied in cases of second-degree burns, as it furthers the regeneration of the skin without leaving scars. Take gem essence (at the beginning, 5-7 drops every 15 minutes; later on, 3-7 drops every hour; after the second day, 3-7 drops, 3 times daily). Also, if possible, bathe the burned area with cold water that contains gem essence (20 drops in 1 litre of water).

Gem water can be applied in the same way (drink up to 2 litres in sips over the course of the day). The wound can also be bathed with this water, in cases of larger burns, before a compress is applied.

Rhodonite should be applied subsequently – or, in cases of first-degree burns, immediately – so that the wound can heal completely. Just as with Blue Tourmaline, it is applied both internally and externally. With small burns, moistening a polished crystal and holding it on the burned spot may be sufficient.

Cancer

The overall and common term "cancer" is used to describe malignant diseases involving tumour formations. If not treated thoroughly and professionally, most end fatally.

Tumours occur because of the unrestrained growth of the body's own tissue. Unlike cancerous forms, so-called "benign" tumours remain largely disassociated from the surrounding tissue and only "crowd it out". In other words, they do not invade into the surrounding tissue or blood vessels and, therefore, only become a problem if they occur in adverse locations (e. g. the brain). In contrast, malignant tumours break through into other tissues and vessels, destroy them and – in addition – generate metastases. These are offshoot tumours, which spread through the lymphatic and blood systems and via other vital body channels. It is these tumours and their effects that are generally referred to as cancer.

When the malignant tumours are generated, the nature of the original cells and their metabolism also changes. In the human organism, every cell is different and specific, i. e. it develops according to its own task and has its own special functions. If such a cell becomes cancerous, it then becomes a non-specific, one-cell organism. It takes on the metabolic process of all one-cell organisms that live without oxygen and adopts the typical one-cell survival programme that seems deeply rooted in our genes. In other words, its function and behaviour is simply that of "reproduction, reproduction, and reproduction". The cell leaves its previous "home" tissue – akin to its "social group" hitherto – and commences dividing wildly. Thus, the malignant tumours begin to grow and spread rapidly.

So, what are the factors that make cells feel so threatened that they relapse into the archaic one-cell pattern of survival? Certainly, they include chemicals that attack the normal genetic inheritance of the cell. Called carcinogens in general, they can include pesticides, fertilisers, food colourings and additives, heavy metals, asbestos fibres, etc. In fact, a huge range exists and can even include some medicines. Others include cigarette smoke, excessive alcohol, hormonal additives in meat and drinking water, some viruses, long-lasting inflammatory conditions. Especially causal is the effect of radiation, whether in the form of X-rays, technological radiation and other types of radioactivity, or even natural radioactivity in certain regions. Indeed, it is worth stating that an investigation of the place where one lives, works or sleeps is always recommended whenever cancer has been diagnosed!

However, it is not only such external risk factors that can lead to the formation of tumours. There are also a number of internal (endogenous) contributory factors. Cancer can also be caused by parasites. In truth, most people live with many forms of parasite in their system without even knowing and without their necessarily causing problems. Yet, if the efficiency of the immune system has deteriorated as a result of continuous stress, chronic inflammatory conditions, toxification or other factors, it can no longer cope with some types of parasites, which then start attacking specific cells. This continues at an increasing rate (i. e. by being absorbed by the cells), and cells try to manage the situation through faster division. At first glance, this process of division seems beneficial, as it reduces the number of parasites per cell by half; but it creates a situation of initial conflict and so can have a truly fatal outcomes

There has been a long and heartfelt debate about the causes of cancer in the context of the overall condition of the human body, life style, and so forth. It is a discussion that continues to this day, as it is less easy to identify causes, which are not obviously external (as explained above). Nevertheless, there can surely be little doubt that the continuous stress of modern life has a "burn-out" effect on our adrenaline production. In turn, this leads to a weakening of the immune system and creates toxic build-up as a result and with one's own metabolic products sometimes also playing an important role.

There are serious schools of thought that continuous high consumption of sugar and wheat flour in particular will, at some point, lead to the consequence that the existing amount of sugar can no longer be metabolically processed. Consequently, the body's sugar storage capacity is exhausted. This problem, which can also cause the so-called age-related diabetes (see Diabetes), can also lead to cell division at an increased rate as well as to cells adapting to the sugar-consuming metabolism. Once again, this can be fatal for eventual survival.

As mentioned elsewhere (see Detoxification), our connective tissue in particular is an intermediary "storage space", where substances that cannot be excreted, are stored "temporarily". Unfortunately, these "stores" increasingly become final repositories because of our modern nutrition and life habits, i.e. they become blocked with ever more amounts of waste products. Eventually, they suffer from lack of oxygen and nutrients and can no longer get rid of the toxic waste products. The effect is that the stores eventually starve and suffocate in

their own waste! It is no wonder then that one or the other cell eventually "panics", goes its own way and activates its emergency survival programme. Its faith in the community of the organism is lost, its need for air, water and nutrients are apparently no longer being met – so it is as though the cell decides to take the matter into its own hands!

I am convinced that the reduction of stress, a diet with a reduced consumption of sugar, wheat flour and animal protein and detoxification and metabolic regulation are, therefore, most important measures to take. Further, in the context of external causes such as radiation and pollution, I recommend strongly examining where one sleeps, lives and works – and changing any of these factors if you are sufficiently concerned or worried.

Of course, I am aware that advocating such a philosophy can certainly involve some very disturbing questions. For example, what about your nutrition? Does your diet include organic, energising, easily digestible, vital food – as opposed to merely filling, so-called "fast food", manufactured with too many additives and chemicals? What do we drink? Good water – or what I would term a liquid that is full of useless substances such as sugar, alcohol, artificial aromatic substances and stimulants? How do we treat our body? How much rest, sleep, care, and beneficial activities do we offer it? How much strain and effort do we demand from it? How many unpleasant situations and discomforts do we expect it to put up with? And so on…

I am convinced that these are questions that we should ask ourselves much more often than is the case. At the very least, becoming ill in any form – but especially with cancer – must surely raise questions about one's entire lifestyle. So, whilst nutrition, sleep and time for regeneration are the basic pillars of life, any condition that affects these pillars will very quickly throw up questions about our work, spare time, life rhythms, habits and vices, stress, desires and frustrations.

I believe that we have to ask questions about how we really live our lives. Is it as part of a community, of nature and of the whole of the cosmos? Or do we behave as a mere individual, as if we were unconnected with the rest of the world? So, in questions about our health, are we not, therefore, faced with much bigger questions about ourselves, our homes and families, about our inclinations and interests, beliefs, convictions, philosophy of life, hopes and yearnings, *joie-de-vivre*, the meaning of life, and our overall goals, successes and failures? After all, these things have an impact on us as holistic beings, with a spirit, soul, mind and a body with its finely adjusted internal teamwork right down to the individual cell and its efforts to survive.

Thus, I am adamant that the asbestos fibre, pack of cigarettes, or even our genes cannot to be wholly to blame if we develop cancer. Rather, I consider that any cancer is the consequence of an individual, multi-facetted development, which takes as its starting point our physical, emotional and mental state. Not everyone can or will agree with this statement, but I sincerely feel that it is not the cell itself that is the "evil", which must be fought by radiotherapy, by chemotherapy, with is often highly adverse side-effects, and by the oncologist surgeon wielding a scalpel. A cancer cell is, on the contrary, the victim of a derailed organization in the body! The body's tissue, lymph, blood, digestion, detoxification, excretion and regenerative ability must all be helped as quickly as possible, so that one-cell survival programmes in the body become superfluous.

So what does this mean concretely? I can only note here some purely *personal* observations and conclusion. So, these considerations are nothing other than just that, and are thus not based upon any conventional medical profession or expertise. Nevertheless, I think it valid to cite here three observations I have made in all the people I know who have survived cancer – and who today enjoy optimal health:

1. They submitted to a radical physical health cure. Holistic treatments were carried out consistently; the body was detoxified; the metabolism was reorganised to include consideration of improved nutrition and care, tissue de-acidification, colon

therapy; drainage of toxic substances, homeopathic therapy.

2. Their outlook became more "life-friendly". Harmful habits were abandoned, regeneration (sleep and rest), strengthening and training (sport and exercise) became a part of their daily life; and their life rhythms became more structured. In addition living areas, especially for sleeping, living and working, were thoroughly examined for radiation and negative biological influences – and all the necessary changes were actually carried out!

3. Conflicts were resolved through counselling or therapy; important and unimportant issues of life were identified, this was often connected with changes at work, socially and in relationships; original life goals were re-evaluated – and, last but not least, lifestyles were adjusted according to desires for happiness and the fulfilment of wishes.

Of course, there cannot be any guarantees, especially with something as invasive as cancer and depending upon the type of cancer and its spread within the human organism. Nevertheless, as with all ailments and illnesses, changes in the way of life and environment, resolution of emotional and mental conflicts must all be positive steps for anyone. (The latter – resolution of conflict – is particularly important, as it is often overlooked! Yet, it is known even in traditional medical science that long-term, smouldering conflicts are the psychological

seedbed for long-term smouldering conflicts in the body. And who can say that the consequence of this may well not be that a cell decides, at one time or the other, to survive by becoming "egoistical"?)

Becoming ill with cancer demands that we change our life. Thus, whilst relying upon the latest advances in medical science, undergoing an operation, having radiation treatment and chemotherapy to treat the cancer, we then continue with life, supported by competent and professional advice – but now also with the extra help of whatever alternative natural and therapeutic measures used in order to obtain a holistic cure.

Cancer is no longer a death sentence! Take as your role model all those people who have overcome it and who today enjoy the best of health! Their paths to success can be the guiding principle on how one can cope with cancer oneself.

It is in this light that I recommend the following crystals be used. Obviously, no crystal or associated therapy can cure cancer. Rather, within the framework of an individually tailored holistic therapy, which includes body, mind and soul, crystals can make a valuable contribution to overall well being; and this has to be beneficial in any circumstances and for everyone.

Noble Opal reminds one of one's original goals, the colourful, creative ideas of one's life dream. In this way, it will touch on a key point from which many conflicts arise, e. g. how do I really want to live my life? In reminding oneself of this, the necessary changes become self-evident. Opal also helps one regain enthusiasm and *joie-de-vivre*, and the most importantly the motivation to become sound and healthy once again. On a physical level, it ensures that tissues and lymph are cleansed, thereby improving the supply of nutrients to the cells and the removal of waste substances from them.

Wear a bracelet, a necklace or a pendant with body contact, or place it in your surroundings, so that it can be seen and it is, at the same time, close to the body. Also, take gem essence (3-9 drops, 3-7 times daily) or gem water (200–300 ml taken in small sips over the course of the day).

Ocean Jasper is the healing crystal associated with tumours as many of its varieties have the signature of individual cells or the "ball-and-cluster-like" signature of cell communities. As a type of Chalcedony, it also stimulates the cleansing of the tissues and lymphatic system, as well as being a detoxifier, having an anti-inflammatory effect and strengthening the immune system. It furthers the regeneration of cells and tissue and regulates the metabolism. In this way, it works as an optimal "re-organiser".

Emotionally, it provides hope, the courage to live, and the desire for a new beginning. Under its influence, changes do not become a burdensome, necessary duty, but instead a new opportunity to be happy.

It improves sleep and the power of regeneration and speeds up many healing processes.

A circle of crystals placed around the bed will be especially supportive in this way. Orange Jasper can be worn in the form of a bracelet, a necklace or a pendant. It can be taken internally in the form of either gem essence (3-9 drops, 3-7 times daily) or gem water (200–300 ml taken in small sips over the course of the day).

Green Tourmaline contains the metallic elements chromium and vanadium, which creates a strongly detoxifying, anti-inflammatory and regenerative effect. The metal vanadium is especially powerful in the processes of degeneration and, in this case – in accordance with the principle "like heals like" – it neutralises destructive processes.

As Tourmaline also improves the energetic processes and the information flow within the body, affected cells can be integrated within the organism once more. Additionally, it also furthers the dissolving of emotional conflicts and leads to a more positive attitude, improving general *joie-de-vivre* so that regeneration can occur. Finally, it also helps one to find one's bearings in new phases of life, and brings forgotten goals back into the light.

It is most effective if worn as a bracelet, necklace or pendant. It can also be taken as gem essence (3-9 drops, 3-7 times daily) or gem water (200–300 ml taken in small sips over the course of the day). It is also possible to place a slice/section of Green Tourmaline in front of a strong torch and to point the beam at the affected areas. This action will transmit the healing information of the crystal to the correct location.

The latter treatment has a very intense effect and should therefore only be increased slowly (3 times 5 minute sessions on the first day, 3 times 10 minute sessions on the second day, and so on).

Carpal Tunnel Syndrome

The carpal tunnel is located in the wrists, on the underside of the carpal bones and tendons. The flexible sinews of the fingers and the forearm nerve, which control the muscles of the ball of the thumb, all run through the carpal tunnel. The carpal tunnel can become narrowed because of chronic inflammation in the wrist, or because of damage from a sprain or undue strain or twisting. As a result, the forearm nerve becomes trapped in the carpal tunnel. This, in turn, leads to feelings of coldness or numbness in the fingers – especially in the index and middle finger. There are then problems with gripping or holding objects, particularly first thing in the morning.

In addition, the patient may also suffer pains in the arm at night – which can reach right up to the shoulder – along with pains and prickling in the hand. Although massaging or shaking the hand gently may bring relief, this will not be sufficient in the long run. If carpal tunnel syndrome occurs over an extended period, the muscles of the thumb will shrink considerably.

Carpal tunnel syndrome is often caused by inflammation, particularly in cases of rheumatism. Another cause is wrist sprain, e. g. adopting an awkward body position whilst writing or using the hand. It can also be caused by displaced body equilibrium in connection with spine problems.

A holistic professional diagnosis should be obtained – as conventional medical science still believes in the existence of carpal tunnel syndrome without any known cause! Naturally, if the cause is more of a rheumatic nature, a course of detoxification is important (see also Detoxification and Rheumatism); but if the cause is of a more ergonomic nature, a holistic body therapy is recommended (e. g. cranio-sacral therapy).

Of course, crystals can be helpful in both cases: **Amazonite** and **Green Tourmaline** are the most important healing crystals for carpal tunnel syndrome. They help both with the causes – which are a consequence of an inflammatory state – and with the consequences of overstraining. As a feldspar rich in lead, Amazonite helps with many kinds of tissue shrinkage and Green Tourmaline stimulates the regeneration of the squashed nerve.

Chrysocolla, Heliotrope, Emerald and **Turquoise** help especially when inflammation and/or rheumatism are the background cause. In addition, they are detoxifying crystals, which means that the syndrome's real causes are also dealt with.

Amber, Dumortierite, Lavender Jade and Sugilite help with the consequences of both sprains and bad body postures – both of which cause the symptomatic mechanical narrowing of the carpal tunnel. Dumortierite is especially good in this case, as it has a rapid pain-relieving effect and gets rid of bad posture habits. It also rebalances the whole body along with providing emotional ease.

In each case, wear a bracelet directly on the wrist or affix a flat, raw or tumbled stone with a linen bandage or similar binding.

It is also possible to take gem essence (5-7 drops, 3 times daily) or gem water (200–300 ml taken in small sips over the course of the day).

Cataracts

A cataract is a blurring of the eye's lens. It can be caused by a gradual deposition of the body's waste substances (a form often referred to as age-determined), metabolic diseases (e. g. diabetes), prenatal infections, or the consequences of injuries, radiation, heat, blinding (lightning), poisoning and other eye diseases. A cataract leads to a decreased ability to focus sharply and an increasing deterioration of vision that can progress all the way to total blindness.

In mainstream medicine, cataracts are treated by an operation in which the lens of the eye is partially or even totally removed and replaced by a lens-implant, contact lens or cataract eye glasses.

In alternative medicine, in which the application of healing crystals also plays a part, there are precautions one can take that can bring to a halt the usually progressive continuation of blurring – or can at least can reduce the speed of this deterioration process. In such treatments, detoxification, metabolic regulation – as well as treatment of the causal diseases or injuries – are highest on the agenda.

See also: Acidification; Detoxification; Diabetes; Eye Problems; Liver Health; Lymphatic Health; Sight Problems; Thyroid Problems

Rock Crystal has been applied for centuries in cases of cataracts. It helps particularly in the early stages, where the lens starts to become blurred. One places either a small crystal or a tumbled stone directly on the closed eyes. The clear, bright, so-termed 'Herkimer' Diamonds are especially suited.

Diamonds themselves can also be helpful in the later stages. Their best effect can be obtained when the cataract is a result of deposition of waste body substances Take gem essence (3-7 drops, 3-5 times daily) or gem water (200–300 ml daily, taken in small sips over the course of the day). A gemstone can also be placed directly on the eyes, or between the eyebrows on the so-called "third eye".

Obsidian also helps, in particular with the consequences of injuries, when it should be applied as fast as possible. Depending on the type of injury, place a flat crystal directly on the eye, or use a segment of obsidian over the eye but without direct contact. Some further curative effect can even be obtained by the calm and relaxed contemplation of a mirror-like polished section of this mineral.

Emerald helps with a cataract resulting from a metabolic problem. (In the broadest sense, poisoning and previous infections also belong in this category.) Place the crystals (preferably simultaneously) on the eyes and on the liver. Also wear a necklace or a pendant and take gem essence (5-9 drops, 3-5 times daily) or gem water (200–300 ml, taken in small sips over the course of the day).

Cellulite

Cellulite is the physical evidence of a structural change of the subcutaneous tissue, where fat deposits are formed which results in irregularities on the surface of the skin ("orange peel" skin). These skin changes have nothing to do with the true medical condition of cellulitis, an inflammation in the skin cell tissue. Cellulite, the cause of which is often incorrectly referred to and ascribed as being age-related, is caused (as are many diseases of the skin and tissues) by waste deposits and accumulation of lymph. The breakdown of such waste deposits and toxins is furthered by many crystals, e. g. **Blue Chalcedony** and **Chrysoprase**. (See also: Detoxification)

Furthermore, exercise, healthy nutrition, massaging the skin and showering with alternating hot and cold water all help alleviate this condition. Until now, however, only two crystals have turned out to be suitable for a true regeneration of skin that is affected by cellulite.

Ocean Jasper stimulates regeneration and reorganization of the tissues after intensive detoxifying cures. It can, therefore, be applied as "preparation" before using **Brown Tourmaline (Dravite)**, if the latter does not have an immediate effect.

Take gem water (200–300 ml taken in sips during the course of the day).

Dravite Tourmaline, which is rich in magnesium, furthers the cleansing and the detoxification of the connective tissue and deeper layers of skin and their structural regeneration. The cellulite's fat deposits are dissolved in this way, and the small dents and bumps on the surface of the skin disappear.

To this end, Dravite Tourmaline should be applied in two ways. On the one hand, take gem essence orally (3-5 drops, 3 times daily) or gem water (200–300 ml taken in

71

sips during the course of the day), which generally cleanses the skin and tissues. On the other hand, Dravite crystals or tumbled stones are placed on the affected areas of the body. This will focus the effect on those areas.

Childbirth

Birth is a complex physical activity involving a wide range of emotional and psychological experiences consisting of a number of demanding phases. As a consequence, a wide range of crystals is required in order to support the mother or the child – especially in the case of any difficulties.

However, it should not be forgotten that in spite of the effort and pain, childbirth is an entirely natural phenomenon and not something to be considered a medical "problem".

So, the use of crystals should remain in the background and they should only be applied when they are really needed. The following table summarises and sets out all those crystals that support birth. In presenting the information in this way, it is hoped that it will become easier to select the right crystal and to apply it correctly.

Before and During Birth

Crystal	Effect	Practical applications
Carnelian	Gives power and courage before the birth	Wear as a necklace or a pendant
Magnesite	Has a relaxing effect and removes resistance or birth crises	Wear as a necklace or a pendant or if necessary take gem essence (7 drops)
Chrysocolla	Has a relaxing effect helps dilation	Wear as a necklace or a pendant or if necessary take gem essence (7 drops)
Heliotrope	Protects against infections	Take gem essence (if required, 5-7 drops every two hours)
Biotite-Lens	Brings on labour; has a relaxing effect; encourages an easy birth	Hold in the hand. Place on the pubic bone in order to support contractions.
Malachite	Stimulates the contractions and relieves pain	Hold in the hand. Place above the pubic bone in order to support contractions. To relieve pains, if necessary, also take gem essence (7 drops).

➤→

Immediately After the Birth

Crystal	Effect	Practical applications
Kunzite	Aids acceptance of the child-and-mother role	Wear as a necklace or a pendant
Blue Tourmaline	In cases of grief or emotional crises	Wear as a necklace or a pendant or, if necessary take gem essence (3-5 drops)
Epidote	Regeneration when exhausted	Wear as a necklace or a pendant or if necessary take gem essence (5 drops)
Topaz	Helps find one's identity	Wear as a necklace or a pendant
Blue or pink Chalcedony	Furthers milk production.	Wear as a necklace or a pendant.

Later Post-natal

Crystal	Effect	Practical applications
Agate	Helps the uterus return to normal size and condition	Place a tumbled stone with uterus signature on the body
Rhodonite	Heals scratches or cuts	First take gem essence (5-7 drops, 3 times daily). Later, when all bleeding has stopped, place a tumbled crystal in briefs.
Pink Agate	For any kind of inflammation	Place a tumbled stone with a signature that looks like the inflamed spot on the body
Moonstone	Helps with the hormonal changes	Wear as a necklace or a pendant
Mookaite	Stabilises physical health	Wear as a necklace or a pendant

Children

Crystal	Effect	Practical applications
Amethyst	Eases the child's "arrival" into our world	Place a tumbled crystal or small crystal in the child's bed.
Rutile Quartz	Helps to overcome birth traumas	Place a tumbled crystal or small crystal in the child's bed.
Calcite	For stable development	Place a tumbled crystal or small crystal in the child's bed.
Aquamarine	Soothes eczema in cases of hypersensitivity	Place a tumbled crystal or small crystal in the diaper.
Citrine	For digestive problems	Place a tumbled crystal or small crystal in the diaper.
Emerald or Peridot	Stimulates the break down of bilirubin. Apply Peridot only for cases with very strong yellow discolouration of skin	Place a tumbled crystal (Peridot) or small crystal (Emerald) in the diaper.

Circulation Problems

Circulation problems occur when the flow of blood through any of the veins and arteries is partially or completely impeded. This can be caused by heart problems; high or low blood pressure (e.g. during pregnancy), hormonal changes (e. g. during the menopause), infectious diseases, and general weakness in the autonomic nervous system or blocked or imperfectly functioning blood vessels. The latter is particularly important, for whilst the heart's action contributes to the transportation of the blood, adequate elasticity, tension and cooperation of the muscular arteries are also essential for proper circulation The arteries transport blood pumped from the heart by the means of a circular contraction of their muscles (see also Blood Circulation)

Chinese medicine formulates the connection between the heart and circulation very clearly, as follows:

The heart is the emperor who provides the tone

The circulation is his first civil servant who does the work – and woe to the emperor whose civil servants are idle!

A thorough investigation of weak circulation will usually reveal specific phenomena such as such as deposits in the blood vessels and their walls, a narrowing or enlargement (varicose veins) and inflammatory states – which are a consequence of tissues containing toxic deposits. Detoxi-

fication is therefore absolutely necessary in order to prevent circulatory problems (see Detoxification). A diet without animal protein and general nutrition rich in vitamins (especially C and E), sufficient physical exercise, rest, sleep, and time for regeneration are all good preventative measures.

Circulation problems often occur as sudden changes in blood pressure and pulse rate. This, in turn, causes inner unrest, tiredness, pallor, dizziness, fits of unconsciousness, cold sweats, shaking limbs and – in extreme cases – circulatory collapse. As immediate first aid, raise the feet above the head and apply cold water to revive the person; but professional medical advice or assistance should be sought in all cases, in order to identify the cause.

The problem can also often be caused emotionally by stress and difficult situations. Obstacles or resistance to one's inner wishes and intentions appear to be reflected in fluctuations of blood pressure. The feeling of failure, total overburdening and lack of energy often exist side-by-side with circulatory problems, and are often caused by lack of enjoyment and enthusiasm. Thus, a change of direction is often needed, in order that personal aims and goals can be rediscovered – and with this an associated new enthusiasm for life, which is still the best medicine for the circulation!

Many crystals described elsewhere (see Blood Pressure; Heart Problems) can also be applied in order to stimulate or calm the circulation. The following are therefore the crystals that really can stabilise the circulation and have a possible effect.

Garnet Pyrope is best for stabilising the circulation. It helps rapidly with circulatory problems, can prevent circulatory collapse (if applied in time), and, as a metabolism stimulating crystal, it can also further the cleansing of and improves the vitality of the blood vessels.

Emotionally it helps to overcome resistance, mobilises essential energy reserves and assists with perseverance.

Haematite and **Tiger Iron** help with weakness, dizziness and brief attacks of unconsciousness – especially if they occur in the morning, when one rises too quickly, or due to pregnancy.

Emotionally, both crystals help one to become dynamic and full of life. Especially Tiger Iron which rapidly removes tiredness and lack of strength.

Ruby stimulates the circulation and helps with tiredness, pallor, dizziness, cold sweats and shaking limbs. It also prevents circulatory collapse, if applied in time.

Emotionally, it enhances passion and enthusiasm – not just temporally, but also as long-lasting fervour.

For all of the of the crystals mentioned above, wear a necklace or a pendant above the hip in such a way, that at least one of the crystals is hanging over the pubic bone.

Garnet Pyrope, Ruby or tumbled stones of Haematite and Tiger Iron can also be placed or stuck on (with sticking plaster) the pubic bone on a regular basis. It is also possible to take gem essence internally, but only in small quantities (2-4 drops, 2 times daily). The same goes for gem water (100 –200 ml taken in small sips during the course of the day.)

Colds

The so-called common cold manifest itself with the classic symptoms of a cough, head colds and hoarseness, all of which are often characterised as flu infections although they do not have much in common with genuine influenza.

See also: Flu; Head Colds

As the name indicates, a cold can, on occasion, be traced back to exposure to cold. Such exposure can actually weaken the immune defence structures in the mucous membranes of the airways. On the other hand, it can only really spread throughout a body that has already been stressed (by toxins or waste etc).

In most cases however, a cold is a form of virus in which the tissues and cells are infected with waste substances that make the virus spread and thus hamper the activity of the immune system. Colds can be prevented by generally "toughening up" the body. This includes regular exercise in fresh air (in all kinds of weather!), sleeping with an open window, ending one's daily shower with cold water, and with regular detoxification. In particular, dairy products should be abandoned as they increase the tendency to getting a cold, a sore throat, bronchitis, and sinusitis (see the relevant chapters).

Further protection can also obtained by rinsing the mouth and teeth with organic, cold-pressed sunflower oil for 10 to 20 minutes every day. **Do not swallow the oil under any circumstances**; but spit it out afterwards and rinse the mouth thoroughly with tepid water! This oil absorbs toxic substances and waste, and supports the healing of colds.

Direct cooling down of the airways (e. g. if you breathe through your mouth), indirect cooling of the whole body (because of inadequate clothing) and cold feet can play a role in triggering the effects of a cold. Cold feet especially cause a reflex decrease in the blood circulation in the mucous membranes of the nose. Therefore, colds tend to occur particularly during cold and wet transitional phases and, to a lesser degree, in a dry and cold winter. In summer, it is mainly cold drinks that have an internal cooling down effect and cold draughts which play an important role in so-called "summer colds".

However, as stated earlier, a cold is actually a viral disease. Viruses that are already in the mucous membranes, or that have been inhaled, exploit the actual weakness of the immune system and where they can propagate very suddenly. Typically, this leads to catarrh, an inflammation of the mucous membranes.

As the immune system becomes even more burdened, there will often also be a subsequent influx of bacteria, which can lead to inflammation and the formation of pus. Fever, in connection with a cold, is an important part of the body's defence mechanism and should **not** be suppressed too early, in order to avoid complications. Any of the following parts of the body and additional symptoms can be regarded as a complication of a cold:

- the nose – head colds
- the throat– cough, hoarseness
- the bronchia – deep cough, breathing difficulties
- the lungs – weakness, lack of appetite, high fever, night sweats, breathlessness
- the heart – acute heart problems
- the sinuses – aching that is intensified by pressure and leaning forward
- the middle ear – earache, fever
- the meninges – headache, vomiting, suddenly rising fever, shivering, disturbed consciousness

A simple cold, cough or hoarseness can be treated quite easily with crystals. However, if the symptoms persist and seem to progress to other parts of the body, e. g. towards the sinuses or the bronchia, a doctor or an alternative practitioner should be consulted. Even here, though, crystals can be applied to complement the professional approach, using safe monitoring and treatment over the course of the illness and a successful cure. In most cases, however, a cure proceeds by reversing the process or direction of the original causes or origins

As with so many other ailments, it is just as important with a cold to consider any emotional background to the illness – personal relationships, ones lifestyle and environment, grief or depression (especially in cases of bronchitis).

The same crystals that are used with cold symptoms can also be applied to deal with any associated emotional problems.

Heliotrope can be applied at the beginning of a cold, when the first sensations of feverishness, head cold or soreness in the throat are experienced.

It should be placed immediately on the thymus gland (between heart and throat), in the form of a tumbled stone or a thin section or taken in the form of gem essence (5-10 drops every hour); or take as gem water (100–300 ml taken in small sips over the course of the day. Necklaces or a pendant can also be effective.

Heliotrope works by initially backing up the body's non-specific immune reaction that attacks all foreign bodies in the same way. This defence mechanism is normally successful in warding off infection and so forth – but where it fails, a disease will progress. Parallel to its physical effect, Heliotrope also increases the ability to defend oneself on an emotional level.

However, if the cold is in its full-blown form, Heliotrope becomes ineffective as the body's attempt at limiting infection has been overcome.

Sardonyx should be then be used if there are feverish symptoms.

Red Chalcedony is the alternative if there is no fever,

Both forms encourage the feverish high temperature, which the body needs naturally in order to hold the disease in check, at least, until it has been identified and neutralised by the specific immune defence. In fact, a high temperature should never be lowered too early when you have a cold, only if it reaches life-threatening levels of 41°C (105°F), or more, should you should intervene.

The crystals can also be applied until the illness has reached its climax and the fever drops again. (By the way, the crystals help one emotionally to confront unpleasant things and to overcome difficult situations). A sign that the illness has been overcome is that the limbs, and the hands and feet in particular, suddenly become hot, after they have been cold, in spite of the high temperature. This indicates that the body is trying to get rid of the heat. In order to assist in lowering the fever, cold compresses can now be wrapped around the calves.

Blue Chalcedony, **Moss Agate** or **Ocean Jasper** can also be applied along with the cold compress as each of them stimulates the lymph flow. In this way the cleansing of the infected areas can be completed. Emotionally, they are also useful for encouraging feelings of relief and for promoting general detoxification.

Blue Chalcedony can be applied if the fever falls rapidly, whilst Moss Agate or Ocean Jasper can be used if the temperature falls gradually. Occasionally, though, it may also rise again through the actual process of detoxification. The selected crystal should be applied until the temperature has fallen to a normal level of about 37°C (99 °F). During this period, bed rest is advised in order to ensure a cure.

When the fever has subsided and a symptom-free state has been attained, apply Brown Chalcedony for another week or two in order to avoid a relapse or complications, as this crystal helps support the immune system over a longer period. Furthermore, emotionally, it heightens one's powers of observation.

(As an aside, at the end of such an illness. it always advisable to take one extra day off for full recovery before going back to business as usual. This "extra" day was once part of any doctor's standard recommendation. However, in today's ever-more complex world, it is usually ignored, as almost every one has major commitments. Nevertheless skipping that extra day off is one of the most common causes of a relapse with complications, or even of a much more severe illness.)

Epidote and **Zoisite** can help if there still is a definite feeling of weakness after a cold. These crystals are regenerative in effect and Epidote particularly can be combined with the Chalcedony already mentioned.

Hold a tumbled stone in the hand or place/fix it on the thymus gland (between the heart and the throat). It is just as effective to wear a necklace or a pendant and to take gem essence (5-7 drops at least three times daily up to a maximum dose of once an hour depending on the intensity of the illness. Also, try gem water (200–500 ml) in small sips over the course of the day.

Cold Feet

Chronically cold feet are caused by inadequate blood circulation which, in turn, is caused by narrowing of the blood vessels (see also Arteriosclerosis) or an imbalance of the "triple warmer" – the system that is responsible for an equalised energy balance in our bodies (see also Blood, Circulation).

It should be noted here that although the triple warmer is connected with the ring finger and that silver rings that are worn on this part of the body have a cooling effect, they should NEVER be worn in cases of cold feet, as they may decrease the effect of the healing crystals listed below.

Further, no one should expect miracles from the crystals mentioned. After all, any inappropriate footwear or a temperature of -20 °C (-4 °F) will naturally result in cold feet, even if one fills up one's boots with crystals! However, crystals can be a great help if feet will not warm up even after having been in a heated room or a bed.

Garnet Pyrope stimulates the general energy distribution for this condition. It strengthens the triple warmer and, therefore, in the long run, also provides for better blood circulation in the feet and a constant supply of heat to them.

Wear a necklace or a small pendant with body contact or put a small tumbled stone or a small crystal into the socks/stockings. Take gem essence (3-5 drops, 5 times daily).

Obsidian heats up chronic cold feet very quickly.

Place a small tumbled crystal into the sock/stocking or a flat cabochon into the shoe.

If cold feet are the only problem, do not take as a gem essence, as Obsidian has a far-reaching effect on other parts of the body. However, gem essence from both crystals can be combined in an ointment (put 10 drops of essence into 10g of ointment base), which is then rubbed into the affected spot. For the ointment base, use a mixture of one part of beeswax and 4-5 parts of jojoba oil. This ointment will help even in minor cases of frostnip.

Concentration Problems

Problems with concentration are quite common and need no special treatment –

apart from rest and recreation, especially if you are tired, stressed or have not slept for several nights. So, do not even attempt to apply crystal therapy as a first option; rather see to it that you get enough sleep and recreation.

If concentration problems continue to occur, even if you have had adequate sleep and free time or if the condition becomes a permanent one, crystal treatment can then be initiated.

Psychologically, concentration problems are usually identified as being either concentration impairment, which is innate, or lack of concentration, which is the consequence of an unprocessed flood of information. Crystal use is helpful in both categories.

However, whilst it is important to have confidence in the effect of crystals, there is also a need to eliminate the circumstances or factors that lead to concentration problems. Overall, the treatment should introduce a positive atmosphere that will improve concentration and so it is important at the outset to be consistent and ensure completion of tasks or assignments, etc. If not, any accumulation of loose ends leads once again to a lack of concentration, distraction or even confusion. The positive steps might advisably include a radical reduction in any such things as background noise, excessive TV viewing, alcohol intake, drugs use, strip lighting and any other negative or distracting ambience.

Recommended positive activities include spending time outside and being aware of the natural world – listening consciously to the wind, water and sounds of animals – walking in the dark and being aware of silence. In addition meditation and exercise such as yoga or Tai Chi will assist, as will artistic occupations. Last but not least, ensure that you sleep for longer periods than was previously the norm.

All of the above, if these changes are carried out, without any severe achievement-orientated approach, they can then become a natural part of ones life. The results may well be surprising, with a sudden enhanced ability to concentrate!

Chrysoberyl helps maintain concentration in cases of stress, tension, tiredness or difficult long-term circumstances. It helps with both poor concentration and lack of concentration. In particular, it is valuable in helping children who have problems in school as a result of achievement demands. Chrysoberyl assists in maintaining emotional and mental focus, whilst still being able to develop new ideas, visions and opinions. In other words, it makes us more conscious of our own thoughts and actions.

Diamond furthers a logical way of thinking, perseverance and self-awareness. It helps avoid becoming distracted and speeds up the rapid processing of received information and sensations. In this way, it affords better control of inner feelings and moods. Diamond improves concentration from a position of inner strength, enabling specific and required concentration on new tasks.

Fluorite helps to create order and to concentrate the attention when there is distraction caused by any "loose ends" or unfinished matters. It enables concentration to be focussed on the present matters in hand, avoiding the aforementioned distraction that continue to occupy the mind – such as uncompleted homework, lesson assignments, overspill task brought home from work, etc., things not fully understood at the time and anything skipped over during lessons, briefings, meetings and the like. Fluorite helps one to identify all of these and is, as a result, useful and, therefore, also a good crystal for all learning situations (see also Learning Problems).

For all three crystals, wear as a necklace, or a pendant for a longer period of time. As alternatively, take as a gem essence (3-5 drops, twice daily) or gem water (taken in small sips over the course of the day).

Constipation

Constipation is the delayed emptying of the intestine and bowel, which is then often hampered by hard stools. As a purely temporary condition, it can be caused by constipating food, changes in eating habits (for example, during journeys) or a heavy loss of fluid.

Continuous constipation, however, is often caused by a lack of exercise, regular suppression (or delay) of visits to the toilet and a diet that is too low in fibre. It also has emotional causes – such as having apparently insoluble problems, difficulties in making decisions and involvement in worrying situations from which there seems no real escape.

A lack of appetite and/or a feeling of having over eaten often accompany constipation. This can become dangerous if the intestine is "sealed" and not emptied for any length of time.

If constipation coincides with paleness of complexion, colic, nausea, a distended or bloated stomach and a rapid deterioration of general health, seek a doctor's advice **immediately.**

Otherwise, constipation can normally be treated by drinking lots of fluids, or using an enema or mild laxative as necessary.

However, as an overall remedy, cleansing the large intestine is strongly recommended. This can be done through diet and colon therapy, adopting a fibre-rich diet and exercise on a regular basis (e. g. daily walks).

Whatever else, it is important to address and solve any of the problems or conditions described above so as to ensure relief from constipation.

If necessary, this can be with the help of a therapist if the causes are emotional or psychological; with a doctor or alternative practitioner, if clearly physical.

Furthermore, the following crystals may also help.

Calcite (**Orange** and **Green**) together with **Amber** – for example, as a necklace or a pendant – aids intestinal function and helps ease constipation.

Rutile Quartz can be applied if constipation and diarrhoea seem to be alternate conditions.

Pink Moss Agate helps with stubborn, chronic constipation – especially if the intestine has already lost it normal action because of overlong (several years) or heavy dosages of laxatives. Here, Pink Moss Agate can sometimes achieve what might seem like small miracles, because of its cleansing, lymph stimulating and detoxifying qualities.

Place a crystal in water for one day and then drink this over the course of the following day. Also, a polished stone or crystal can also be placed or fixed on the stomach, or worn as a necklace or pendant.

Black Tourmaline eases constipation that occurs on journeys, in other changed personal circumstances or arising from eating too much constipating food. It stimulates intestinal activity and quickly helps restore the overall status quo. In using Black Tourmaline, either on the body or carried in a trouser pocket, always ensure that the crystal is pointing downwards, on the left side of the abdomen (where the large intestine travels downwards).

If there is access to a couple of crystals or crystal rods, these can be placed on the abdomen, pointing clockwise and following the course of the large intestine (see Fig. 5). The crystals should point upwards on the right side of the abdomen, go to the left over the abdomen and then point downwards on the left side.

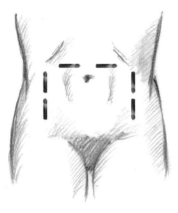

Fig. 5: Arrangement of Tourmaline crystals or crystal rods when treating constipation.

Less complicated, but also effective, is the wearing of necklaces or pendants – and taking gem essence (3-7 drops, 3 times daily), or gem water (200–300 ml taken in small sips over the course of the day).

Conjunctivitis

Red eyes, swollen eyes, increased secretion (sticky eyes), a burning and itching feeling, a sensation of having a foreign body lodged in the eye and light sensitivity may all be signs of conjunctivitis.

This can be caused by reduced tear flow, foreign bodies in the eye, vapour and gasses, ultraviolet radiation, allergic reactions and infections. If conjunctivitis manifests repeatedly, there may be a connection with a heavy accumulation of toxins and waste matter in the tissues, a weak liver and anger or disappointment about things we cannot "bear" to look at. In order to relieve inflammation, one should drink lots of fluids (not coffee) and eat food that is rich in vitamins.

See also: Eye Problems

Agates that contain an eye signature, particularly those with naturally red colours, relieve all kinds of conjunctivitis. Place either small section/slices or tumbled stones on the closed eyelids.

Blue Chalcedony helps particularly with reddish, burning eyes that secrete an insufficient amount of fluid. As Chalcedony also stimulates the lymph flow and detoxification, necklaces or pendants of **Blue Lace Agate** worn for a longer period also helps reduce a general tendency towards conjunctivitis.

Heliotrope is particularly helpful with conjunctivitis, where there is a heavy secretion, i. e. with sticky eyes and strong itching. Place a polished crystal or a flat section/slice directly on the closed eyelids.

Ocean Jasper helps with very stubborn conjunctivitis that is otherwise treatment-resistant. As it has a very strong detoxifying effect, strengthens the immune system and stimulates the lymph flow, it also helps reduce the tendency towards conjunctivitis.

Place a polished crystal or a flat section/slice on the eyes; or wear it around the neck in the form of a necklace or a pendant.

Emerald is particularly helpful with conjunctivitis that develops simultaneously with, or is caused by, infected airways.

Place small crystals or tumbled stones on the eyes or place a tumbled stone in the mouth. Alternatively, take either gem essence (5-9 drops, 3-5 times daily), or gem water (100–300 ml taken in small sips during the course of the day). Emerald water that has been slightly warmed can also be used to bathe the affected area.

Contusions

A contusion is compressed or squashed tissue caused by a blunt impact, such as a blow or a fall. It can affect the skin, subcutaneous tissue, muscles, periosteum or bones. Contusions are often connected to severe tension pains and can cause subcutaneous bleeding. (See also: Bruising)

Because it leads to a kind of "shock" on a cellular level, an awareness of what caused the actual contusion can in itself lead to a distinct improvement in the condition.

For this purpose, go through the whole event once more – exactly as it happened, where it happened and as quickly a possible after the incident (of course without hurting oneself again!). If one has fallen down, take up the exact position once more. Sometimes it is necessary to repeat the respective movement sequence several times, until the pain from the blow briefly increases and then decreases. This is the moment to stop. This process of raising one's consciousness focuses one's attention and one's life energy on the affected spot and thus accelerates the healing process.

Afterwards the damaged spot can be treated with cold arnica poultices, internal homeopathic arnica remedies or with the following crystals,

Amethyst provides for the rapid relief of any residual pain and helps dissipate any tension that may have arisen because of the blow. If it is applied immediately, major swelling is prevented so that only minor bruising will result.

Prase helps when immediate treatment has not been possible. It relieves pain and reduces swelling. It also speeds up the renewal of affected tissue.

Rhodonite is especially useful to alleviate bruising more quickly. It has a pain-relieving effect and helps dissipate any shock resulting from painful contusions. Another advantage is that it is just as effective in both short and long treatment

For all three of the above, place a flat tumbled stone or a section/slice on the affected spot, securing it there with sticking plaster or inside a bandage. Alternatively, or in addition, take gem essence (if necessary, 5-9 drops, 3-5 times daily) or gem water (200–300 ml taken in small sips over the course of the day).

Coughs

A cough is simply a sudden, albeit somewhat noisy, expulsion of air. In most causes, we cough in order to free the throat of mucus, foreign bodies or other sources of irritation. A cough can be triggered by inflammations of the throat, the larynx or the bronchi, as well as by irritating gasses, smoke, dust or ingesting food into the airways ("going down the wrong way"). However, a cough can sometimes have an emotional cause, such as nervousness and tension. (See also: Colds; Bronchitis; Flu)

As long as a cough is cleansing the airways by loosening mucus, it should not be suppressed. Rather, it is the underlying illness or irritation that should be treated and this alone will often make the cough disappear. However, if coughing is so heavy or continuous that it becomes disproportionately annoying – for example, when preventing or interrupting normal sleep – it should be relieved in some way. Classic household and folk-based remedies, such as onion poultices, can actually be quite effective, as can the following crystals.

Aquamarine relieves coughs caused mainly by allergies, colds, nervousness and stress. In particular, it is helpful when there seems to be no involuntary cough-provoking irritation, but coughing continues as a need for clearing the airways.

Chalcedony and **Noble Opal** provide rapid relief from all kinds of coughs, including the so-called "smoker's cough" or a cough resulting from some emotional cause. Both crystals encourage expectoration, especially when this otherwise proves difficult, and they relax the throat and chest.

Fluorite helps particularly with dry, irritable coughs, whether they are caused by external irritants (gasses, dust, smoke) or in connection with a cold.

Moss Agate and **Ocean Jasper** help first and foremost to relieve continuous coughing attacks. They help both with smoker's cough and with colds, especially when the latter seems to linger or when the healing process is extremely slow.

Rutile Quartz relieves coughs connected with bronchitis. It also helps to relieve tightness in the chest and alleviates breathing difficulties, relaxing the bronchia and the chest.

For all the above, place a polished crystal or section on the chest and also wear as a necklace or a pendant on the throat or chest. Take gem essence if required (5-7 drops, every hour) or gem water (200–300 ml taken in small sips over the course of the day).

Cramp

Cramp, especially in the calf muscles, can be very painful, but it usually occurs only in one leg at any time. It may result from a sudden lack of magnesium (caused by, for example, night-time urination or during pregnancy). More rarely, it is caused by a lack of calcium and potassium, by an excess of acid in the body; by a large and sudden fluid loss (e.g. diarrhoea), shock and resulting upsets in circulation (for example swimming in cold water).

Recommended therapies include hot baths, massage (for blood circulation and the metabolism) and use of magnesium-based crystals.

Magnesite and **Serpentine**, as crystals rich in magnesium, seem to achieve the best results. They can be placed against the calf for relief or worn in the form of bracelets, necklaces, or pendants with direct body contact, in order to increase the magnesium metabolism. In addition, they help not only in cases of cramp, but also have a general alleviating effect, supporting the body's metabolism and, to a minor degree, blood circulation.

Cuts

Small cuts can heal within a couple of minutes using healing crystals.

Rhodonite or **Mookaite** as tumbled stones or in the form of a section/slice, moistened with one's own saliva if necessary, are pressed, directly onto the point of bleeding. In fact, clean, minor cuts sometimes heal so quickly that a plaster will not be needed.

In cases of larger cuts, one should apply the necessary first aid and make a bandage. After that, it is recommended to repeat the accident using the same cutting instrument but without the actual contact. In so doing, the "cell shock" caused by the injury is dissipated. This has all to be carried out exactly as it took place, where it took place and as quickly as possible after the incident. Whilst no further injury must be caused (for example, lightly holding the offending knife close to, but not touching, the cut) it might still be necessary to repeat the exercise a couple of times – until the pain suddenly increases, after which it decreases. This is the point to stop.

The exercise is one of consciousness-raising and which directs our attention and, consequently, our life energy, towards the affected spot to further the healing process.

Obsidian can also help if the above is not possible. Hold a tumbled piece of Obsidian in the hand or place it close to the cut, in order to dissipate the "cell shock". After this, place a tumbled stone or a slice of Rhodonite or Mookaite on the injured spot. One can also take gem essence (5-9 drops) or gem water (100–200 ml taken in small sips over the course of the day); or carry a necklace or a pendant of Rhodonite or Mookaite.

Cysts

Cysts are cavities in the tissue, comprising one or more chambers and containing fluid. They can occur in many organs, including the kidneys, liver, lungs, glands, mucous sacs, ovaries, etc. In very many cases, they remain harmless and so require no therapy, unless they are caused by diseases (e. g. parasitic attack)

However, a cyst can sometimes be detrimental to the normal functioning of a neighbouring organ, through direct pressure or partial displacement. In these cases, the cyst should be examined by a doctor; and if it proves impossible to shrink in any other way, it will have to be removed surgically.

See also: **Ganglia**

Many people live with cysts for a long time without even noticing them. They are often discovered by accident and should not cause either worries or fear. Most cysts are benign and can appear and then disappear again.

Problems with the supply of tissue nutrients or the removal of waste seem to favour the formation of cysts. Thus, detoxification and regulation of the metabolism also play an important part in shrinking a cyst (see Detoxification). Further, benign cysts are not aggressive, unlike cancerous tumours.

Holistic therapy recognises a connection between cysts and so-called "encapsulated" pain from former injuries that cannot be resolved emotionally or psychologically and so manifest themselves physically. In this case, the answer is that if the corresponding problems are resolved in some way (even by therapy), then the related cysts will also disappear.

Agates with a relevant internal signature (e. g. Water Agate) have a positive effect upon many cysts.

Ocean Jasper is equally effective, as it has a structure similar to the cavities in cells or tissues.

As chalcedonies, they both further the supply of the tissue with nutrients and oxygen and the removal of waste and other metabolic products. This speeds up and eases the shrinking of cysts. Ocean Jasper is especially valuable as it also supports the resolution of emotional conflicts and strengthens against potential diseases.

Place slices/sections or flat polished crystals of the above as close as possible to the location of the cysts, fixing them in place with sticking plaster if necessary. As a supplementary application, wear the crystal as a bracelet, necklace, pendant, or a gem crystal, on the body; or create a circle of crystals around the bed (this is more effective for Ocean Jasper).

If necessary, also take gem essence (5-7 drops, 3-5 times daily), or gem water

(200–300 ml taken in sips during the course of the day).

Dandruff

Dandruff is caused by metabolic and excretory disturbances and consists of the flakes or platelet-like skin cells that are easily loosened or cast off. It usually occurs as a result of dry skin, particularly on the head, but can also occur in connection with skin diseases with a defective keratin formation (psoriasis, seborrhoea, etc). Because of its underlying causes, colonic therapy and detoxification (see Detoxification) are measures that can really help on a fundamental level.

Further relief in cases of dandruff formation on the scalp can be obtained with the help of the following crystals:

Aventurine detoxifies and regulates the skin's supply of nutrients and the removal of waste substances. It thus has a direct link to the skin (see also Sunburn) and dandruff; especially the form containing silver-coloured Fuchsite mica inclusions that provide a clear signature corresponding to dandruff.

Wear it as a necklace or a pendant, it is also possible to rinse the hair with gem water. Alternatively, take gem essence (5-7 drops, 3 times daily), or gem water (200–300 ml taken in small sips over the course of the day).

Amethyst helps in the form of Hildegard von Bingen's Amethyst Water (see page 25) to relieve dandruff formation. After a gentle hair wash, rinse thoroughly and let the hair dry naturally, preferably in the open air.

Antimonite is also helpful in preventing heavy dandruff formation. Place Antimonite into some clean water for a day and then add sulphur essence at 20 drops per litre of water. Apply this as a hair rinse at least once a day.

Defective Vision;

see Ametropia; Eye problems; Eye Strain

Depression

Being depressed means feeling downhearted or dejected. These definitions are very important in realistically understanding the term "depression", as there can be no experience of depression without dejection, or even feelings of repression and suppression. Accepted medical science distinguishes between endogenous (inner, and possibly unrecognisable, genetic causes), and acquired causes (physical diseases, personal loss, conflicts, crises, failures, or humiliations). However, it can be argued that medical science overlooks the fact that there is a "dejection factor" at the beginning of, or before, every case of depression. Such a state can arise from many circumstances, but the most common tend to be as follows:

- other people – parents, teachers, work superiors, partners, etc.
- general social, family and personal situations – loss of job, problems with personal relationships, separation, loss etc.
- other life circumstances and health – diseases, disabilities, obstacles, etc.
- lifestyle and personal attitudes – too narrow minded a philosophy, antipathetic moral attitudes, seemingly life-threatening stances, etc.

This "dejection factor" is often ignored, as depression does not normally develop spontaneously, rather it emerges gradually. Thus, the original cause may often lie far in one's past. Sometimes, depression can be triggered or activated again when experiencing a situation or meeting a person similar to those in the original, causal situation. This leads to the totally wrong conclusion that a feeling of depression has developed without a recognizable cause. When this happens to us, the worst thing about is that such a diagnosis aggravates the affected person's feelings of hopelessness and impotence. Further, in today's professional, so-called, "therapy treatment" with its tranquillising psychoactive drugs, everything is intensified once more. This can indeed be a truly vicious circle!

Real help can only be given for depression by discovering the dejection factor and finding an appropriate solution – either by learning to live with it, or by liberating one-self from it. During this process, some outside therapeutic help is usually necessary, as the depression itself impairs our ability to think clearly and to solve our own problems. However, any depression can be cured using therapy without the involvement of any psychoactive drugs, given the therapist's knowledge of depression. There is always the proviso, of course, that one displays the necessary openness needed in order to throw light on all aspects of one's life. Then, together with the skill of the therapist, the dejection factors can be identified.

Crystals can be of help precisely at this juncture, as they encourage openness, the ability to think, create the right mood, the ability to confront unpleasant things, and the willingness to work on oneself. Rather like taking a walk in sunlight, or using St. John's Wort preparations (but please notice that St. John's Wort makes the skin hypersensitive to sunlight!), the following crystals do not replace the essential therapy needed for depression, but make it easier to go through the process.

Amazonite helps with severe despondency and feelings of impotence, especially if one feels a victim of some overwhelming fate. It encourages a healthy belief in life and stimulates the concept of taking one's fate in one's own hands.

Citrine helps against depression caused by overwhelming outside influences and whenever there are feelings of having had enough of everything.

Dumortierite makes it easier to cope with depressive situations. It is especially important, however, for helping one to talk about the feelings of depression and its causes. This makes it one of the most important crystals to accompany any form of therapy.

Opal brings *joie-de-vivre* in hopeless circumstances – and, in particular, when any kind of physical or mental activity seems incredibly difficult, totally meaningless and joyless. It brings hope and motivates us to take care of oneself and one's life.

Rutile Quartz helps one to be open to any helpful influences from outside during a depression. It lifts the spirits and makes us ready to talk and admit fear and weaknesses – things that are usually kept strictly under wraps. Quite simply, Rutile Quartz is a "sunbeam" in the midst of deepest hopelessness.

Golden Topaz helps with all depression, no matter what the cause. It strengthens self-confidence and the ability to express oneself. It also enables you to regain control of those parts of life that you might believe are lost. It helps with living one's own life and sticking to one's own ideas, wishes and ideals.

Wear the above crystals on the body for long periods, in particular on the solar plexus. Necklaces, pendants, tumbled stones with a hole bored through them, and ornamental crystals are all suitable.

Gem essence (5-7 drops, 3 times daily) or gem water (200–300 ml) taken in sips during the course of the day.

See also: Melancholia

Dermatitis

Dermatitis – more correctly called neuroermatitis – is a chronic inflammatory skin disease with eczema-like lesions. The condition often starts on the cheeks, and then spreads over the elbow joints, the hollows in the backs of the knees, the buttocks, neck and face and – finally – to the whole body.

Because perspiration and the normal operation of the sebaceous glands are impaired, the skin becomes very dry and irritated, producing skin flakes and dandruff. Painful itching attacks are experienced (especially during the night). Dermatitis is often connected with other allergic problems and the best cures are usually obtained when the condition is treated consistently as an allergic reaction (see also Allergies; Hay Fever; Bronchial Asthma).

In all cases it is important to try and find out what might be causing any stress, whether this stress results from actual substances, radiation effects, food allergies – or a combination of these problems. In addition, try to reduce any overall emotional pressures, conflicts and fears – if necessary, with the help of a therapist.

In cases involving children, any seeming "loss of security" is also a very important factor. It may even have its origins before birth, at a time when the mother may have had worries during pregnancy, for example if going through a divorce, fears for the future, and so forth. In order to ensure feelings of security in infancy, even traditional medical science advises breast-feeding for as long as possible, if one's child has dermatitis.

Detoxification regimes, such as colon therapy, and healthy, toxin-free nutrition are other important measures to take in order to avoid stress and the conditions that can be a cause of dermatitis. Regular breaks from oppressive urban environments – in the country, mountains or at the seaside – can also have a healing effect.

Dermatitis should only be self-treated in association with an alternative practitioner as I consider traditional medical science is unable to offer any treatment other than cortisone or antihistamines. I have seen individually targeted homeopathic and alternative therapies show good results, especially when regular energy clearing procedures, and technological checks of the medication combinations were involved. It is only within this sort of regimen that healing crystals should be used.

Amethyst is especially helpful to deal with itching. This is very important in cases of dermatitis, as areas that have been scratched raw often are exposed to second-ary infections (staphylococci and similar). Amethyst also contributes to the cleansing and healing of the skin Hildegard von Bingen's Amethyst water (see page 25) is especially effective (see Skin Care).

Aquamarine is useful in dealing with dermatitis, particularly in association with hay fever, asthma or other kinds of allergies – and when the symptoms are aggravated by increased lifestyle demands and overall stress. Emotionally it helps deal with these stresses and encourages a lightening of attitude and relaxation.

Chrysoprase is the most effective crystal in cases of dermatitis, as it detoxifies the system very effectively. This is especially important if a large amount of cortisone has already been prescribed and applied. Additionally, Chrysoprase helps identify the potential emotional causes of disease, such as grief, jealousy or feelings of a loss of security. In so doing, it helps to resolve internal conflicts or crises with one's surroundings.

Emerald assists as a remedy for dermatitis. As a mineral in structure akin to Aquamarine, it can also be applied for treating many allergies; and, like Chrysoprase, it furthers detoxification. However, Emerald is particularly effective in the cleansing of the intestine – this is often very important with cases of dermatitis.

Emotionally, Emerald helps with a loss of bearings; also with perplexity, confusion and despair. It brings the new hope and the strength that is needed in order to endure what seems to be unbearable.

Ocean Jasper with a predominantly green signature helps with dermatitis. It also contributes to cleansing the body, harmonising the immune system and to clarifying conflicts. Beside that, it brings new hope and the will to be cured in connection with very stubborn and continuous diseases. Ocean Jasper prevents further infections e. g. herpes viruses, to which one is particularly sensitive in cases of dermatitis.

Wear a bracelet, a necklace or a pendant of any of the above. Also, take as a supplement or as an alternative, as gem essence (3-9 drops, 3-5 times daily) or gem water (200–300 ml) taken in small sips over the course of the day for a longer period.

Detoxification

Detoxification has nowadays come to be regarded as one of the most important factors in the cure of many diseases, particularly as we are subjected more and more to denatured food, toxic substances, radiation and stress to a much higher degree than in previous times. Overeating, particularly with a high content of animal protein (in particular cows' milk; see below) also leads to similar "pollution".

This harmful bombardment forces our bodies to work extra hard in order to stay healthy. Further, it tends to transform systematically our connective tissues, in particular, into a regular "waste disposal site". This occurs because all the substances that our bodies cannot adequately transform or excrete will be deposited temporarily within our connective tissues. In principle, this is a sensible and useful process, as such substances actually only remain there until they are released later – so that during a rest and recuperation phase they are then excreted.

Too much stress, a general lack of recreation and too little sleep, all combine to prevent many of us living in the westernised industrial nations from obtaining these beneficial rest periods. In this way, the tissues become a kind of "memory store" of the absent metabolic processes, and the body reacts with evermore sensitively to its increasing pollution by substances that are already present to excess in the tissues. The result can be hypersensitivity, acidification, allergies, a tendency to infections, metabolic and blood circulation problems, and diseases of the heart and circulation. Many of these phenomena are the desperate attempts by the body to defend itself, to digest and to excrete.

Alternative practitioners are noticing a distinct decrease in the number of "normal" illness such as common colds with a strong immune reaction (fever, cough, mucous secretion etc). Instead, there seems to be a distinct increase in the number of "creeping" and chronic illnesses, such as stuffy noses and blocked sinuses that last for weeks and continuous irritating coughs. In addition, whilst there may now be a lack of any accompanying fever, the condition and a general feeling of weakness are lasting for weeks. As an alternative practitioner once put it, all this is due to the fact that, "we are overloaded with toxins right up to the eyeballs".

So, detoxification is an extremely important term and will often be mentioned in these pages as being central to healing. There are many ways of detoxifying the tissues, of which the following have been tried out successfully:

- annual cures using spring herbs
- regular curative fasting
- diet, especially reduction of animal proteins
- salt baths (e. g. with natural, high-quality, unprocessed salt)
- sauna treatment
- intestinal cleansing
- drinking plenty of good quality water
- wholesome nutrition based on organic food

In particular, one ought to give up, or at least avoid, cow's milk. Nowadays, cow's milk lacks the normal enzymes and tends, for example to contain numerous antibiotics. This milk is only partially digested by our digestive system, which leads to deposition of the bovine drugs within the human body.

Furthermore, it is a good idea to exercise restraint with any use of painkillers, sleeping pills, powerful medicines, alcohol, tobacco, drugs, coffee and sweets.

Finally, the mental aspects of detoxification also need to be addressed, i. e. processing and releasing of incidents and situations that "poison" our lives: problems, conflicts, anger, loss, grief, guilt, bad conscience etc., for which therapeutic help may be required.

Having agreed on all the methods for detoxification of the body with a doctor or an alternative practitioner, when poisonous toxic substances and "waste' are released from the tissues, the body must be in a position to excrete them! Otherwise, the increased "pollution" will actually lead straight to some form of illness. The diet should be adapted to the individual circumstances. The latest dietary craze or trendy diet in the latest magazine will rarely fulfil this purpose.

Crystals are able to support the processes of detoxification in two ways: firstly, they support the purification of the tissues of wastes and toxins; and secondly, because they encourage the excretion of these substances respectively through the liver and the kidneys, the intestine and the skin. Chrysoprase and Green Tourmaline are ideal in this context, as they are supportive on both fronts.

Chrysoprase is the optimal crystal for detoxification. As a nickel-containing mineral, it helps purify the tissues of polluting substances and (as a Green Chalcedony) excretes these via the lymph system, liver and kidneys. Mentally, it also liberates us from strain, grief, worries, etc.

Blue Chalcedony improves the elimination of toxic substances and waste via the lymph system and their excretion through the kidneys. It should be the crystal of choice in cases of acute illness, during the period when further polluting substances are not to be released from the tissues. Moreover, Blue Chalcedony is always a sensible choice when the level of excretion through the skin (foul smelling sweat) and the intestine (diarrhoea) is too high. As an ancient Chinese saying puts it:

What the kidneys do not excrete,
* is excreted by the intestine.*
What the intestine does not excrete,
* is excreted by the skin.*
What the skin does not excrete will kill us.
Emotionally, Blue Chalcedony is helpful for stress, depressing conflicts and grief. It offers lightness and confidence and enables some freedom of discussion about any such worries.

Ocean Jasper is a type of Chalcedony that improves the discharge of waste and toxic substances whilst, at the same time, furthering a gentle, continuous detoxification of the tissues. Therefore, it can be applied optimally both for acute diseases and prophylactic cleansing diets. Crystals that are predominantly green in colour are the most suitable.

Peridot on the other hand, stimulates first and foremost the purification of the tissues, eliminating waste and toxic substances and their processing through the liver. Peridot has a very strong effect and so sometimes causes violent physical reactions and emotional outpourings of any accumulated annoyances and deep-rooted frustrations. Consequently, it should only be applied by the physically and mentally stable who want to detoxify thoroughly.

Green Tourmaline helps principally with degenerative processes in the tissues, the nerves or the joints that are caused by the deposition of waste products. This crystal also furthers both purification and the excretion of these substances. Emotionally, Green Tourmaline encourages patience, an open mind, honesty and sincerity.

Wear as a bracelet, a necklace, a polished crystal with a hole, or a pendant for long periods and place or fix a crystal (tourmaline), a polished stone or a segment on the liver in the evening. It is also possible to take gem essence (3-7 drops, 3 times daily), or gem water (100–300 ml taken in sips during the course of the day; with Chrysoprase, however, only 20–100 ml).

Diabetes

There are two basic types of the condition referred to under the general term of "diabetes".

Type 1 diabetes is the form that is normally understood by "diabetes" (medically, it is called diabetes mellitus, form the Latin "honey-sweet flow"), is an intrinsic condition characterised by high blood sugar levels and sugar in the urine. Diabetes mellitus manifests mostly (but not always – see age-related diabetes below) as a result of a lack of insulin, a hormone produced in the pancreas (in the Islets of Langerhans). Insulin is responsible for the cells absorption of sugar as glucose and the formation of the starch-like substance glycogen from the excess sugar. This is normally then stored in the liver and the muscles. However, if there is a lack of insulin in the body, sugar levels in the blood rise, until the kidneys no longer retain the sugar and excrete it in the urine. This leads to increased loss of fluid and minerals.

The lack of absorption of sugar into the cells and the subsequent loss of fluids and salts cause a weakening of the blood circulation and the muscles, accompanied by a general decrease in energy levels. Initially, typical symptoms are increased thirst, dryness of the skin and the mucous membranes, frequent urination (including during the night), tiredness and loss of weight – and all this in spite of hunger, and an increased consumption of food. At a later stage, there may be itching, skin complaints, lack of appetite, slower healing of wounds, eyesight trouble and sexual problems. If the disease is not treated, or when

there is a sudden onset, metabolic problems such as nausea, stomach ache, increased respiration, dizziness, and mental disorientation right through to unconsciousness (diabetic coma), and collapse of the heart and the blood circulation may also occur.

A slower course of the disease is more common, however, and with inadequate treatment this may result in gradual damage that become apparent later on. Along with this, changes in the composition of the blood and its degree of viscosity cause high blood pressure and diseases of the blood vessels (e. g. arteriosclerosis), which, in turn, lead to other symptoms.

Type 2 diabetes, or "late onset" (age-related) diabetes, has to be considered separately. In this type of diabetes, both the level of insulin and blood sugar levels are high. High levels of blood sugar are not caused by a lack of insulin, but by the defective absorption of sugar/glucose by the body cells. Causes of this type of diabetes may include a clogging of the tissues, this is caused by (among other things) the consumption of too much animal protein. This, in turn, may cause problems within the blood vessels and with the supply of nutrients to the cells. The latter need constant supplies of nutrients – hence the high level of insulin – but do not receive the ready store of sugars. Quite simply, this occurs because "access is blocked". Type 2 diabetes can, therefore, actually be cured completely with a healthy diet that is devoid of animal protein, accompanied by thorough detoxification (see Detoxification).

Nevertheless, all kinds of diabetes should always be treated under professional and qualified medical guidance. The right balance of therapeutic measures is absolutely essential and, if necessary, a supply of insulin and a special diet. Crystals that are able to stimulate or further the production and effects of insulin – and, if necessary, detoxify and cleanse the tissues, or relieve the above-mentioned symptoms and side effects – can be applied as a supplement.

In order to access the psychological background of the disease, one should bear in mind that diseases of the pancreas are sometimes caused by a feeling of not being able to understand certain things, i. e. experiences and life situations, in particular personal loss. This unfulfilled wish to understand often creates mistrust and bitterness, i. e. one loses "the sweetness of life" (the sugar). Of course, this is not always the case, but in many instances, an examination of such circumstances has lead to unexpected improvement in many suffers.

Amber helps with diabetes, especially when excess weight or obesity and continuous frustration with oneself are connected with the disease, or are evident at the same time. Amber furthers a feeling of freedom from care and enhances a move to having a happy attitude overall.

Chalcedony stimulates the production of insulin in the early stages of diabetes and the cleansing of the tissues in Type 2 diabetes. Furthermore, it helps relieve many of the accompanying symptoms, such as disturbances in the balance of body fluids, skin complaints and the mucous membranes, high blood pressure and impaired vision. It also helps us understand and solve the conflicts that have caused the disease. Blue and Pink Chalcedony are best suited for this.

Citrine stimulates the production of insulin, thereby helping with all symptoms and effects of the disease. Citrine improves an existing sense of well being and helps "sweeten" one's life.

Ocean Jasper stimulates the production of insulin, the cleansing and regeneration of the tissues and regulates the balance of fluids. It can, therefore, be applied for both types of diabetes. Furthermore, it stimulates the recognition and solution of conflicts that are causing the condition.

Place or tape each of the crystals mentioned above on the pancreas, regularly and over a long period. Apply raw or tumbled stones and flat sections or segments.

If necessary, take gem essence (3-5 drops, 3 times daily) or gem water (100–300 ml) taken in sips during the course of the day.

Diarrhoea

Diarrhoea is the term used to describe excessive, mostly liquid and frequent stools, which are caused by an inadequate water re-absorption or over-secretion of fluids into the colon. It can have many causes. Disturbances within the self-cleansing mechanisms of the intestine, infections, inflammations, problems with the digestion of or allergies to certain foods, toxification, a hyper-active thyroid gland and various kinds of digestive disturbances are only some of the possible physical causes. Moreover, there may also be nervous complaints, feelings of guilt, fear, excitement, or emotional and mental confusion. Diarrhoea that lasts for longer periods should not therefore be ignored, but be investigated by a doctor or an alternative practitioner, before further complications can occur caused by a continuous lack of fluid and salts (electrolytes) in the system.

In order to prevent matters from going this far, diarrhoea can be relieved by eating bananas, blueberries or grated, raw apples (use a shredder made of glass). Heilerde (a fine healing clay rich in minerals that soothes stomach problems), charcoal tablets, plenty of liquid and replacement of the lost electrolytes (e. g. by taking high quality salt and proprietary remedies will also help stabilise the intestine again. The crystals mentioned below also have a relieving effect. In order to ensure a complete cure, however, the physical or emotional causes must also be identified and treated.

Amethyst furthers water re-absorption in the colon and is therefore particularly helpful in less severe cases of chronic diar-

rhoea. It is also very helpful when grief and confusion accompany the diarrhoea.

Wear a necklace or a pendant for longer periods or regularly place a crystal or a polished crystal on the stomach every morning. It is also recommended to take Amethyst as gem essence (2-5 drops, 3 times daily) and as Hildegard von Bingen's Amethyst Water (see page 25), but no more than one liqueur glass daily.

Dumortierite helps with diarrhoea that is caused by problems with certain foods, minor cases of toxification, or problems that accompany fear or continuous emotional discomfort. Use in the same way as Amethyst.

Jet relieves all forms of diarrhoea.

In acute cases, place a crystal on the stomach and one in the mouth at the same time. However, for continuous treatment, wear a necklace or a pendant while also taking gem essence (3-7 drops, 3-5 times daily).

Serpentine helps when diarrhoea and constipation alternate, or when there are digestive problems with cramp-like pains.

Place a polished stone on the stomach when necessary; or wear a necklace or a pendant for longer periods. Alternately, take gem essence (3-7 drops daily).

Ear Problems

see Middle Ear Infections; Hearing Problems

Energy Loss

see Tiredness

Eye Problems

There are many kinds of eye problems as well as actual diseases These range in form from innate sight defects (short and long sightedness, weak sightedness, nystagmus, squinting) through acquired problems (age conditioned long sightedness, tired eyes, increasing ametropia, blurred eyes and others), to diseases or the result of diseases (inflammation, glaucoma, cataract, detachment of the retina etc.). Despite of all the different backgrounds and connections between our sight organs, nerve system, blood circulation, fluid balance and musculature, the same crystals can be used time and again in order to treat nearly all cases of eye problems.

See also: Ametropia; Cataracts; Conjunctivitis; Eye Strain; Nystagmus; Sight Problems; Squinting

In principle, appropriate home and workplace lighting is very important, especially if you suffer from an eye disease that is becoming progressively worse. It is better to use flicker-free "daylight" lamps (i.e. with a full light spectrum and not strip or fluorescent lighting), to take plenty of liquid (preferably non-carbonated, acid-free, good quality water), adopt a diet rich in vitamins and minerals (particularly vitamin A, selenium, and high quality salt), boost your liver function (see Liver Health) and ensure that you get sufficient sleep. All these factors will always be beneficial in effect. However, if you simply cannot avoid working for long periods in front of a computer screen, or in artificial light, it is important to take regularly outdoor walks in order to try and restore some overall balance to intense working conditions.

Of course, emotionally and psychologically, many eye diseases are often connected to the fact that we can neither see, nor want to see, certain things; or are trying to avoid a certain point of view, etc. Nevertheless, it is rare to obtain any resolution to this state of affairs and so fretting away over what you do not want to see is pointless. After all, if we knew what the problem was, no doubt we would see! Instead, far more effective is to make a general effort to gain new perspectives and points of view. Try to adopt a broadened horizon, with more tolerance and understanding, in order to try and gain a new sense of spiritual freedom. In this way, a new and different point of view may also have a positive influence on your eyes and vision.

Of course, with many eye and sight problems, there is a complexity of interacting causes, i.e. genetic or inherited factors, lifestyle, diet and nutrition, eye-strain, stress, ailments such as allergies, emotional upsets, and so on. Usually, there is also a close connection with the state of the liver

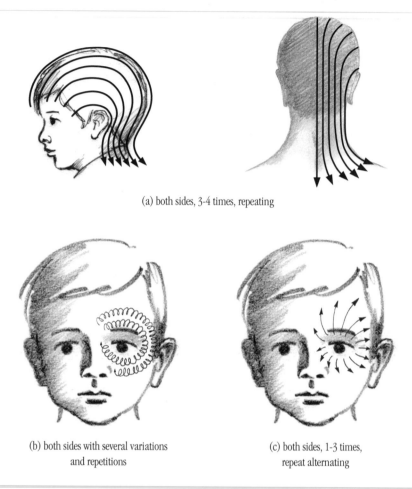

(a) both sides, 3-4 times, repeating

(b) both sides with several variations
and repetitions

(c) both sides, 1-3 times,
repeat alternating

Fig. 6: Treating eye problems with Amethyst.

and the eyes (see Detoxification; Liver Health).

As a general rule, the most effective solution is one in which all possibilities are considered – ideally with an experienced consultant, therapist, doctor or alternative practitioner – treatment is then applied that is appropriate to the individual case.

If this is done and combined with certain exercises, you can obtain improvements even with seemingly innate eye problems (and even with those that often are

98

regarded as incurable). Extensive literature is available on such eye exercises and about centres with courses for improving the sight. However, crystal therapy can also have a supportive and complementary effect, helping to, relieve problems and stabilise the condition once an improvement has been achieved.

Agate, especially when containing inclusions of an eye signature, is always the first choice of crystal for organic eye problems. For dry, burning eyes, Agate of a blue-grey natural colour is best; with inflammation in the tissue or in the inner eye, use the pink natural form, (if possible, a crystal that includes a signature resembling the choroid, the area of small blood vessels at the rear of the eye); and for retinal diseases, a detached retina or changes in the refraction of the lens and cornea, use Agate with a Rock Crystal centre. Tumbled stones or section/slices should be placed on the eyes regularly for a quarter of an hour (at night for the best effect).

Amethyst relieves many eye diseases that are connected with eyestrain or nervous problems, such as tired eyes, nystagmus, ametropia, reduced sight, squinting, etc.

First, relax the whole head with Amethyst in the form of a piece of a druse the size of a hand. Use it to stroke the head as if using a brush, but without touching the head. Move the crystal with even strokes from the forehead, over the head and upper rear of the neck downwards (see Fig. 6).

Four or five parallel strokes like this are needed from the line of the parting to the ear; then three or four times on both sides. After that, massage the area around the eyes gently with a light, polished Amethyst, applying circular movements. Finally, stroke the area around the eyes, moving outwards in a radial movement, touching the skin very gently with the crystal.

This procedure can also be carried out prior to placing other crystals on the eyes as part of a further treatment (e. g. Rock Crystal, Aquamarine, Emerald or Sardonyx).

Polished Amethyst can also be placed on eyes that are pressure-sensitive, watery, or where the sight is blurred. A compress moistened in Hildegard von Bingen's Amethyst Water (see page 25) may also help when placed on the eyes.

Aquamarine belongs to the Beryl group of minerals, which are among the most important crystals for healing eye problems. They relax the area around the eyes and improve muscle tone. In addition, all forms of Beryl have a positive influence upon the nerves; Aquamarine itself is applied particularly in treating nystagmus, ametropia, squinting and weak sightedness and when other eye conditions have deteriorated after strenuous work. It is also among the most important crystals for eye diseases caused by allergies. Spiritually and emotionally, Aquamarine also aids in the broadening of ones horizons.

Place either a small crystal or a tumbled

stone on the eyelids; or wear as a necklace or pendant. Alternatively, take either gem water (200–300 ml taken in small sips during the course of the day), or gem essence (5-9 drops, 3-5 times daily). It is often helps to rinse the eyes with Aquamarine water.

Rock Crystal has been used for centuries in cases of cataracts and other diseases that blur the vision. In addition, Rock Crystal can have an improving effect on short and long sightedness and squinting.

Place a small crystal or a tumbled stone directly on the closed eyelids. The brightly shining "Herkimer Diamonds" are particularly suitable forms to use. Treatment with Rock Crystal seems to be especially effective if complimented by the Amethyst treatment described above.

Blue Chalcedony helps with reddened, burning eyes and also with conjunctivitis. As Chalcedony stimulates lymph flow and detoxification of the tissues, it is often applied in cases of glaucoma, blurred vision and infections of the retina and the choroids.

Crystals can be placed upon the eyelids or worn as a necklace or pendant of Blue Lace Agate. Also, try taking as gem essence (5-9 drops, 3-5 times daily), or gem water (200–300 ml taken in sips during the course of the day).

Chrysoprase, as a Chalcedony that is rich in nickel, has a similar effect to Blue Chalcedony. However, it also helps with rapid detoxification, which often has a positive effect on eye diseases. Unlike many other detoxifying crystals, it is often best to place it directly over the liver, as the latter has its own inner energy connection to the eyes.

Diamond reduces the deposition of toxins in the eye. It is most effective if taken as gem essence (3-7 drops, 3-5 times daily), or gem water (200–300 ml taken in small sips during the course of the day).

Diamond also has a direct effect on the optic nerve and the sight centre of the brain. This makes it an important crystal in cases of weakened vision, cataracts, clouding of the vitreous humor in the eye itself. It can be placed directly on the closed eyes, or between the eyebrows (on the so-called "third eye"), as a supplement to taking as gem water or essence.

Dioptase is applied in anthroposophic medicine and as eye drops for eye pain, burning and reddened sore eyes.

Place a crystal or a crystal cluster on the closed eyelids. Alternatively, take gem essence (3-5 drops, 3 times daily). Beside that, Dioptase has a positive effect on the liver and can be placed directly on the liver in cases of weak sightedness.

Emerald, like Aquamarine, belongs to the Beryl family of minerals. It is one of the most important crystals for treating ametropia, squinting and tired eyes. It relaxes the area around the eyes, stimulates the nerve function and has a positive influence on the eye musculature. In addition,

Emerald helps alleviates instances of poisoning or toxins, improves the metabolism, fights infections and reduces inflammation (e. g. associated with glaucoma, blurred vision, cataracts, wakened sight, etc.). It is particularly effective with eye diseases that are caused by inflammation of the airways.

Spiritually, Emerald has a "broadening" effect on any existing narrow point of view or limited horizons.

Place small crystals or tumbled stones directly on the eyelids and the liver (preferably at the same time). In addition, wear as a necklace or a pendant. Finally, also take as gem water (200–300 ml taken in small sips during the course of the day), or gem essence (5-9 drops, 3-5 times daily).

Emerald water is good for eye rinsing, too.

Noble Opal improves and regulates lymph flow and so helps, just alike Chalcedony, in treating inflammation of the eye, glaucoma, blurred vision, and with infections and diseases of both the retina and the choroid. It is applied as for Chalcedony.

Ocean Jasper is also a Chalcedony, which regulates the fluid balance of the eye and simultaneously strengthens the body's immune defence system. It is, therefore, used for inflammation of the connective tissue and in the inner eye, as well as for the resulting conditions of glaucoma, loss of vision, and damage to the retina or choroid. Ocean Jasper can also be used to treat blurred vision and a crystal containing an eye signature is especially effective.

Place a tumbled stone on the eyelid. Alternatively, wear as a necklace or a pendant around the neck. Alternatively, place a crystal on the liver; or take gem water (200–300 ml taken in small sips during the course of the day).

Sardonyx is one of the best crystals for treating the eyes. This is due to the fact that its constituent part of Chalcedony (the light areas) furthers fluid regulation, its Onyx content (black areas) aids detoxification and the Sard (red areas) improves the blood circulation. Thus, it also helps with nystagmus, ametropia, squinting, reduced sight, sight problems in twilight conditions, diseases of the retina or the choroid, disturbances of the sight nerves and the sight centre.

Place a raw or a tumbled stone directly on the eyes. Alternatively, take gem essence (3-7 drops, 5 times daily), or gem water (200–300 ml) taken in small sips during the course of the day.

Sodalite is another very good crystal for the fluid regulation in connection with the eyes – both externally for dry eyes and for any lack of internal eye fluids. Consequently, it has a strong, preventive effect with many choroid and retinal problems (e. g. a detached retina).

Place a tumbled stone on the eyelids and take gem water (200–300 ml taken in small sips during the course of the day). In addition, wear as a necklace, pendant or gem crystal around the neck.

Tourmaline, with its different coloured varieties (Blue, Pink, Green and Watermelon) helps especially with eye nerve problems or eye diseases caused by injury (squinting, reduced vision, etc.).

Place either crystals or tumbled stones directly on the eyelids; or take as gem water or gem essence (dosage as outlined above for Emerald).

See also Nystagmus, Eye Problems; Eye Strain; Ametropia, Glaucoma, Cataracts; Squinting

Eye Strain

Tired and strained eyes are very common nowadays with increased TV viewing, working with computer monitors and in artificial light. A feeling of pressure around the eyes, mild pain, a burning sensation, red skin, dryness, blurred sight and temporarily reduced vision during reading are typical symptoms in this context. In order to avoid long-term damage, ensure that your diet is rich in vitamin A, drink plenty of pure water and always solve the problem at a causal level. More efficient light sources, shielding of monitor screens, etc., naturally make more sense than just applying the following crystals.

See also: Ametropia; Eye Problems; Sight Problems; Squinting

Agates as small section/slices or tumbled stones, especially those containing

eye-signatures, can be placed upon the eyelids in cases of dry or burning eyes.

Amethyst is effective with pressure-sensitive, watery eyes and blurred sight (see Sight Problems). Place either tumbled stones or compresses moistened with Hildegard von Bingen's Amethyst Water (see page 25) on the eyes.

Aquamarine as tumbled stones or crystals can be placed on closed eyelids after tiring work, especially if an already existing eye disease has worsened. Rinsing the eyes with Aquamarine water also brings about fast relief.

Dioptase helps soothe painful, burning and reddish eyes. There are commercially available Dioptase eye drops for this purpose. You can also place crystals or crystal clusters on closed eyelids.

Emerald relieves tired eyes, especially if it is of a beautiful Emerald green colour. You can also place a crystal or a tumbled stone on closed eyelids.

Exhaustion

Exhaustion occurs because of excessive strain or – looked at differently – through a lack of recovery from an illness. It signifies that one's available energy resources are totally used up.

If exhaustion occurs without any apparent cause and within an otherwise normal, healthy state, then one's energy must have already been decreased by some other factors, e. g. some undetected physical illness or emotional burden. Such exhaustion "without apparent cause" does nevertheless have a cause and it should be investigated without fail – consulting a doctor or alternative practitioners if necessary.

See also: Tiredness

Crystals can also be applied in order to overcome exhaustion and help one "bounce back" faster. For short-term exhaustion, which is caused by physical strain, an old home remedy can be applied, which is closely connected to the crystal therapy – a pinch of table salt on the tip of the tongue!

Bronzite helps with exhaustion that is caused by the "energy-robbing" stress of every-day life. As a mineral rich in both iron and magnesium, Bronzite is active externally whilst simultaneously calming internally. It is especially helpful when no actual recovery seems in sight for a quite long time.

Epidote helps one to recover after an extreme effort and severe illnesses. It is particularly suitable when feeling totally drained and incapable of performing even the smallest activity.

Garnet Pyrope helps in maintaining a positive attitude in difficult times, when there seems little hope of change but where it is vital to continue doing what has to be done. It mobilises energy reserves in precisely the right amounts, and so that they are longer lasting. It also stimulates the metabolism, regeneration and reconstruction processes within the body.

Rhodochrosite has a rapid animating and stimulating effect and helps overcome exhaustion quickly. However, it should not be applied for too long a period, as energy reserves are used up quickly under its influence – and, ironically, an even greater loss of energy occurs.

Ocean Jasper helps in particular when exhaustion is caused by either internal inflammation or chronic illness. It furthers the healing of these conditions, improves the removal of waste and toxic substances that have been produced in this connection, and revives the metabolism. In this way, it provides a new source of physical energy. On the emotional front, it also helps one emerge from a feeling of resignation, periods of despondency and other negative states – and therefore brings hope, confidence, vitality and drive.

Tiger Iron creates new energy in cases of weakness and exhaustion as it boosts the iron metabolism. It has a slow, but lasting, strengthening effect. Other than being avoided in cases of inflammatory diseases have caused exhaustion, it is quite aptly called "the tiger in the tank".

Zoisite (like Epidote) helps regenerate and recover after severe illnesses. The most suitable crystals are Zoisite minerals that contain Ruby.

All the crystals mentioned can be worn

for body contact in the form of bracelets, necklaces or pendants. Alternatively, they can be taken internally in the form of gem essence (5-7 drops, 3-5 times daily) and gem water (100–300 ml taken in small sips over the course of the day).

Whilst Rhodochrosite should be removed fairly soon, all the other crystals can be worn or applied for longer periods.

Fatigue

see Tiredness

Fear

Fear is an emotion common to all of us and is experienced as a state of anxiety, alertness, and awareness in dangerous situations. It is a natural, basic reaction that serves to enables us to act quickly. This is all connected with the instinctive, automatic and natural secretion of adrenaline from glands into the body – as a result of which, our general readiness for action is increased. So, rather than being a negative emotion, fear is actually appropriate and essential for survival, sharpening the senses and providing an immediate focus on what is happening.

However, a fearful response is not really appropriate when there is no acute danger. Nevertheless, many people live in a permanent state of fear of possible dangers. On the one hand, this condition is based upon a wide range of past experiences. On the other hand, it can also be fostered by a daily stream of negative information with which the mass media supplies us so abundantly. It is in this latter case that fear has a clearly negative effect. In other words, we can believe that we are in a dangerous situation even when this is not the case. The result is that we can end up acting inappropriately most of the time. Indeed, in extreme cases, this can even result in compulsive behaviour or disturbing physical symptoms, e. g. excitement, anxiety, palpitations, difficulties in breathing, and so forth.

However, lesser kinds and degrees of fear can be overcome. If you can determine just what makes you afraid – even if this is a fear of the unknown – you can then face up to it and confront it. Nevertheless, this all has to relate to something that you recognise.

In the condition referred to these days as "panic attacks", or in cases where there is no apparent cause for fear, the previously described course of action cannot really apply. Here, fear is the result of having experienced a range of different situations that have led to a "passive" way of life – one characterised by excessive caution. In such cases, the past has to be confronted and (by means of therapy if necessary), a way has to be found that will dissipate the impairment that is a psychological state caused by previous negative experiences. In the long term, this is the only way in which irrational attacks of fear be cured. In effecting such a resolution, complementary therapeutic process also requires a certain degree of motivation and ability in order to confront such difficult issues.

To summarise, chronic and irrational attacks of fear can only be resolved through raising self-awareness – if necessary, with the additional help of a therapist. Crystal therapy cannot achieve thus alone, but will ease the process by increasing ones inner ability to confront difficult issues. Indeed, the supportive nature and effects of crystal can be very helpful with the process.

Amazonite helps with suddenly occurring attacks of fear. It is particularly good whenever there is a feeling of being the victim of some overwhelming fate. Amazonite stimulates self-determination and an overall trust in life.

Dumortierite helps with minor attacks of fear. It communicates feelings of relaxation and ease and makes it possible to see stresses and strains in a less threatening and intimidating light.

Rhodonite helps in dealing with fear that arises in connection with fatalities, personal loss, injuries, violence, acute danger or death. It relieves any excessive, though irrational, attacks of fear, typical signs of which are a need for protection or talking a great deal about present fears, yet without experiencing any relief.

Rutile Quartz helps with fear that exposes your own faults, inadequacies or harmful acts. It also helps when there is a feeling of losing control, or of suppressing fear and maybe withdrawing into yourself.

Sugilite helps with any kind of fear, even in its strong and irrational forms. It provides the courage needed to confront unpleasant feelings or situations and makes it easier to recognise unconscious causes of that fear. Furthermore, Sugilite helps to resolve conflicts, but without any feelings of having been unduly compromised, so that any insights gained can also be translated into positive action.

Wear any of these crystals for longer periods in the form of bracelets, necklaces or pendants. Whilst fear will usually not disappear suddenly, given time, the effects in healing effect of these crystals and a sense of greater awareness will be become apparent.

Fertility Problems

A few crystals are said – known, even – to stimulate fertility, i. e. the procreative capacity of men and the ability of women to conceive. The more certain you can be about the cause of reduced fertility, the more purposefully and effectively these crystals can be applied. But, as ever, the cause should always first be clarified by a specialist or doctor wherever practical.

Possible causes for female fertility problems are functional disturbances in the ovaries, hormonal disturbances (of the pituitary gland and thyroid gland), blocked Fallopian tubes (e.g. following inflammation) or a disease of the uterus.

Some parallel causes of male fertility include impotence, trouble with sperm production or difficulties with the sperm-conducting channel – such as inflammation of the testicles, the epididymis, prostate or the urethra.

In many cases, all of the above causes can be eliminated, and yet fertility still appears impaired. Here, it may often be helpful to look for emotional and psychological causes. An unconscious desire not to have children can often have the same obstructing effect as a strong but contrary desire for children, combined with high pressure to "perform" the relevant gender roles. Personal problems within a partnership and/or sexuality may also frequently be a hindrance to reproduction.

Crystals can be a wonderful help with any impaired fertility that arise from both organic and emotional causes. However, they cannot provide a substitute for an open dialogue or a healing heart to heart interchange between the affected partners. In cases of impaired fertility, a search for whose "fault" it all is can be extremely damaging within a relationship. In contrast, mutual support between the partners is definitely beneficial, whether the desire to have children is fulfilled or not.

For Men

Ocean Jasper improves the procreative capacity. It either leads to increased sperm production or improved viability of the sperm. The precise background to these processes has still not been clarified; but a speedy fulfilment of the long-cherished wish to have children, has been confirmed many times over. Maybe this is not surprising as "fertility" is one of the emotional qualities of this life-affirming and life-supporting crystal.

Thulite helps with impotence and infertility that have no clear cause. It furthers lust, sensuality and interest in sexuality. Physically, Thulite furthers regeneration of the genitals after an inflammation.

Zoisite is often even more effective. It stimulates the formation of sperm and regeneration of the genitals after inflammations. It can help with all causes of impaired fertility. Particularly effective are Zoisite crystals containing Ruby.

For Women

Chrysoprase helps with impaired fertility that is not a result of any organic damage that might have been caused by previous illnesses, medication, or hormonal contraceptive aids. Chrysoprase can also help clarify the situation within a partnership, assisting honest discussion and opening up both partners emotionally to help each other with their wish for a child. This is especially useful when conflicts between the partners relate directly to the desire for children. (Chrysoprase is, of course, also useful for men in connection with this context.)

Moonstone helps with infertility caused by hormonal disturbances and unidentified emotional tensions between the partners. If Moonstone is worn for a longer period and the curtains in the bedroom are not drawn at night during that time, the hormonal system may – under certain circumstances – readjust to the Moon's cycle, so that there is a possibility of conceiving at the full Moon.

Rose Quartz helps with organically-caused infertility. It improves blood circulation in the genitals and assists in their regeneration after an illness. It thus helps overcome many disturbances. Emotionally and psychologically, Rose Quartz furthers warmth and romance between partners.

Golden Topaz is the most successful crystal for infertility, no matter what the cause. It helps with functional disturbances in the ovaries, hormonal disturbances and organically-caused blockages. Emotionally, it encourages happiness, security, sexual self-confidence, self-determination and self-realisation within the partnership.

With all of the above, wear a necklace or a pendant with direct body contact, preferably on the abdomen. Also, take gem essence (3-5 drops, three times daily) or gem water (50–200 ml taken in small sips during the course of the day).

Fever

Fever is a defence mechanism of the human organism, in which the body temperature is raised to values above 37.5 °C (99.5 °F). This also increases the metabolic rate along with acceleration of the pulse and breathing rate. Accompanying phenomena are lack of appetite, dullness, dizziness, headache, and restlessness and – in extreme instances – feverish hallucinations or delirium. In most cases, the occurrence of fever serves to support the body's immune defence system and it's cleansing us of toxic substances and waste products. Therefore, as a rule, fever should not be suppressed, unless it reaches 41 °C (106 °F) or more and thus becomes life threatening. Too rapid a suppression of fever often impedes a thorough cure and so may lead to a relapse and transform an acute illness into chronic one.

With a harmless course of the fever, fever-lowering remedies should not be implemented until the peak has been passed and the fever curve is on a downward course. The patient should be able to feel the change between a rising and a falling temperature.

In order to promote temperature rise, the body concentrates its own energy within the main torso of the body – so that the extremities, in particular hands and feet, are chilly to the touch. The skin and muscles may even remain chilly, tremble and shiver. In order to lessen the fever symptoms, the energy is spread over the skin and into the body's extremities, where it is dispersed and released more easily. This then makes hands and feet become warmer, the general feeling of the fever is increased and perspiration begins in order to cool the body down. This lowering of the fever temperature can now be enhanced by cold compresses wrapped around the calves

Alternative therapy advice is that these compresses will have an even better effect if you add Bach Flower Rescue Remedy, ethereal eucalyptus oil and gem essence from Moss Agate to the water.

Conventionally, the recommendation is to rest, preferably staying in bed and drinking plenty of water or tea (herbal if possible) in order to offset the loss of liquid caused by the perspiration that accompanies any high temperature. Depending on the underlying illness, fever-stimulation or fever-lowering remedies must be coordinated with a doctor or the alternative practitioner – most particularly with a truly high temperatures or fever lasting for a long time.

This is the stage where crystal therapy can now assist the healing process as many have a fever-stimulating or fever-lowering effect.

Fever-stimulating crystals may be applied in order to raise fever, but only if that is necessary for the recovery process and the following selection have all proved to be reliable and to have a measurable effect as fever-stimulating crystals.

Carnelian has a strong fever-stimulating effect without actually raising the temperature too much. Apply it if there is seems to be a general tendency of no increase in the fever temperature.

Ruby has an even stronger fever-stimulating effect than Carnelian. It can be applied whenever fever stimulation is vital for the healing process to be initiated.

Sard only stimulates fever slightly. It can be applied in a complementary role in order to start the healing process and if there is already a slightly raised temperature that then remains constant.

Crystals with an observed effect in reducing fever are as follows:

Rock Crystal can be applied in the form of the so-called "generator crystal", in order to reduce the fever and lower a dangerously high temperature as fast as possible. Stroke the space around the patient with the largest pointed surface of the crystal, using gentle motions from above and downwards over the forehead, face, neck, body, arms

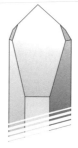

Fig. 7: Use of the Generator Crystal

and legs. If you do not have a generator to hand, you can carry out the same exercise with a broad tumbled Rock Crystal.

Blue Chalcedony, Moss Agate and **Ocean Jasper** lower temperature and can be applied when the fever has passed its peak. Blue Chalcedony helps with an easy, fast reduction, while Moss Agate and Ocean Jasper help with a slower lowering, or if the temperature curve goes up and down.

Chrysocolla has a lowering effect dependent on the actual course of the fever. So, it can be applied at any time and is especially recommended in cases of emergency or extremely high temperatures.

Hold a tumbled crystal in the hand or put it on the thymus gland (between the heart and throat) or wear a necklace or a pendant directly on the body. Also try gem essence (5-10 drops) as required, from three times daily to once an hour.

Financial Worries

There is a suggestion, as yet totally unproved, that the best way to relieve financial worries is to gaze, in a contemplative frame of mind, upon one's own diamonds in the safe! However, this author's assumption is that it only works if the diamonds have been fully paid for! (See also: Worry.)

Dumortierite, the "take-it-easy-crystal" is a better choice in more normal circumstances.

Opal can also help in cases of hardship and worries — even if its application does not lead to a cure of the root cause of the problem.

Flu

Flu — being the commonly used, shortened form of influenza — is often equated with the common cold or related illnesses. However, it is a virus-based disease that spreads epidemic-like through infection. Its symptoms appear rather like those of the common cold, but are usually much more aggressive. The sufferer very soon has a fever-like state, with a high temperature of 39-40 degrees Celsius (about 100 Fahrenheit), accompanied by shivering, the feeling of having been knocked out, pains in the head, the eyes, the chest, the back and the joints — and sometimes conjunctivitis, nausea (children also often have stomach and intestinal problems), blister-like eczema and reddened skin. Later, inflammations follow in the tonsils and the airways, with a dry cough and hoarseness, a slow pulse and falling blood pressure. Never underestimate a bout of genuine flu. One should stay in bed under medical supervision in order to cure it and avoid further complications!

As with colds, any kind of continuation of the illness into the inner parts of the body should be regarded as a complication. Such complications can lead to:

- Pneumonia (weakness, lack of appetite, high fever, night sweat, breathlessness)
- Heart and circulation problems (disturbed heart rhythm, heart injury, collapse of the circulation)
- Sinusitis (pain that feels worse when nasal pressure is applied, or if one bends forwards)
- Inflammation of the middle ear (earache)
- Cerebrospinal meningitis or encephalitis (head ache, vomiting, further temperature increase, shivering, loss of consciousness, hallucinations)
- Stomach and intestinal illnesses (inflammation, serious cases of diarrhoea)
- Liver and spleen swelling
- Kidney damage

Symptoms such as weakness and problems with the heart and circulation may continue up to one month after abatement of the actual case of flu.

The intensity of the flu and the increased danger of complications (compared to a common cold) demand a more careful application of crystals. It is also helpful to rinse the mouth and teeth with organic, cold-pressed sunflower oil for 10 to 20 minutes every day. In this way, waste and toxic substances, which impede the immune system, are drawn out of the tissue. However, the oil should NOT be swallowed under any circumstance!

Heliotrope can be applied at the beginning of a bout of flu as the body's first non-specific immune reaction is strengthened by it. In many cases, it succeeds in warding off the virus before it can spread on a larger scale. Parallel to its physical effect, Heliotrope also furthers our mental and psychological ability to ward off infection or seriously limit the effects.

Place or fix a polished crystal or a flat section on the thymus gland (between heart and throat). Take gem essence (5-10 drops per hour) or gem water (up to one litre taken in sips over the course of the day). The wearing a necklace or a pendant of Heliotrope has also proved to be effective.

Moss Agate, however, should be used if the flu actually breaks out, with a raised temperature and all the above symptoms. It is important that the flow of lymph and the continuous cleansing of the areas affected by the disease be kept going, as toxic substances that have accumulated after the disease, in particular, can lead to the complications mentioned above. Use Moss Agate – which also represents emotional cleansing and relief, should therefore be applied until the illness has clearly abated.

Chalcedony can then be applied as a replacement for the Moss Agate and in order to continue detoxification via the lymph channels at a more slowly, thus removing stress from the whole organism. Chalcedony furthermore brings some light relief emotionally and psychologically, that being one of its typical properties! Apply it until temperatures have fallen to a normal level.

Nevertheless, one should stay in bed until fully cured. In other words, at least one symptom-free day of rest and regeneration is essential before daily activities are resumed. Nowadays, this vital day of rest and recuperation, previously a basic recommendation of nearly all doctors, is all too often skipped. Therefore, it worth bearing mind that missing out that extra day of recuperation often causes a relapse with complications and an even more severe bout of flu.

Emerald should be applied for at least one week when the fever has abated finally and a symptom-free state has been achieved. It will prevent relapses and complications – and also helps to continue the detoxification process, to keep the immune system stable and, eventually, re-establishes the body's overall harmony.

Epidote or **Zoisite** can be applied in order to overcome the typical weakness and exhaustion after a bout of flu. Epidote is especially regenerative and can be combined together with Blue Chalcedony in the last phase of the illness. If the flu affects the heart and circulation, you can apply Pink Chalcedony which re-establishes full health particularly on this area.

To use Moss Agate, Blue Chalcedony, Emerald, Epidote and Zoisite, hold a tumbled stone in one hand or put it on the thymus gland (between heart and throat). You can also fix it there with a first-aid sticking plaster. In addition, you might wear a neck-lace or a pendant with body contact and/or take gem essence (5-7 drops if required, from 3 times daily up to once an hour).

Foot Problems

Feet that have become tired as a result of standing for at long time, or that hurt in some other way, can be refreshed with crystals and proven remedies such as cold rosemary foot-baths. However, there is nothing better than physical exercise, which re-establishes the overall harmony of the body. Take a walk in comfortable shoes or – even better – without any footwear at all. There is little use in applying crystal therapy alone without exercising at the same time.

Blue Chalcedony has a cooling effect and relieves pain quickly. It also ensures that any retained fluid is drained.

Place a crystal into a little water for at least 24 hours and use the water for a footbath.

Alternatively, massage the feet with a tumbled stone. Gem essence can also be used for a footbath (30 drops in 5 litres of water).

Magnesite has a refreshing effect on tired feet, as is releases tension.

Use a tumbled stone for foot massage; or take as gem essence (5-7 drops once); or place a necklace around the ankles while putting up one's feet for a short while. If you want to test the effect for yourself, wrap the Magnesite necklace around only one ankle.

A distinct difference in the feet will become apparent after only 10 minutes.

Moss Agate and **Ocean Jasper**, as Chalcedony variants, likewise have a cooling and relieving effect, as they eliminate accumulations of fluid. Apart from this, they have an even more activating, stimulating and refreshing effect than Chalcedony itself. They are applied in the same way as Chalcedony (see above).

Forgetfulness

See Memory Problems

Fungal Infections

Fungal infections generally affect the skin (including hair and nails), the mucous membranes, the colon and the lungs. However, fungal spores from outside the body can only "take root" and spread if they find an appropriate environment – the right "breeding ground", as it were. No fungus really has much of a chance to survive in a healthy human organism, unless its body tissue is already heavily laden with toxic deposits and waste substances. When this happens, our body will try to excrete such contaminants by other means – through the skin, the mucous membranes, the intestine and the lungs. All become weakened by this process and this constitutes an environment in which the fungi can thrive.

See also: Athlete's Foot

There appears to be a connection between heavy metals and fungal infections. Most heavy metals (e.g. mercury, cadmium, etc,) are normally highly detrimental to the body, thus there are some cases where fungal infection is not actually bad for us. In these cases, fungi help bind the heavy metals and thus make it easier for the body to deal with them, resulting in less damage. However, the fungal infection is in itself a drain on the system, producing its own, injurious metabolic products.

There is then a state of trying to "cast out the demon with the devil", so to speak, as it becomes clear that it is not just the fungal infection that has to be counteracted and removed. If it is only the fungi that are dealt with, the problems they have caused are simply replaced by the problems caused by the toxic presence of the heavy metals. Therefore, it is important that all waste and toxic deposits are removed from the tissue. After all, if the tissue is in an unhealthy state, it is the very thing that makes a fungal attack possible in the first place.

In contrast, healthy, detoxified tissue offers no food value to invasive fungi, which will then disappear completely by a natural process. It is pretty clear then that a diet low in or without animal protein, along with colon therapy and further detoxifying remedies (see Detoxification) are highly important measures to take in order to avoid fungal infections.

Household remedies which seem to relieve fungal infections, include tea tree oil. However, this should only by applied externally, e. g. in a 10% solution and/or as an ointment. In addition, the following crystals can also be used in full confidence in all cases of severe infection, although their use is only complementary, as they cannot alone ensure a lasting cure.

Chrysoprase and **Smoky Quartz** in combination are the most efficient remedy against fungal infections. It is thought that the detoxifying Chrysoprase and the dissolving Smoky Quartz provide beneficial complementary effects.

Firstly, take Chrysoprase in the form of gem essence (5-7 drops, 3 times daily) or gem water (20 – 50 ml taken in small sips over the course of the day). At the same time, wear it in the form of a bracelet, a necklace or a pendant (in cases of localised infections, place a tumbled stone on the affected spot). After two days, apply in addition Smoky Quartz, to be worn continuously as a necklace or pendant. This treatment should continue for several weeks, but will then produce good results

Ocean Jasper or **Agates** containing within them signatures of a localised fungal infection can provide soothing relief. Primarily, they contribute to the relief from the consequences of fungal infections, such as inflammation, diarrhoea, etc. They stimulate the metabolism and aid in further detoxification of the tissue. However, they

are by no means as effective as Chrysoprase and should be applied mainly in cases of localised, external fungal infections (e. g. on skin, nails, etc.)

Place a tumbled stone or a section/slice onto the affected spot. Alternatively, take gem essence (3-7 drops, 3 times daily) or gem water (200–300 ml taken in small sips over the course of the day).

Fluorite is very effective if the mucous membranes are also subject to fungal attack (e. g. thrush), as it generally stimulates the cleansing and regeneration of mucous membranes. It can often be applied successfully when the combination of Chrysoprase and Smoky Quartz appears to have no effect.

Wear as a bracelet, necklace or pendant, or take gem essence or gem water (dosage as above, for Agate). In an emergency, place a tumbled stone into the mouth for a while – taking **great** care not to swallow the stone inadvertently!

Gall Bladder and Gallstones

Nearly all problems with the gall bladder are often not recognised specifically or directly as such. Nausea, which is triggered by secreted gall, can originate from the stomach or the pancreas; and dull pains in the upper part of the stomach may also originate from either the stomach or the intestine. Only the symptom of acute gall bladder colic is unambiguous that it is evident immediately for what it is.

Gall bladder problems more often manifest themselves indirectly, e. g. as pains between the right scapula (shoulder blade) and the spine, as a one-sided headache or as a decreased ability to digest fats and general distaste for fatty food. Thus, always consult a doctor or an alternative practitioner at the slightest suspicion of gall bladder problems in order to clarify the causes.

Bile itself is produced in the liver and contains – beside water and salts – the gall dye (bilirubin), which has been derived from disintegrated red blood corpuscles, bile acids, cholesterol, lecithin, and other fat-soluble substances. All must be excreted from the body (along with drugs, a range of hormones and various metabolism products). The bile fluid is then accumulated in the gall bladder and, when necessary, flows on into the duodenum. There, it serves the digestion of fats, breaking down fats in the food into tiny particles. These themselves are then acted on by adipolytic enzymes and can at last be absorbed into the blood.

Apart from that, bile contributes in two ways to the cleansing and detoxification of the body: Firstly, it carries fat-soluble wastes and toxic substances from the liver into the intestine (see above). Secondly, it also dissolves similar substances in the intestine, so that they can then be excreted. The bile itself is so precious that only 10% of it is released with the stool 90% being re-absorbed in the colon and transported to the liver for recycling.

Gall bladder problems may arise when an already weakened gall bladder is overworked (e. g. because of food that contains too much fat); when there is an inflammation; or when gallstones have been formed. Such stones irritate the gall bladder or the gall channels, respectively. In the worst case, they can even cause a blockage.

Similar problems may also arise when the gall bladder is under too much pressure through emotional strain or suppressed anger. Basically, an attempt (possibly a failed one) to control one's emotions or deal with those of others may thus lead to gall bladder problems.

Looking at gallstones specifically, they occur when the composition of the gall fluid is not optimal because of an inappropriate diet, (e. g. not enough fruit and vegetables that are rich in enzymes, too much denatured food, etc.), metabolic problems, an overworked liver or the emotional problems described above. Then, not all of the substances remain dissolved, but bind together instead and become crystallised. Fortunately, the crystallisation process can be reversed in some cases as when the gall fluid regains its correct composition, the stones may then re-dissolve.

Gall stones are responsible almost exclusively for the most violent and acute gall bladder problems, called gall colics These are very severe cramp-like pains in the right upper and central part of the stomach (pains that also radiate into the spine and the right shoulder), restlessness, nausea, vomiting, cold sweats, painful pressure in the upper part of the stomach and defensive tension. They are also sometimes accompanied by a fever and collapse of the circulation. Depending on the intensity and gravity of the problems, **seek medical advice immediately** or go directly to hospital. On the way, amber or other crystals can be applied, but otherwise do not hesitate!

Healing crystals serve as an accompanying therapy to medical help; but only apply them after securing a professional diagnosis, and as a supplement to the prescription of a doctor or alternative practitioner.

Amber is the most important crystal for gall bladder problems. It has a pain-relieving effect for colic and will improve the composition of the gall fluid, dissolving many gall stones. Emotionally, it helps with the consequences of grief and fears. These affect not only t the stomach, but sometimes also the gall bladder − in particular, in cases of helplessness, impotence and aggression caused by the latter and that is directed inwardly against oneself.

Chrysocolla helps with both inflammation of the gall bladder accompanied by a high fever, and with the consequences of violent emotions or suppressed anger.

Chrysoprase helps with accumulations in the gall system, with nausea caused by an irritated or overloaded gall bladder and,

with any latent aggression resulting from a troublesome conscience or unresolved conflicts.

Dumortierite relieves cramps, pains and nausea caused by gall bladder problems. Furthermore, as the "take-it-easy-crystal", it helps alleviate possible disease sources, such as strain, suppressed anger, exaggerated control etc.

Emerald helps with colic, as well as with inflammations, that are a consequence of stress, or (perceived) injustice. Emerald is also a helpful crystal for any gall bladder problems that seem to appear when other people (members of the family, subordinates, colleagues etc), start to 'get on your nerves".

Heliotrope is applied for acute inflammations of the gall bladder and system. Emotionally, it helps with general irritability caused by too many interruptions and other external influences.

Magnesite relieves gall bladder colic and also helps dissolve some gallstones. Furthermore, it helps with nausea accompanying severe emotional strain, excitement and stress.

Malachite helps with gall bladder colic and releases suppressed feelings, repressed irritations, anger and aggressions. Therefore, it is particularly good when gall bladder problems occur as a consequence of such suppression and external psychological and emotional pressures. It helps one avoid unnecessary argument, but also enables us to tackle the unavoidable ones both courageously and emphatically.

Ocean Jasper with a predominantly green colour helps with acute and chronic inflammations of the gall bladder and with the consequences of strain, unresolved conflicts, lack of recovery and disturbed sleep.

Peridot supports the long-term regulation of the gall fluid, so that gallstones are no longer formed. In order to reduce existing tendencies of gall stone formation, it should be applied regularly for several months. It can be placed in something like high quality sunflower oil, which is later used for salad dressings, etc. As this Peridot oil detoxifies very gently and improves the metabolism, the whole family can participate in this "cure".

For all the above, place or fix a crystal directly over the gall bladder; or wear a bracelet, a necklace, or a pendant on the body. You can also take gem essence (3-7 drops, three times daily), or gem water (100–200 ml taken in small sips during the course of a day.

Ganglia

A ganglion is a non-malignant abscess, which, in most cases, appears on the back of the hand, the foot or in the hollow of the knee. It is a form of cyst or protuberance of the internal skin tissue of a joint, sinew or the tendon sheaths. It has a gel-like content and is caused by degeneration of the connective tissue.

In general, although it may be unsightly, the visible, taut, elastic bulge that is a ganglion causes no problems, but it can cause undue pressure, pain and sense disturbances if a nerve is trapped by the ganglion.

Seemingly, ganglia are caused by an interplay and interaction of different factors. All the way from overstrained joints or sinews, through bad posture, to misaligned vertebrae. Additional causes can be an inadequate supply to and/or cleansing of the connective tissue – as a result of accumulations of toxins and waste, post-injury defects in blood vessels, general stress or metabolic problems.

See also: Cysts

The traditional medical treatment for a ganglion is physical exercises, in order to strengthen the musculature; or surgical removal.

Alternative treatments tend to be more comprehensive (see Detoxification) in order to improve the supply of essential nutrients to the tissue. Any such treatment is best complemented by therapeutic corrections to posture and the spinal column (e. g. craniosacral therapy, osteopathy, Dorn-Breuss method, etc.).

It is worth considering other factors too. It is a fact that a ganglion mostly occurs between the ages of 20 and 30, precisely that phase of life when there is still the youthful ambition and drive but also the start of other commitments (house, family, job, business, etc.). Therefore, whilst still fed by that early youthful energy, we still believe we can accomplish everything through effort and sheer will power. However, this increasing tension between two aspects of life is the precise recipe that can cause a ganglion to appear. Always take into account – the pressure, effort, and emotional and psychological stresses – when dealing with a ganglion.

Based on all of the above it becomes possible to influence the shrinking of the ganglion with herbal applications of comfrey and rue, homeopathic remedies or crystals.

Fluorite is by far the best healing crystal for treating ganglia. Also called "calcium fluoricum" in homeopathy, Fluorite regulates the supply of energy to the tissue and aids removal of toxins and waste. Being composed of calcium and fluorine, it induces a more relaxed, open and flexible attitude. As a mineral with a natural cubic crystal configuration, it boosts our capacity to become more flexible emotionally, especially if we end up with heavy commitments too early in life. Its calcium content also helps with rebuilding of joint and sinew tissue.

Apatite is the second choice. As a crystal of calcium phosphate, it has a wide range of influence on bones, joints, sinews and muscles. In homeopathy, Apatite is referred to as "calcium fluoricum" and with its hexago-

nal crystal configuration; it encourages an "upright" or "straight" attitude, both mentally and physically. Beside that, being also a phosphate, it helps in the development of the energy we all need for the tasks of life. Whilst relieving stress and worry, Apatite simultaneously strengthens the musculature. In turn, this eases any strain on sinews and joints. Finally, Apatite also improves the supply of tissue nutrients as a direct result of its calcium content, and also furthers rebuilding of joint substance and sinews.

Place slices/sections of crystals, or flat tumbled stones, as close as possible to the ganglion, fixing them there with a sticking plaster or bandage. It is also possible to wear the crystals as bracelets, necklaces, or pendants – in which case, this should be worn twenty-four hours a day for the best effect.

As a supplementary treatment, or as an alternative, take as gem essence (3-9 drops, every hour), or gem water (100–300 ml taken in small sips over the course of the day). Both fluids can also be rubbed into the affected skin.

Amazonite, **Chrysocolla**, **Ocean Jasper** and **Green Tourmaline** are also recommended although work with them in this context is till in its early stages. (See: Joint Pains; Synovitis; Tennis Elbow)

Glaucoma

Glaucoma is the result of a high inner pressure in the eye. This curbs the blood circulation in the optic nerve head, thereby reducing the field of vision. In the worst case, it leads to permanent damage of the sight nerve and to blindness. It can have many causes; blocked channels that drain fluid from the eye, diseases of the heart and circulation, severe nearsightedness, severely hardened eye muscles, chronic inflammations in the inner eye, and formation of cysts among others.

Glaucoma often develops rather slowly and insidiously. However, sometimes there can be an acute attack, which is often accompanied by considerable pain, severe reddening, an enlarged pupil and palpably hardened eyeball. In this case, a specialist or doctor should be consulted immediately.

Raised pressure in the inner eye fluid (the aqueous humour), is the common factor in all cases of glaucoma, this can be treated immediately. Traditionally, the pressure is regulated by the use of medication and surgical procedures. Nevertheless, glaucoma can also be dealt with by means of alternative treatments and the application of crystals.

In addition to these measures, one should first and foremost also treat the causal factors or those likely to lead to a progression of the disease – such as regulation of fluid in the eye (which is improved significantly through detoxification), inner tensions (fear, stress, etc.), heart diseases, circulation problems and, of course, any other eye complaints.

Chalcedony and **Noble Opal** improve the regulation of the fluid in the eye as well as overall lymph flow. Provided that a therapy addressing the causes is initiated at the same time, both have an immediate relieving effect and can be applied for longer periods leading to a permanent improvement.

Chrysoprase, like Chalcedony is rich in the metal nickel. It has the same effect as Chalcedony and Opal, but is also a strong aid in detoxification, which always has a positive impact on glaucoma. Contrary to

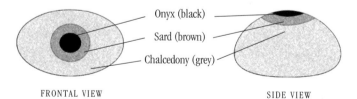

FRONTAL VIEW   SIDE VIEW

Fig. 8: Sardonyx that has been polished especially for healing eye complaints.

the other mentioned crystals, it is often better to place it on the liver, which has a close holistic energy connection with the eyes.

Ocean Jasper is also a Chalcedony and so regulates the fluid balance and, at the same time, relieves inflammatory states. Consequently, it can also be applied for acute attacks of glaucoma, when the inner eye is inflamed simultaneously.

Sardonyx is also one of the best crystals for use in cases of glaucoma. It improves fluid regulation because of its Chalcedony (light areas) content, encourages detoxification via its Onyx (red areas) content and the blood circulation due to Sard (red areas). This combination of different varieties of Chalcedony also leads to improvements on a causal level. Particularly good results may be obtained with Sardonyx, which has a natural eye signature, or with crystals that are ground like a cabochon. In that form, the black Onyx is in the centre of convexity, like a pupil, which again is surrounded by Sard (like the iris), which again is surrounded by the grey chalcedony corresponding to the eyeball (see Fig. 8).

In most cases, unpolished or tumbled stones are placed on the eyes (except for Chrysoprase) and either gem essence (3-7 drops, 3-5 times daily) or gem water (100–300 ml, taken in small sips over the course of the day) is taken with Chrysoprase, however, 20–50 ml is the correct amount to take.

All of these crystals mentioned are Chalcedonies or akin to Chalcedony (Noble Opal), so their use and application can also be combined and, for example, be worn in the form of a necklace.

Goitre

see Thyroid Problems

Graves Disease

see Thyroid Problems

Grazes

see Abrasions

Grief

Grief is the emotion that occurs with of the loss of a loved one, loss of security or important possessions, broken relationships, rejection, unrequited love, disappointments, being ignored (in particular with children), a feeling that one has not understood something specific, or that one is being misunderstood.

Put another way, in principle, a state of grief is bound to exist when we can no longer reach, touch or hold on to somebody or something precious to us, or be in touch with them any more

Tears bring about the fastest relief and, as far as is possible, should never be suppressed.

However, one of the greatest helps in connecting with grief is an attentive, unobtrusive listener – someone to whom one can talk about everything that is causing the suffering. This way, it becomes easier to identify the true causes of what is really hurting. Even if the painful circumstances do not change as a result, the feelings of grief should then be less overwhelming. Talking it through seems to take away some of the "enormity" of the emotion, thereby once more creating "space" for the everyday aspects of life.

See also: Stress

Crystals can support the process of overcoming grief in many ways. They help tears to flow freely, aid in accepting the inevitable, assist in talking to others about the grief, or to just enable the rediscovery of what otherwise makes one happy. In summary, the following crystals can help change our state of health and stimulate us to regain control of our life.

Amethyst helps one to overcome grief that occurs with loss, particularly that of loved ones. It encourages a degree of objectivity, to recognise the meaning or significance of events and to find comfort in this understanding.

Noble Opal makes it easier to come to terms with grief and to let go of a fixation with its cause – so that it becomes easier to refocus on other areas of life. Nobel Opal makes it possible to find beauty and enjoyment in life once again, and to find happiness therein.

Dumortierite makes it possible to talk openly and honestly with other people about grief, deep sadness and fears. In this way, it brings relief, comfort and helps one to re-establish courage, a confidence in the future and other people – and to regain a new, positive attitude towards life.

Jet helps one to overcome the blows of fate and to pass through deep grief, in particular when the latter is also associated with feelings of guilt. Beside that, it helps alleviate the inner, useless se elf-pity – the spurious self-justification, blaming other people, and explaining away things – and to accept the inevitable, reopening oneself to real life.

Rhodonite helps to overcome the kind of grief that seems to imprison us and not let go of emotional pain. It takes away the feeling of martyrdom, ideas of having been treated unfairly, and aids wholehearted forgiveness of others. Thus, Rhodonite lifts the spirits, brings about a new readiness for life and helps one out of seemingly hopeless situations.

Blue Tourmaline eases the ability to cry freely, thus bringing great relief, particularly if one has not been able to cry for years. Beside that, it can help unburden the heart by talking about the grief.

Hold a crystal (Amethyst, Tourmaline), a raw stone (Noble Opal, Jet), or a tumbled stone in the hand; or wear as a necklace or pendant for a longer period of time.

Growing Problems

Disruption or disturbances in the natural growth rate and condition of children can have many causes. These range from a psychological or emotional basis of simply "not wanting to grow up", through physiological or inherited development retardation, to lack of nutrition or consequences of illness. Each has to be considered as more than one factor may be relevant with every single case.

Emotional growth obstacles can occur as the aftermath of a severe disease, or by some trauma through which the child is severely and semi-permanently stressed or feels subject to some undue responsibility. A resulting decision, conscious or subconscious, might then be made "not to grow up," or not to become a grown up – and this can actually lead to a slowing or even cessation, of the body's natural growth process. If this happens, it is important to identify the serious incident or set of circumstances that lie at the root of the problem. If necessary, this can be done with therapeutic assistance, or talking it through under methodical supervision, in order that the child's psychological decision can be retracted.

Crystal therapy is a valuable ancillary treatment in the above.

Larimar helps create a feeling of openness and assists in changing firm decisions.

Rhodonite will help in the healing of the effects of any traumatic experiences.

A lack of the appropriate mental stimuli (e. g. isolation, too little contact with the real world or with nature, too much viewing of the "virtual reality" of computer games or television and not enough social contact) may play a role in growth disturbance.

If this is the case, it is important to encourage as much positive outside contact as possible for the child (e. g., play activity with other kids, helping other children, caring for pets and wild animals and being aware of nature). Beside that, it is important to build emotional security by means of activities that stimulate the developing senses and the emotions – socially, intellectually and physically (fewer computer games!).

There are several crystals that can be applied in order to boost this process.

Agate will encourage contact and a sense of protection.

Chrysoprase and **Golden Topaz** help to enhance feelings of safety, openness, and self-awareness.

Tourmaline in all of its varieties aids the natural process of overall development.

Inhibited and disturbed growth and development arising from a physiological cause s often regarded as irresolvable. However, it can still be extremely stressful, especially when the unfortunate child also feels inferior compared with its surroundings, siblings or friends, or if he or she is not treated appropriately.

However, what is sometimes seen as a predisposition to restrict growth can also represent mere "possibilities", which can be activated or balanced. In this case, there are several crystals that stimulate growth where development appears to be impeded.

Apatite speeds up growth and is also included in homeopathic remedies to "build up" calcium in the bones.

Calcite, is another calcium-based mineral, also furthers body development and is also used like Apatite in homeopathy "calcium carbonicum".

In contrast to slow or restricted growth is the phenomena of growth being too rapid, or occurring in what are often referred to as sudden growth spurts. Associated problems here are usually pains in the bones, joints, back, ribs, etc.,

Aragonite, another calcium-containing mineral, often called "onyx marble", will help with a re-harmonisation of growth

Fluorite may also help in pain relief and with normal growth regulation.

Hormonal disturbances, especially a lack of the growth hormone somatropine in the pituitary gland or of insulin (as in diabetic conditions) and hormones of the thyroid gland can also lead to growth disturbances. Crystal therapy is helpful in such circumstances.

Aquamarine and **Moonstone** are good for treating the pituitary and thyroid glands.

Citrine or **Ocean Jasper** and **Tourmaline** (multicoloured forms) help with insulin-related conditions and help in achieving a proper hormonal balance in the body (see also: Diabetes).

It is worth noting here that traditional Chinese medicine identifies metabolic diseases and liver inefficiently or malfunction (see Liver Health) as a loss of body energy in the form of a weakening of what it alludes to as the element "wood" – which is also analogous to the body's growth and development.

All growth problems arising from these conditions should be examined and clarified by a doctor, or an alternative practitioner (especially one who works with acupuncture or Traditional Chinese Medicine – see above).

In this context, crystal therapy will assist and complement any treatment.

Amazonite will assist in cases of reduced growth caused by metabolic problems in the liver.

Dioptase furthers the body's natural growth or "building up" processes.

Emerald furthers growth and regulates the metabolism.

As mentioned previously, the effects of chronic diseases can also impede growth. Here, there are so many possible causes (e. g. rheumatic diseases, heart defects, kidney break down, inherited diseases, skeletal defects, poor digestion in the intestine, inefficient breakdown of nutrients, etc.) that specific causes need to be clarified and treated professionally.

Provided that such a treatment is carried out on a causal level, one can then also apply crystal therapy.

Emerald is useful for the after effects of chronic inflammatory conditions such as rheumatism.

Epidote and Zoisite are important, overall regeneration crystals.

Finally, it is unfortunate that in modern westernised society, under-nourishment still has to be taken into account as a recurring cause of growth disruption. Whilst it can be considered almost a crime that true malnutrition is still rife throughout much of the world, it remains relatively rare in our part of the world – but only relatively!

Unfortunately – almost as much damage can be caused by the wrong diet or by unbalanced nutrition, than by a serious need of food. Apart from a lack of vitamins and minerals, sugar (as the so called "calcium thief"), is also often implicated in growth problems. Despite a growing awareness of the damage it causes in recent years, sugar is still consumed by children in the form of sweets and soft fizzy drinks at far too high a level.

Osteoporosis and associated developmental disruptions are being identified in young people today. In such cases, of course, only a proper whole-food diet, with a reduced sugar content will help.

Apatite, Aragonite, Calcite and Fluorite are all recommended. In addition, being a cubic crystal, configuration Fluorite

helps one "let go" of detrimental habits.

Wear the crystals as a raw or a tumbled stone, or as a bracelet, necklace or pendant 24 hours a day. As a supplement, or as an alternative, take gem essence (3-9 drops, every hour), or gem water (100–300 ml taken in small sips over the course of the day).

Gout

Gout is caused by problems with the body's uric acid metabolism. When too little uric acid is secreted by the kidneys, uric acid salts are deposited in joints, in mucous bags, in the skin or in the inner organs. These deposits often remain unnoticed, until an infection, injury, hypothermia, excessive alcohol consumption or strongly acid-forming food triggers an attack, of gout pain in a joint. Such painful attacks occur typically at night or early in the morning and can result in a raised temperature, a racing heart, general feelings of being unwell, problems with the joint(s) and severe pain and sensitivity to touch.

As a rule, only one joint is affected by the first attack. In most cases, this will be the basic joint of the big toe, the foot or the knee joint, or the basic joint of the thumb. There may be long periods without problems after the attack. This should not lead one to believe that new uric salt deposits are not being created. Indeed, new attacks may

123

only occur after several months, even occurring in parts of the body previously unaffected. If the gout becomes chronic, knots and abscesses are generated, which gradually become stiff. If there are similar deposits in the kidneys, there can also be inflammation, high blood pressure and – in the worst case – kidney failure.

Gout can only be healed through a consistent diet, which contains few animal proteins and very little alcohol. Furthermore, one should undergo a thorough detoxification (see Detoxification), take plenty of fluid (tea or water!), plenty of rest and enough sleep. In acute cases, the affected joint should be kept still and cooled with compresses. However, regular, but moderate, physical exercise – such as walking – is necessary between the attacks. Of course, all these measures should be carried out under the supervision of a doctor or an alternative practitioner.

Crystals and other remedies can support such measures – and, indeed, without them, the crystals will have no lasting effect! As gout is a disease that is very aggressive, it is also helpful to consider if there are areas of one's life, where anger, impatience or aggression remain unexpressed, being bottled up and so 'gnaw' away at you inside. If this is the case, therapeutic help can also indirectly contribute towards relief.

Amber has a relieving effect on acute rheumatic attacks, pain, and sensitivity to touch, raised temperatures and inflammation. Raw or polished amber helps relieve damage following acute gout and should, therefore be placed on the tender or painful areas as quickly as possible. It furthers a calm mood and a sunny outlook, and thereby helps to relieve the rheumatic attack, physically as well as emotionally.

In order to relieve symptoms that follow an attack, place a raw or a polished crystal on the tender areas as quickly as possible and wear a necklace or a pendant with body contact. Also, take gem essence (4-6 drops every half hour) or gem water (300 ml taken in small sips over the course of the day).

Chrysoprase can be placed on the tender area together with Amber when an attack of rheumatism occurs. Besides that it can be worn even when there is no pain, in the form of a necklace or a pendant with body contact.

You can also take gem essence (3 drops, 3 times daily) or gem water (20-50 ml taken in small sips over the course of the day). In this way it furthers detoxification of the tissues and helps heal the body of the gout. Emotionally, it helps bring grief and suppressed anger into one's awareness and even helps one to 'let go' of these things. It is one of the few crystals that can help with jealousy.

Diamond has a relieving effect on the rheumatic attacks of chronic gout, if it is applied properly. Place small raw diamonds into 100 ml of water or (diluted) white wine for this purpose for at least 24 hours. Drink the water, or the wine, over the course of the following day, while the next batch is made ready (Hildegard von Bingen's recipe). Carry on for several months, until all rheumatic symptoms have vanished.

Diamonds bring order and clarity, without compromise, into one's life; they cleanse and remove what we do not need and thus help us to discover even the most hidden causes of disease – and then eradicate them.

Fluorite helps dissolve uric acid crystals in joints in cases of advanced problems. It makes one conscious of suppressed feelings and helps one emotionally to release old burdens.

Place Fluorite on the tender areas whilst also taking gem essence (5-7 drops, 3 times daily), in order to focus the effect. It can also be worn in form of a necklace or a pendant with body contact for longer periods of time.

Gum Disease

Bleeding and inflammation in the gums is often caused by metabolic upsets, which, in turn, are caused by tissue becoming full of toxins and waste matter. A lack of vitamins (especially vitamin C) or hormonal changes at puberty or the menopause can also be a cause.

Of course, this assumes that there is otherwise good dental hygiene and that any gum problems are not caused by actual injuries or lack of such hygiene (see Detoxification).

Periodontosis is a form of gum disease where actual shrinking of the gums occurs that is caused directly by inflammation. Again this can be the result of a defective supply of nutrients or toxification of the gums. As with all serious oral problems, consult a dentist as soon as possible and before the teeth become loose.

Apart from the above, the most effective treatment for gum disease is to rinse the mouth and the teeth regularly with organic, cold pressed sunflower oil, for some 10 to 20 minutes a day. **Under no circumstances swallow the oil** but spit it out afterwards and rinse thoroughly with tepid water!

The oil absorbs toxic and waste substances. In addition, the rinsing will produce a rapid improvement in a very short time.

Jet, Amber and **Rhodonite** are particularly helpful in dealing with bleeding and inflammation in the gums and with periodontosis.

Place a tumbled stone in the mouth, take gem essence (3-5 drops, 3-5 times daily), or gem water (200–300 ml taken in small sips over the course of the day).

Haemorrhoids

Haemorrhoids are bulging, sometimes knot-like, expansions of the network of blood vessels above the rectal muscle. They are caused by weak connective tissue, which has, in turn, been caused by chronic constipation and pushing hard during a bowel movement, a lifestyle that includes sitting down a lot, or in connection with pregnancy. Haemorrhoids first manifest themselves as an itching, stabbing pain or bright-red blood in the stools. Later, these may also be cracks in the skin, as a result of permanent inflammatory states, abscesses and the occurrence of extremely painful thromboses in the affected veins. In such cases, seek immediate help from a doctor.

To avoid letting matters get that far, haemorrhoids should be encouraged to shrink as soon as possible. For this purpose, exercise such as regular walks, a diet rich in fibre and – if necessary – treatment of the intestines to prevent constipation are all recommended.

Agate in various forms but with a vein signature is particularly recommended for use in connection with haemorrhoids. These can be agates with circular, concentric rings (so-called Eye-Agates) that resemble cross sections of veins or the Mexican Crazy Lace Agates with red markings, which, so to speak, visually display the entire network of veins in the rectal area

perfectly. Agates can be affixed above the rectum or worn in one's underwear for an external application. For an internal application, one can drink water, in which the crystals have been placed for one or two days.

Amethyst may help relieve the itchiness and can be worn in one's underwear or be applied externally in the form of Hildegard von Bingen's Amethyst Water (see page 25)

Heliotrope is advised when there is inflammation. It is best to apply it both externally and internally. Externally: place a tumbled stone in one's underwear or apply gem water.

Internally: Take gem essence (3-7 drops, 3-5 times daily) or gem water (200–300 ml taken in small sips over the course of the day.

Rhodonite is applied in the same way as Heliotrope where minor bleeding occurs. It furthers both the healing of the wound and shrinkage of the haemorrhoids.

Hay Fever

Hay fever is an allergic reaction to certain types of flower, grass and tree pollen. It occurs at the flowering time of the specific plants to which the sufferer is allergic and is result of irritation of the mucous membranes of the upper respiratory tract (sinuses). Typical symptoms are swelling and inflammation of the nasal mucous membranes, attacks of violent sneezing, a runny nose, painful sinuses – along with an itching, burning and watering of the eyes. Severe cases may even produce a high temperature and irritation of the mucous membranes of the mouth, throat, or even of the bronchia – as well as asthma attacks.

Most cases of hay fever can be treated successfully with healing crystals – although, as with all other types of allergies, a regime of thorough detoxification is also recommended as a supportive measure.

Diet is also an important factor here and it is advisable to have a doctor, specialist or alternative practitioner test for possible food allergies. In addition, rest and the right amount of sleep will encourage overall regeneration.

Finally, in many cases, it is always worth considering the emotional side of things as a contributary cause.

In addition to therapy using the crystals described below, black caraway seed oil has also proved to be a great help in treating cases of hay fever. Take a teaspoon of the oil three times daily, or according to requirements.

See also: Allergies; Asthma

Aquamarine is the first crystal of choice for treating hay fever as it is most commonly used for allergies that show serious reactions in the respiratory system. For sufferers of hay fever, Aquamarine should be applied before the beginning of and during the entire pollen season. Emotionally, Aquamarine encourages a sense of lightness and a relaxed attitude, especially when there is a feeling of having to fend off too many annoying and irksome external influences.

Landscape Jasper is also a great help in treating hay fever. It cleanses the tissues of toxins and waste metabolic products, and so should be used for at least a month before the onset of pollen distribution. Landscape Jasper has a calming effect in cases of nervousness and excitement and helps to reduce stress.

Ocean Jasper with a green and white markings, or with clearly visible inclusions of pure Chalcedony (the transparent parts), is also helpful in cleansing the body and regulating the body's immune system. It reduces any tendency to allergies and so helps with hay fever, if employed early enough. It also encourages a new, positive attitude towards springtime and to nature and all other areas of life which otherwise might be associated with the worry – even a dread – of another annual bout of hay fever.

These crystals should be initially worn as a bracelet, necklace, or pendant, as a drilled and polished stone or as a piece of jewellery. When the pollen season begins, also take them internally as gem essences (5-7 drops, 5 times daily) or gem water (200–300ml taken in sips during the course of the day).

Headaches

Headaches are in general a sign of stress, tension, overtiredness, or various kinds of illnesses. (After all, a big problem is often referred to as a "major headache") They can originate from the muscles, blood vessels, nerves or the brain's membranes. If there is no obvious external cause (such as a blow to the head, etc.) the causes are usually inflammation, blood pressure or other changes in the composition of the body's fluids.

Any one of these can arise from one of the following, or from any combination:

- Tension, particularly because of bad posture (tension of the back and the back of the neck when driving) or eyestrain (reading in bad light, working for long periods in front of a computer monitor)
- Feverish illnesses (colds; flu; sinusitis; conjunctivitis; cerebrospinal meningitis or encephalitis, etc.)
- Hormonal changes (e.g. before menstruation)
- Changes in the blood pressure (blood circulation disturbances in the brain, high blood pressure, falling blood pressure in connection with migraine).
- Metabolic and digestive disturbances (hunger, feelings of "an empty stomach", or low blood sugar)
- Hypersensitivity in connection with changing weather (e.g. in connection with hot autumnal winds, poor air quality with lowered oxygen content, etc.)
- Problems with the cervical spinal column
- Nervous and emotional causes (major problems, things on one's mind)
- Severe general diseases (e.g. kidney problems)

In all practicality, such a wide range of causes means that a doctor should examine any one with a headache that lasts for more than 24 hours.

One part of any headache cure is to remove earrings, hair slides hair bands and necklaces. Then, stroke the forehead gently with the fingers or fingernails, over the head and towards the back of the neck. This should be complemented by other activities and treatments: taking physical exercise in fresh air; applying cold compresses to the forehead and/or the back of the neck; having a foot massage; taking alternate hot and cold showers or baths.

The combination of calming and stimulating essential oils in an aroma lamp (e.g. lavender-lemon grass) will also help.

Se also: Migraine.

Any application of crystal treatment must depend on the diagnosed cause. A headache that occurs only once, and the cause of which is well known (tension headache, migraine, seasonal headache, etc.) will have its specific remedial treatment. However, the following have all proved be helpful.

128

Amethyst is very beneficial for tension headaches having their origin in eyestrain and from tension in the back of the neck or the spine (see above listing).

Take a druse the size of a saucer and, as with brush, without touching the body, stroke from the forehead over the top of the head to the back of the neck (see Fig. 9). If you make 4-5 parallel strokes from the front hairline to the ear, on both sides repeat this 3-4 times, the headache will, in most cases, disappear.

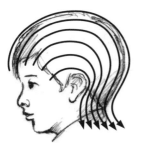

Fig. 9: Treatment with an Amethyst for tension headaches.

Rock Crystal in the form of small "Herkimer Diamonds" will relieve headaches without any obvious causes – and all types of headaches that occur as a consequence of blood pressure changes, hypersensitivity to changes in the weather, or of general disease.

Make an isosceles (three-equal sided) triangle of three small Herkimer Diamonds pointing upwards and outwards on the forehead. As a rule, the headache will then decrease in intensity, even within a couple

of minutes. If necessary, vary the size of the triangle.

Amber helps alleviate headaches that are caused by hormonal changes (e. g. premenstrual tension and so forth), by metabolic and digestive problems, or by nervous or emotional causes. Wear a necklace (for best results) or a pendant with direct body contact. Alternatively, take gem essence (7-10 drops when required) or gem water, if essence is unavailable.

Emerald helps with headaches associated with inflammation and feverish illnesses. In such cases, place or affix a crystal or a polished gem on the forehead; or wear a necklace (as the best choice) with direct body contact – or a pendant for a longer period.

As an alternative, take gem essence (3-9 drops, 3 times daily) or gem water (200–300 ml taken in small sips over the course of the day).

Magnesite and Rhodonite are helpful with all headaches. In a glass of water, mix the gem essence from of the crystals with Bach flower rescue remedy. Drink this over the course of the day along with lots of other (non-alcoholic) fluids.

Smoky Quartz, like Amethyst, relieves tension headaches. Most effective is to wear it as a necklace, preferably of amber (why amber?) beads. It has a permanent relieving effect on the specific causal tension and can, therefore, also be worn along with Amethyst after treatment.

Head Colds

A head cold is an acute or chronic inflammation of the nasal mucous membranes and sinuses, which is accompanied by increased secretions from the nose, sneezing, and a runny or stuffy nose. It is mainly provoked by viral infections. Infection and cold temperatures "catching a chill", are the external factors that cause a head cold. Internal factors are the accumulation of lymph and tissues laden with toxins and waste, especially because of cow's milk [dairy] products, which make the spread of viruses possible. Milk cows are nowadays kept in a way that is, targeted towards mass production of milk this means it is difficult for our bodies to digest their milk, this in turn leads to the above-mentioned pollution of the tissues. The factors that lead to problems with dairy produce are, among others, lack of enzymes and residues of medicines and other harmful substances. This pollution of the body impedes the activity of the immune system and, in this way, opens the floodgates to disease and germs.

See also Colds; Flu; Sinusitis

The same precautions generally applied against colds should be taken to prevent a head cold – regular physical exercise in fresh air (in all kinds of weather), sleeping at night with an open window, ending any bath with a cold shower, foregoing dairy products, colonic therapy and regular detoxification (see Detoxification). In addition, rinsing the mouth and teeth with organic cold-pressed sunflower oil for 10 to 20 minutes every day is effective. **Under no circumstances swallow the oil**; but move it around the teeth and spit it out afterwards, then rinse thoroughly with tepid water!

Crystals that have a generally healing effect on colds can also be applied against head colds. Two of them, in particular, have proved to have an outstanding effect.

Heliotrope is most effective against acute head colds, especially when additional bacterial infections have caused the formation of heavy mucus.

Place a flat tumbled stone or section/slice at the right and left sides of the nose and below the nose, or place in the mouth. It also helps to take gem essence (5-7 drops, 3 times daily, or when required), or gem water (200–300 ml taken in small sips over the course of the day).

Emerald is helpful with chronic head colds, those that drag on, and when the nose fails to start running in order to clear the infection. It hinders inflammation of the mucous membranes in the nose and halts its progress to the sinuses and relieves already manifesting sinusitis (see Sinusitis).

Emotionally, Emerald brings greater clarity of thought and orientation in any confusing life situations that cause loss of perspective, a condition that often manifests itself physically through a stuffy nose.

Place one Emerald on the bridge of the nose, another under the nose and/or a third one in the mouth. Also, take gem essence (5-9 drops, 3 times daily or when required) or gem water (200–300 ml taken in sips over the course of the day).

Hearing Loss

Sudden loss of, or severely diminished hearing, tends only to occur in one ear, although it can lead to sudden deafness. Its direct cause is almost certainly disturbances in blood circulation of the inner ear, which, in themselves, may have various causes. These include deposits in blood vessels, cramp in blood vessels, and any problems with the neck or spinal column. (See also: Hearing Problems.)

On the other hand, many cases of a sudden loss of hearing cannot be explained adequately. However, there are certain measures that can be adopted immediately. Drink lots of clear fluids and, if necessary make and drink herbal infusions in order to alleviate the condition as quickly as possible, so that the acute loss of hearing does not become permanent hardness of hearing, or deafness. Above all, though, a doctor should treat any acute loss of the hearing **immediately**.

Hardness of hearing – a gradual deterioration of hearing – can occur as a result of infections in the middle ear, viral infections and disease of the hearing nerves such as shingles, or degenerative processes (so-called age-dependent hardness of hearing, which is probably caused by chronically impaired circulation). Deposits in the blood vessels may also be responsible. (See also: Middle Ear Infections.)

All types of ear problems have in common the important part played by the circulation. Any upsets with blood flow are, in turn, connected with infections, deposition of toxins in the tissues and deposits in the blood vessels. Detoxification cures are, therefore, very important as preventive measures (see Detoxification).

For immediate treatment, however, crystal therapy that aids the circulation and prevents inflammation is a good stand by. The following can be applied on the way to the doctor or as a supplement to the resulting treatment. – Although one should refrain from self-treating without adequate knowledge.

Sardonyx is the most important crystal for all kinds of ear problems. It helps in many cases, from increasingly impaired hearing, through to hardness of hearing. If it is applied immediately, it may also help, quickly and efficiently, in cases of a sudden loss of hearing. Its wide-ranging effect is probably due to the fact that it stimulates both blood and lymph flow.

In acute cases, place or hold a tumbled stone or a section/slice on the affected ear. In addition, take gem essence as a supplement (to begin with, 15 drops, later on 5-7 drops, 3-5 times daily); or drink gem water (up to 1 litre over the course over the day).

Garnet Pyrope is best as second choice in connection with ear problems. It helps with both blood circulation and repair of an infected inner ear. In cases of a sudden loss of hearing, hold or place a tumbled stone or a crystal, directly on the affected ear – or wear it as a necklace or pendant

It is also helpful to take gem essence (3-7 drops, 3 times daily) or gem water (200–300 ml taken in small sips over the course of the day).

Heliotrope helps above all with noises in the ear (tinnitus) and impairment of the hearing, in particular when infections and inflammation have preceded the problem, or are still present.

Apply the so-called ear-olive, which is carefully introduced into the outer ear. These ear-olives have a little eye in one end, to which a small string is attached, which can be used to draw it out of the ear again.

Rhodonite, Ocean Jasper, Turquoise and **Black Tourmaline** also sometimes have a positive effect on noises in the ear (tinnitus) and gradual impairment of hearing right through to definite hardness of hearing. This may be caused by an improvement in the blood circulation (Rhodonite), stimulation of the lymph flow and detoxification (Ocean Jasper), relief from acidification and poisoning (Turquoise), or by an improved energy sup-

ply to the ear (Tourmaline).

Place a tumbled stone or a slice/section of Rhodonite, Ocean Jasper, Turquoise or Black Tourmaline on the ear or wear as a necklace or a pendant. Alternatively, take gem essence (3-9 drops, 3 times daily) or gem water (200–300 ml taken in small sips over the course of the day).

Hearing Problems

Apart from inflammation (see Middle Ear Infections) noises in the ears, sudden loss of the hearing and acquired hardness of hearing are amongst the most frequent ear and hearing problems.

Noises in the ear – generally called tinnitus – are usually experienced as a continual ringing, humming, roaring or buzzing in the ear – especially at night or when the surroundings are quiet. It is a highly irritating problem and causes great discomfort on the sufferer.

Tinnitus was previously considered mostly to be the result of ear diseases. Nowadays, it appears increasingly that it has no single identifiable cause – although blood circulation problems or damage to the hearing nerves can definitely contribute to the condition, which has also been observed in connection with acidaemia and poisoning. Nevertheless, both traditional medical and alternative practices still remain more or less perplexed

Of course, like so many other ailments, noises in the ears can have an emotional origin. It could be even, literally, that things, which sound annoying – situations that one might describe in exasperation as "a constant yakking in the ear" – or that one does not want to hear can be a cause. However, such connections are still highly speculative.

Some crystal have proved helpful in dealing with tinnitus – but as there are still mysteries surrounding the origins of these noises, it is not possible to state clearly which specific crystal will be the most effective. It can often be a simple case of trial and error, with the following being recommended. (See also Hearing Loss.)

Garnet Pyrope helps with both blood circulation and repair of an infection of the inner ear.

In cases of a sudden loss of the hearing, hold or place a tumbled stone, or a crystal, directly on the affected ear – or wear it as a necklace or pendant in cases of noises in the ear.

It is also helpful to take gem essence (3-7 drops, 3 times daily) or gem water (200–300 ml taken in small sips over the course of the day).

Heliotrope helps with noises in the ear, especially when infections and inflammation have preceded the problem, or are still present.

Heliotrope can be applied in the form of so-called "ear-olive", which is carefully introduced into the outer ear. These are small smooth pieces of the crystal, which a small eyehole pierced at one end, to which a small thread is attached. An ear-olive is introduced with great care and only shallowly into the outer ear, using the attached thread to draw it out of the ear again after treatment.

Rhodonite, Ocean Jasper, Turquoise and **Black Tourmaline** can also have a positive effect on tinnitus that may be caused by circulation problems. Rhodonite can cause an improvement in the blood circulation and stimulate lymph flow Ocean Jasper will also assist in a similar way with detoxification, whilst Turquoise can bring relief from acidification and poisoning and Tourmaline improves the overall energy supply to the ear.

Place a tumbled stone or a slice/section of Rhodonite, Ocean Jasper, Turquoise or Black Tourmaline on the ear or wear as a necklace or pendant. Alternatively, take gem essence (3-9 drops, 3 times daily) or gem water (200–300 ml taken in small sips over the course of the day).

Heartburn

Heartburn occurs, when acidic stomach contents flow back up into the oesophagus. This leads to a burning or rasping sensation, which goes all the way up to the throat. It is caused by acidification and

133

over-extension of the stomach, especially after eating fatty, very sweet, or acidic foods. Sometimes, heartburn occurs as a consequence of a too low a stomach acid content, which then causes a fermentation of the stomach contents. Persistent heartburn can lead to inflammation in the mucous membranes of the throat.

A suitable diet is clearly the best remedy for heartburn on causal level. Such a diet should include limited consumption of meat, meat-based products, eggs, cheese and milk and avoiding coffee, tobacco, sweets and alcohol.

Kaolin, a type of clay rich in minerals that relieve stomach problems, and the juice of half a lemon in a glass of water can relieve acute heartburn.

Diaspor, Magnesite and **Turquoise** have been shown to have good results in relieving heartburn, with Diaspor being the most effective of the three.

Place a crystal (Diaspor) or a tumbled stone (Magnesite or Turquoise) on the stomach; or wear as a bracelet, necklace or a pendant. Alternatively, take as gem essence (3-7 drops) or gem water (50–100 ml taken in small sips over the course of the day).

Heart Problems

Heart problems are usually experienced by the onset of palpitations, painful twinges, and general feelings of unease or oppression, pains, burning sensations, fear and breathlessness. All can be caused by inflammations, arteriosclerosis, a weak heart or other cardiac diseases that must be treated immediately in order to avoid permanent damage to the heart or an acute threat to life.

The first step must **always** be to seek a doctor or a reliable and qualified alternative practitioner. In cases of even more serious problems, call the emergency medical services IMMEDIATELY. Only later, after the professional examination, should any measures be taken that involve the beneficial effect of healing crystals.

Crystals should only be applied **in addition** to medication and applications prescribed by a doctor. Such crystal use is complementary and supportive in and contributing to a normalisation of heart function.

The heart provides the basic rhythm of the human organism and through the circulation; it ensures the supply of blood to all cells, tissues and organs. However, it is not the only organ that is involved with the pumping of blood around the body. Without the active involvement of the muscular arteries, it would not be able by itself to push the total and required volume of blood through the whole system of veins and arteries. Without the integrated mechanism of the whole human body, it would be overwhelmed in the long run. This is where crystals with a beneficial effect on the heart also help the circulation and general efficiency of blood vessels.

Traditional Chinese medicine expresses this connection between the heart and the circulation very clearly, with its symbolism of the ancient imperial state:

The heart is the Emperor who sets the tone;
the circulation is his highest civil servant,
who does the work
— and woe betide the Emperor whose
civil servants are idle!

Unfortunately, modern western medicine often has the effect of over-stimulating the heart when the circulation is seemingly "idle", but is perfectly normal and routine. This is a mistake. Over the short or long term, it can in itself cause heart problems. On the other hand, rather than using modern treatments "off the shelf", as it were, if one looks for the causes for the reduced blood circulation, there are usually contributing circumstances. These can include deposits of toxins and waste products in the blood vessels and their walls; also, a narrowing, widening or inflamed state that have their roots in tissues that have become polluted with toxins and waste products. Detoxification is therefore extremely important, in order to prevent heart problems (see Detoxification).

Specifically, in cases of coronary attacks, the connection between deposits of toxins and arteriosclerosis is clearly evident. Preventive precautions are therefore more or less the same as those applied in cases of arteriosclerosis. In other words, adopt a strict diet, without animal proteins but rich in vitamins (particularly vitamins C and E). At the same time, it is vital to take sufficient physical exercise – and ensure you have plenty of rest, sleep and time for regeneration.

It is now accepted generally that tension, stress, emotional problems and – above all, an overall lack of *joie-de-vivre* – are harmful to the heart. Therefore, it is also extremely important to maintain a positive attitude and beneficial lifestyle. It is always far better to get on with things, whether hobbies, personal ambitions, family life and having friends, rather than giving up on too many facets of life and forever postponing them until later. In summary, "later" should always begin now!

Crystals can support the heart in three ways. They can act preventively by supporting the detoxification process and thereby the circulation; they can relieve acute problems; and they can have a positive emotional input. All of the following are effective at these three levels.

Aventurine enhances the detoxification process within the body tissue, especially in preventing the formation of deposits in the coronary arteries that supply blood to the heart muscle. Emotionally, Aventurine also encourages relaxation, regeneration and recuperation.

Pink Chalcedony relieves symptoms of a "racing heart", an accelerated heart rate, and strengthens the heart itself. It relieves inflammation in an around the heart, particularly in the case of a persistent cold or bout of flu. It supports the processes of cleansing and detoxification and thus increases the flow of blood. In this way, it clearly eases the work of the heart. Emotionally, Pink Chalcedony encourages kindness, cordiality, inner peace, understanding and helpfulness. It also helps in cases of heart neuroses and heart problems without any apparent organic cause but that arise because of any fears about the heart.

Heliotrope relieves inflammation and prevents the further narrowing and formation of deposits in blood vessels. It can also be applied as a preventative for coronaries and in the case of any apparent heart attack (i. e. sudden and severe heart pains), and as an emergency crystal (whilst waiting for a doctor in an emergency). In such circumstances, one should hold a polished Heliotrope section or a flat, tumbled stone over the heart until the crystal fells warm to the touch, i.e. as per body heat. Then exchange it for a new, cool crystal. Heliotrope helps to deal with the unforeseen situation and to maintain necessary control and alleviate feelings of fear or panic.

Rose Quartz helps with disturbances of the heart rhythm. An irregular heartbeat is often connected with an irregular rhythm of life. Consequently, Rose Quartz reintroduces recognition of such fundamental requirements as rest, sleep, recreation, nutrition, closeness, protection and a sense of security. In this way one's lifestyle changes can often be automatically beneficial to the heart.

Rutile Quartz helps any fears that one may have about the heart. It has a relieving effect on feelings of constriction and oppression and helps one find a new sense of *joie-de-vivre*. On the inner by reinforcing important wishes, goals and visions. Rutile Quartz is an anti-depressive and so has a relieving effect in cases of deep grief.

Sard strengthens the heart. It improves the circulation and blood supply, helps with a weak heart and any irregularities of heart rhythm. Sard also stabilises the heart's function in any cases of strain and long-lasting stress It also helps when "we take something too much to heart", are too "soft-hearted" or even suffer from a "broken heart".

Watermelon Tourmaline helps with all kind of heart problems. It enhances patience, loving and tender emotions, relieves fears and prevents any detrimental over-excitement. Place a polished section on the heart (attaching with adhesive plaster) for use as a prophylaxis. In acute cases, wear it in the form of a necklace or a pendant.

Overall, for all of the above, place a tumbled stone or polished section in the general area of the heart. In addition, you can wear a necklace or a pendant with direct body contact over the heart, and/or take gem essence (5-7 drops, 3 times daily) or gem water (200–300 ml taken in small sips over the course of the day).

Herpes

Infection by the herpes virus may lead to a whole range of diseases such as shingles, conjunctivitis, infections of the genitals, etc. This book cannot really cover these illnesses, as they should **always and only** be treated professionally. Consequently, this entry is confined solely with the small lip blisters that are caused by the Herpes simplex virus.

There can often be a relatively long period between transmission of the infection and a visible outbreak. The outbreak can be triggered by such diverse causes as the ultra-violet radiation of strong sun light, colds, seemingly small injuries (cracked lips caused by dry air, etc.), over-consumption of alcohol, exhaustion or general stress. The symptoms are an initial feeling of tightness on the lips, together with slight itching. This develops gradually and becomes a burning sensation, before the blister itself appears. Initially, such blisters are reddish and painful to the touch. After some time, the blister cracks, leaking a yellowish serum. Finally the blister starts drying out and eventually heals.

Unfortunately, anyone who has already experienced herpes has a high probability of getting it again. Alas, in most cases, it cannot be totally eradicated, as the virus remains dormant within the system until one of the triggers mentioned above causes the formation of a new lip blister. These are not the signs of a severe illness, but are extremely unpleasant nonetheless. As they attack the lips in particular, and are therefore highly visible, they are also extremely unattractive. For this reason alone, it is a good idea to take immediate action at the first feeling of discomfort around the lips.

The best remedy for herpes is an extract of lemon balm leaves (*Melissa officinalis*), which is applied to the affected spot immediately upon the first feeling of any tightness or soreness. Essential oils of myrrh and tea tree oil have the same healing effect.

Chrysoprase is the crystal with the best overall effect. Place it in your mouth, like a sweet (using a tumbled stone) while, at the same time, regularly moistening the affected spot with the crystal; the faster you start such treatment, the better.

Lapis lazuli can be used in addition, as a supplement or if you do not have access to Chrysoprase It can be placed directly on the affected area, as either a raw or polished stone. First and foremost, it will relieve the burning sensation.

Rhodonite can be applied if the blisters are open. It supports the healing process but also prevents the formation of the small reddish scars.

You can also take gem essence prepared with the crystals mentioned (2-3 drops per hour). If you apply alcoholic preparations, be careful they not to come into direct contact with the blisters.

Gem water, on the other hand, can both be applied externally and internally (200–300 ml daily, taken in small sips over the course of the day); with Chrysoprase, however, take only 20–50 ml).

Hoarseness

Hoarseness is a coarsening or partial loss of the voice which is caused either by an infection of the upper respiratory tract (see Colds) or an overuse of one's voice. Emotional causes such as excitement, stage fright, last-minute nerves, difficulties in uncomfortable situations, or suppressed anger, can also lead to hoarseness. (See also: Throat Problems)

Amazonite is helpful with hoarseness due to voice strain of any form, when one has "a lump in one's throat", or when one cannot express grief, distress, unhappiness or "bare one's soul".

Aquamarine is particularly effective, when hoarseness occurs in connection with allergic reactions, excitement, nerves or in connection with periods of stress. It helps to assert oneself verbally and thus to be heard.

Blue Chalcedony can be used in cases of hoarseness caused by respiratory infec-

tions or by great stress causing voice strain. It also helps in expressing oneself, and so once had the nickname "stone of the speakers" for several centuries.

Lapis lazuli is a good choice when hoarseness occurs as a result of suppressed anger or difficulties in speaking about unpleasant matters. Furthermore, it helps when the voice has become hoarse – or even loss of voice – because it has been strained.

Sodalite helps with long-term hoarseness when something unspoken gets "stuck in the throat". It also encourages the immediate and conscious statements at the appropriate time

For all the above, place or affix a polished crystal or section, or a crystal on the throat, or wear a necklace, or a pendant with body contact close to the throat. Also try gem essence (3-7 drops, 3 times daily) or gem water (200–300 ml, taken in small sips over the course of the day.)

Homesickness

Homesickness is a strong yearning for ones home, an uncomfortable and often oppressive feeling which occurs together with a strong desire to see once more some familiar surroundings and faces, connected with whatever we feel to be "home" or "our native soil". When we suffer homesickness, we might even experience feelings akin to

138

grief – a sign that we have lost what we are familiar with – a sense of heartbreak, loss of appetite, lack of interest in present surroundings, feelings of loneliness – and many other accompanying phenomena. Indeed, because homesickness is mainly emotional and psychological in character, extreme cases can even assume a psychosomatic character and can lead to real illnesses.

Homesickness has a double effect upon us. On the one hand, we miss our familiar surroundings (depending on the reason, duration and the conditions of the separation), while, at the same time, we find it difficult for to adapt to current, unfamiliar surroundings. Consequently, it can sometimes be helpful to have around you something familiar, something that "carries information" about one's home; but that can also enable us to try and "tune in" to new surroundings. It follows therefore that crystals can fit the bill for both these requirements.

Minerals that occur naturally in the soil of where we consider to be home, and with which we can feel deeply connected to in some way or another, can constitute a kind of "home spirit" for us. Using crystals or unpolished stones of these minerals, we can create a form of energy field by arranging them around our bed, placing them in the corners of a living space or bedroom, or just carrying them around with us. By so doing, we can create a form of spiritual atmo-

sphere akin to being at home, even if it purely in one's mind. Thereby, we carry our home in our heart and so can lessen the feeling of loss and alienation that constitute homesickness. Some very beneficial effects have been obtained by people, homesick and far away from home, say, it in a foreign country, and who regularly used the following crystals.

Chrysoprase is very effective for homesickness. Basically, it has the effect of helping us develop feelings of inner peace and security, so that we can feel the sentiments of actually becoming part of ones "native soil", no matter where we are. It is a particularly good in helping children, who have bee separated from their parents, e. g. at a holiday camp, a school retreat, or the like. A pendant that can be worn around the neck, and also be held in the hand, can be a great help in such cases, when one is really downhearted.

Amber has a similar effect, especially if it is a piece that one has already worn, or been carried or worn by someone we know well, for a long time. As amber is excellent for storing information, it helps capture "home vibrations", this, as well as its typically carefree-cheerful properties make it a perfect personal anti-homesickness crystal.

Apart from these, other crystals too can provide inner peace and be helpful for alleviating homesickness.

Agate can provide inner peace, security and protection.

Amethyst can be worn or carried to overcome the worries associated with homesickness.

Dumortierite will help with any form of worry or stress as a result of its well-known "take-it-easy" properties.

Lavender Jade and Serpentine will contribute to creating inner peace.

Overall, of the above, the best results so far have been obtained with the Chrysoprase and Amber as "homeland" crystals.

For the second aspect of homesickness, using crystals to help adapt to new surroundings, cordiality and contact between people is far the best answer. It is self evident that such interaction is essential if one wants to achieve better contact with current circumstances and surroundings and so overcome the feeling of being a stranger. However, there can often be situations where cultural differences, local customs, physical surroundings, language, climate, life style and overall ethos can seem very unfamiliar to us if away from home or when abroad. For many people, however willing, this is when it is helpful to engage consciously with the unfamiliar and to absorb what one might term its "earth information". Drink local water if known to be safe; eat local food prepared in traditional ways; try tasting the local beverages and drinks; and familiarise oneself as much as possible with the landscape and natural history of the place. In this way, one can become familiar with the new surroundings on many differ-

ent levels – and the feeling of being a stranger will relatively easy to change to one of becoming acquainted with everyday life, customs, and so forth. Then, a far better time can be experienced and enjoyed very soon after being immersed in our new surroundings.

Quite simply it can even be a help to pick up a stone from any new surroundings – preferably in a beautiful or pleasant spot where you feel comfortable and so have positive associations with – and then carry it about on a daily basis. Believe it or not, this can also help with accessing the way of thinking of the region or country and its people. (But take care that your chosen 'stone' does not happen to be a gemstone from a local mine, or an archaeological find – in some countries this could cause you quite a few problems!)

Petrified Wood is one form of crystal that helps one 'take root' rapidly in new surroundings. These minerals occur as a small piece of fossilised tree, of which there are many kinds. It is best to choose a raw or a tumbled stone or a cut and polished section that feels comfortable and helpful to you. Bracelets, necklaces or pendants can also be worn and so enable you to enter into a 'personal relationship' with them and the land.

Noble Opal (curiosity), Fire Opal (enthusiasm), Mookaite (variety/new experiences) Pink Chalcedony (cordial encounters) along with any other form of

Opal are some other crystals that can help in opening the mind and spirit to new surroundings and assist in a positive approach to new surroundings.

In practical terms, it is best to wear them as a bracelet, a necklace or a pendant with direct body contact.

Housemaid's Knee

see Knee Problems

Hyperactivity

The increasingly cited "Attention Deficit Hyperactivity Disorder" (ADHD) and hyperkinetic syndrome are different terms for a phenomenon in children and young adults that is receiving considerable attention these days but that is difficult to understand. For reasons that are explained below and that I as the author hope will soon be obvious, it is easer initially to use just the term "hyperactivity".

Hyperactivity has been increasingly identified over the years and is now understood to be a complex condition that can include such symptoms as unrest of the body's motor mechanisms, concentration disorders and impulsive actions. Yet, that definition itself already shows how difficult it can be in practice to make a distinction between a pathological condition and the normal behaviour of a lively child. It seems as if more and more teachers at schools and kindergartens confront parents with this unqualified diagnosis of "hyperactivity", simply because they cannot cope with the child concerned. But even the medical profession itself and other specialists stress that that one should not apply the term "pathological hyperactive" carelessly or irresponsibly.

It is not so surprising therefore that critics of such 'rushed' assessments therefore quite rightly refers to the fact that at least 90% of the children, who are characterised as "pathologically hyperactive", are actually totally "normal" children by today's standards. Therefore, it is against that background and on that basis that I will first concentrate on "general hyperactivity" – even if, in the end, some cases may be truly pathological.

The general observation is that nowadays many children in westernised, modern society are more restless, lack concentration and have more problems in social areas. There are many possible reasons for this, and I must apologise, in advance, if I appear to dwell at some length on social politics, but the problems of our children are, to a greater extent, of a societal nature, rather than individual ones.

In particular, I would like to draw attention to five essential points, categorised below, which I believe, sincerely, are the main factors that contribute to such "general hyperactivity".

1. Rapid over-stimulation

The modern media to which our children are now exposed (and even overwhelmed), but with which they so like to interact, expose all of us to optical and acoustic stimulation of extraordinarily high intensity and at very high speed. This goes for computer games, music videos, children's films and other associated phenomena. If you compare the modern, electronic-based media with that of an earlier age, there is clearly a tremendous difference. Modern children become accustomed to this speed of presenting information and stimuli – and they adapt to it. In other words, they become restless, nervous, without much concentration and easily distracted. In fact, I venture to say that they represent to the market in general the "ideal future human being", easily manipulated by advertisements and (usually) consumer-based trivial information – and that is exactly what is intended!

2. Reduced experience, inconsistency and disparity

Within the general media especially, there is now a huge reduction in direct life experience. This is accompanied by a disparity between real life and what the media presents. A child at play in the open air can enjoy and use the full range of its senses, motor skills and creativity. This form of activity, through direct involvement and experience, leads to sensory satisfaction –

and, finally, to healthy tiredness. In contrast, children who are over-exposed to television viewing or occupied for most of their time with computer games of one form or another become considerably limited and restricted when it comes to using their motor skills and direct experience via all the senses. To this, then add the minimal mental effort involved in watching the screen, that is paralleled physically only through the movements of the fingers. Yet, simultaneously, on a sensory level, there is a bombardment of contrasting stimulation – but limited solely to visual and acoustic impressions – which has to be digested.

Unsurprisingly, the basic consequences are basically a "stressed out" child, lacking real-life experiences, and who is thus only able release its inner tensions and burdens through uncontrolled (and sometimes totally hysterical) behaviour. Which is why the unfortunate kid is then put back in front of the "goggle-box" again, because the ever-manic screen keeps child "so nice and quiet". Irony upon irony, one might say, if it were not far more important than a mere social observation.

3. Out-of-step development

In addition to all of the above, today's children develop physically and intellectually faster than they do emotionally and socially. Whilst the factors I have listed as 1 and 2 above certainly contribute to this phenomenon, intellectual development is also stimulated by the way the modern media present themselves.

Neither emotional development (which presupposes the full development of the senses and creative play), nor social development (which can only be nurtured through the immediate, physical contact, that takes place between people), are stimulated by the mass media.

Coupled with the above, I think there are contributory factors of an environmental and dietary nature. There have certainly been serious scientific suggestions that the ever-rising residues of drugs and hormones in the water supply might be linked to earlier sexual maturity! Further, the general modern diet is packed with huge amounts of sugar, animal protein, phosphates, acids, etc. As a result, it contains more and more of what I might most easily term as being "accelerating-components", whilst "substance-providing" ones, such as vitamins, minerals, enzymes and basic compounds are more or less lacking. Such an unbalanced mix and disharmony of the vital elements of life create a continuous potential for frustration and inner conflict for the entire period of our development, from childhood, through youth and even on into to adult life.

4. Goal-orientated upbringing

In my view, the climax of all of these imbalances and disharmony, however, is found in the modern upbringing of children in west-

ern society. Increasingly, through official policies and social pressures, intellectual development is pushed at earlier and earlier stages in a child's education with a constant desire for ever-higher levels of achievement. The goal seems not so much to be for the personal and overall enhancement of individuals and society, but the creation of a labour force with a high level of achievement that can be exploited for as long as possible. More and more we are "licked into shape" to fit the requirements at every level of our modern and ever more inhuman industry. Accordingly, the education is adapted to requirements that range from the need for an elite to the basic and acquiescently mundane.

I suggest that it is exactly for this purpose, that intellectual disparity is needed and, as a result, emotional development and social maturity in general will take a downward curve. In many cases, an early alienation from the parents through full-time child-care in large groups further contributes to this downward curve. This is in no way meant to blame parents who, because of economic need, have little other choice. The blame should be directed towards the market-based policies of society which are, thereby, so often deepening the gap between rich and poor. It may seem an irony in the twenty-first century to cite such a phenomena. Yet it is a fact that that many families only can survive with two full-time wage earners. The result of these developments and tendencies is that we see more and more hyperactive children, more and more depressed and suicidal teenagers, and more and more unhappy adults. Surely, our biggest sin of omission is that we do not subordinate all our modern achievements to the larger goal of providing a happy life? Our children are bound to become "hyperactive", if they are to cope with a world filled with the waste and mountains of debt, which they will undoubtedly inherit.

5. A modern collective subconscious – our *zeitgeist*

Factors such as over-stimulation of the senses at exorbitant speed, reduction of direct life experience, disparity with reality, disharmony in development and goal-orientated upbringing all combine to create what is often call a "morphogenetic field", the *zeitgeist* (a valuable German term meaning "spirit of the times") which shapes our modern times. Morphogenetic fields have been explained as being "the developing and evolving mental fields common to all, which influence our formation and behaviour".

That is not necessarily an easy concept to grasp. So, imagine there is a pool of information, where all human experiences are collected and stored, which are then at the disposal of all so that one can learn and continue developing. But this is not a new idea; previously it was referred to as the "Akashic Archives" or "the Akashic Record", as a way of describing the collective subconscious.

What is even more interesting is that the presence of morphogenetic fields can be proven empirically in behavioural research! For example, when many people learn something quite specific, even if they live geographically miles apart from each other and have so have never been in contact, it will becomes increasingly easier for their successors to learn the same thing. This principle is evident very widely in the development of humans, animals, and plants and even in cases of non-organic development processes (a multitude of examples of this type can be found in books by Rupert Sheldrake). According to this principle, morphogenetic fields are the true explanation of our system's motor-driving evolution.

Consequently, this means that the collected experiences of a generation, its overall psyche, intellectual, emotional and social achievements, all flow into the morphogenetic field. From there, they have an impact on the development of following generations. Indeed, we create that very *zeitgeist* ourselves, through our children growing up and developing. Everything that we create on an emotional, spiritual and psychological level is also passed on to our descendants!

I have gone into such detail and background on this, as I am sure that this is also the reason why our children today are affected in their development by the afore-mentioned high- speed flood of information, reduction of experience, etc., while their parents are still trying to find new paths in order to support and raise their family. However, the *zeitgeist*, the morphogenetic influence, is like a maelstrom. In essence, it cannot be avoided and so we must learn to deal with it – for whether we like it or not, our children are born into a field full of unrest, rapid impulses, diversions, disharmony and tensions. In other words, what we term "hyperactivity" is nothing other than our own self-created *zeitgeist*.

Against this background, it is therefore important to consider the following in respect of hyperactivity in children:

a) there are children who, as a consequence of a tranquillity that is rooted in their very essence, are affected to a much lesser extent by this *zeitgeist*; thus cannot truly be considered hyperactive.

b) there are children who show a clear resonance with this *zeitgeist* and therefore become very lively and active – but also jumpy, impulsive and restless; this is a display of normal hyperactivity.

c) there are children, whose predisposition and constitution resonates so strongly with the ruling *zeitgeist* that they suffer a distinct deterioration in their quality of life as a consequence of this experience; this can indeed be hyperactivity considered as "pathological".

Against this background one has to ask what our attitude towards hyperactivity is going to be.

What can we do then?

Firstly, we have to accept that it exists, as times have definitely changed, compared to 20, 40 or 60 years ago! We cannot live in the past or use its outdated perceptions.

Then, we must remind ourselves that hyperactivity is basically not a pathological condition, but simply the 'zeitgeist'. Such children are not ill; and, the most important thing, albeit almost a truism, is that we love them and that is the greatest help that we can give them.

Apart from that, we can ensure that our children can spend as much time as possible accumulating meaningful sensory experiences, in a holistic sense, and engaging in creative play and activities. These include safe but free play, romping about in order to experience the joy of having heaps of energy. There has to be the conscious experiencing and encouragement of physical agility or of any artistic and musical talent, so as to learn how to control different human energies. Direct contact with and experience of the natural world and one's surroundings – seeing and knowing animals, plants, stones and the elements – also play an important part in this process.

If all the human senses really participate in the day-to-day experience and if things that have been created with one's own hands can also be touched or experienced, then the soul can grow and develop. Positive contact with parents, brothers and sisters, peers, adults and other living beings, also assist in the development of necessary social skills.

Giving a child the opportunity for shared games and projects – in whatever " safe haven" is available, where it can play with peers without exaggerated adult control – is far better than simply loading it with a wide range of toys. Give your child a "nest' while it is small; then a playground and a safe place, when it is at toddler age. Later, provide understanding, interest and support, when it first goes to school; then, above all, have an open ear, when the child becomes a teenager. Even if you get an earful of complaints (which is almost inevitable!), it is important that you remain open to what they have to say.

So, give your child a supportive sense of order that it can trust and rely upon along with a regular, daily rhythm of life. Regular sleep, regular and preferably shared mealtimes, and regular bedtimes are part of such a pattern – plus some spare time, during which you can give your child your attention. Such a routine is the best possible basis for a child's emotional and inner stability. Indeed, much more can be said, but that is somewhat beyond the scope of this book.

Encourage your child's natural positive inclinations as far as possible. As parents, we often have to strike a difficult balance.

On the one hand, it is important to keep on motivating the child to persist in a learning situation until real success is experienced (e. g. when learning to play a new instrument). On the other hand, it remains vital not to force a child into doing something it no longer wants to do. Yet, even when true motivation is clearly important as a counter to the short-lived *zeitgeist*, the child's wishes, preferences and inclinations should be given a higher priority than parental ambitions!

We can also emphasise consciously the main points or features in the choice of the child's educational direction. A woodland or green-based playgroup, for example, offering a natural experience of the seasons produces far more input to the senses and creative potential than does a house or totally indoor centre, be it ever so well equipped. The same goes for the policy and facilities of schools, within budget limitations and unavoidable constraints.

Finally, it is also extremely important for parents to support life goals expressed by their children. It may be a truism, but we can only find real emotional and mental happiness, when allowed to develop our own lives. This has to be achieved within ourselves and not by having to follow external edicts, no matter how well intentioned they might be. Thus, the most difficult and yet most rewarding development in any adult-child-relationship is its transformation into a friendship – and one based upon equality between the (by now) young adults and older ones.

However, even with such an overall and encompassing encouragement during the development of our children, there are still bound to be some hyperactive phases. Even with the best of intentions by the caring adults, children can become restless, lose concentration, fail to persevere, have extreme mood changes, become aggressive, experience difficulties socially, etc. As a consequence, they can rob us of many a night's sleep through worry and causing a great deal of perplexity. In the end, though, children have their own will and well-developed obstinacy. Maybe it is lucky that it is not as easy to "train" them, as many psychologists still believe!

One thing we can be sure about, nevertheless, is that the helpful measures outlined below will work much better, on a basis of loving, gentle encouragement, than if we leave the development and the upbringing of our children to television, computers, electronic games and so forth. So, whilst it remains extremely important that they become familiar with modern media and technology, this should happen, wherever possible, within a larger framework – one that offers many other, beneficial and positive experiences and possibilities for overall, sound development.

So, looking again more directly at hyperactivity, it becomes extreme or even "pathological" mainly in cases where there is already some predisposition or inner cause, as well as when influenced by factors previously described and that intensify such behaviour.

Within the framework of crystal healing the basic human constitution is closely connected with the actual physical molecular structure of the minerals – the crystal lattice itself. So, in that context and in cases of hyperactive phenomena, four basic crystal configurations need to be identified:

The triclinic arrangement, which equates with great openness and sensitivity, but also as associations distractedness, confusion and lack of concentration.

Its polar opposite, the hexagonal, which represents goal orientation, concentration and rapid development.

Rhombic' structures, characterised by sociability, affability, empathy and adaptability.

Trigonal configurations, which represents constancy, simplicity, inner peace and contentedness.

All of the crystals mentioned below belong to these four main crystal configurations and can therefore, in addition to their symptomatic indications, be effective on a constitutional level.

Homeopathy suggests and offers the following remedies:

- agaricus (fly agaric)
- calcium phosphoricum (Apatite)
- stramonium (thorn-apple)
- tarantula hispanica (tarantula)

- tuberculinum (tuberculosis bacteria)
- veratrum album (hellebore).

Of course, these are not all the remedies that are readily available. However, it is interesting that a lone crystal appears amid the above-listed poisonous (and partly also hallucinogenic) plant and animal remedies. This is Apatite, which is, in fact, recommended for crystal healing (see below). Homeopathic remedies should only ever be taken after consulting a traditional homoeopath, a radiesthetically-aware or knowledgeable physician, or alternative practitioner has carried out kinesiological tests.

Nutrition and diet are also extremely important in this overall context and the main recommendation is to have a child tested professionally for food allergies. Especially sugar (sweets and all confectionery), phosphates (as ingredients in proprietary and commercially sold sausage and cold cuts, tinned foods, soft drinks and sweets), stimulants such as caffeine (cola drinks, coffee, black tea), artificial colours or flavour substances (e. g. the sweetener aspartame in so-called "diet drinks"), cow's milk products, eggs, tomatoes, and even wheat, should be examined (the once-forgotten grain called spelt is a good substitute for the latter).

If there are signs of food allergy among these or other foods, a changed and appropriate diet is strongly recommended.

In addition, professional tests for electromagnetic pollution and heavy metal poisoning should be carried out. The presence of these metals (lead, mercury, cadmium, etc.) can be detected either radiesthetically or kinesiologically and be eliminated by suitable remedies (see Detoxification); and harmful electromagnetic fields should be excluded with help from natural or technical radiation.

Finally, Bach flower remedies have a role here. Very often, they have been shown to have a very positive effect on hyperactive children. Especially recommended are:

- Impatiens – for restlessness
- Scleranthus (one year old tuber) – for erratic indecision
- Wild Oat – for loss of orientation or changeability.

Generally speaking, the Bach flower essences can be chosen intuitively – by letting the children pick them at random – and their accuracy and the spontaneous effect are often quite amazing. Crystals are often very effective when used in combination with Bach flower essences, as they stabilise permanently the rapid, and occasionally short-term, effect of the latter (see Detoxification).

Amazonite is one of the most important crystals for treating hyperactivity. As triclinic feldspar, with traces of lead, Amazonite helps maintain attention and concentration for long periods. Amazonite also balances the mind and soul, thoughts, feelings, willpower and intuition. It helps hyperactive children acquire an inner calm and to utilise the positive results of this very rapidly. In this way, better self-control results and immediate impulses are no longer blindly worked off. Instead, they are recognised but are expressed in a more normal way or even withheld. Amazonite helps one find a "mental foothold" and to counter the challenges of life with a degree of trust.

Apatite helps with hyperactivity which is much exaggerated or when the child is very irritable and aggressive. As a hexagonal phosphate, it helps to channel superfluous energy into controlled paths, to recognise boundaries and to accept them. It assists in openness and an outgoing nature and thus improves social adaptability. Apatite is also recommended when there is a distinct connection between nutrition and hyperactive phenomena. It has a regulating effect upon the metabolism and therefore helps reduce any consequences of a diet that is not adhered to.

Aquamarine helps with severe motor unrest, i.e. when children are constantly "running on adrenaline", have poor concentration and are easily distracted. As a hexagonal, ring-shaped silicate, containing aluminium and beryllium, it regulates the nerve and brain functions and encourages hormonal balance – especially in respect of the pituitary and thyroid glands. Additionally, Aquamarine encourages perseverance, growth and development, and improves learning abilities.

Chrysoberyl helps with extreme hyperactivity. This can be defined as children who seem to be almost removed from their perception and behaviour, display severe attention-seeking behaviour and, have severe learning difficulties and social problems at school. It is a good choice when one has the feeling of being unable to reach children even when talking with them. As a rhombic mineral, Chrysoberyl improves contact with reality, as well as the conscious ability to maintain attention and connection with one's surroundings. Because of its aluminium and beryllium content, Chrysoberyl also has a nerve-regulating effect. In fact, EEG examinations show that Chrysoberyl helps balance the two halves of the brain. It breaks down stress frequencies there and revitalises inactive brain areas or missing ranges of brain rhythms. In turn this improves concentration and overall achievement, as well as regulating extreme mood swings, irrational fears and lack of self-control. It can also help with impairment of the senses, loss of speech or memory, with reading and writing difficulties, and if the child rapidly runs out of steam when under stress.

Tourmaline may help with hyperactivity as it furthers a holistic and harmonious development of one's whole self. Multicoloured tourmalines, in which blue Indigolith, pink Rubellite and green Meredith appear together, can be applied to this end. If only single-coloured tourmalines are available, the blue form **Indigolith** has proven to be the most effective. As a trigonal ring silicate, Tourmaline helps one find inner quiet, firmness and peace. It reduces inner tensions and helps with self-focus and trust. It furthers awareness, empathy, helpfulness and the realisation of the consequences of one's actions. As mineral containing boron, it also improves self-control. In addition, the coloured Tourmalines have a calming effect on the nerves because of their lithium content. Thus, Tourmaline brings harmony into one's life experience, sensory perception and actions.

For all the above, wear as a necklace or pendant on the thymus gland – and preferably place a crystal on the forehead for 10 minutes once or twice daily. If it is uncomfortable to wear the crystal on the chest or the throat, a bracelet can be worn (usually on the right arm). In addition, take as gem essence (3-5 drops, 3 times daily) or gem water (100–200 ml taken in small sips over the course of the day). As ever, though, Chrysoberyl should preferably be taken in smaller doses.

Hypermetropia

see Ametropia

Iodine Deficiency

see Thyroid Problems

Immune System Health

Bouts of infections and illnesses that seem to recur at short intervals indicate a weakened immune system. It makes sense, therefore, to strengthen one's immune system in order to avoid infections and similar kind of illness wherever possible.

Naturally, a detoxification programme will be required (see Detoxification), as tissue already clogged with toxic waste speeds the spread of disease and makes it harder for the immune system to respond properly. A good nutritional base of organic food and regular cleansing cures (fasting and the use of spring herbs) are highly effective methods. In additional, rinsing the mouth and the teeth with organic, cold-pressed sunflower oil for 10-20 minutes every day also provides good protection. Toxic waste and food debris are concentrated by the oil, which cleanses the mouth, gums, teeth and airways. In so doing it helps prevent colds, etc. However, do NOT swallow the oil under any circumstances!

Beside this, it is very important to increase the body's overall basic resistance. Only a properly trained immune system will maintain its ability to react to attack. Proven every-day and traditional remedies include a number that are clear common sense; physical exercise in fresh air (in all kinds of weather!), sleeping with an open window and taking alternate hot and cold baths. For those who do not have physically demanding work, it is important to allow the body to perspire in the fresh air from time to time. This can take the form of bike rides, walking, hiking tours, the mores strenuous forms of gardening, chopping wood, etc. It is also well worth considering alternative exercise techniques such as yoga, Tai Chi and similar routines in the open air – as well as a regular tapping of the thymus gland (on the breastbone, between the heart and throat). All of these are equally effective in strengthening the immune system.

Of course, lower levels of overall stress and emotional tension also help... There is a direct connection with one's emotional condition and immune system. Any crisis point in life – such as the pains of old age, grief, fear, conflicts and problems – should be resolved wherever this is feasible, if necessary with the help of a therapist.

When there seem to be "something going about" and many friends, family and colleagues are succumbing, or when there is an actual epidemic, protect yourself and your immune system by taking Echinacea-based remedies that are readily available from health stores and alternative treatment outlets.

Crystals can also support and help both for protection against illness and for regeneration of the immune system after a severe illness.

Chrysocolla strengthens the immune system, as it cleanses the tissues and the lymphatic system. It can be applied preventively, if one has a strong tendency towards infections, or in order to speed up the healing process during the disease. It also helps in achieving greater emotional stability in cases of stress, indecision and so forth.

Epidote helps to rebuild the immune defence system after a severe illness and to normalise the body functions. It can be applied, in particular, if one is still feeling very weak some time after an illness. It is also useful for anyone seemingly prone to infection. Emotionally, it helps in cases of stress and in dealing with painful experiences. It eases the overcoming of frustration, grief and self-pity and thus improves the emotional constitution.

Heliotrope helps especially at the beginning stages of an illness or when suffering from inflammation. In both cases, it supports the immune system by neutralising the cause of infection and so helps limit the disease. Emotionally, Heliotrope also furthers psychological self-protection and helps to ward off any unwanted influences.

Ocean Jasper is one of the best crystals for strengthening the immune system. It furthers detoxification of the tissues, the lymph flow and the immune system's ability to react to infection. It can be applied both preventively, when there is a high risk of getting infected, and during all phases of infection from viruses or bacteria. It is particularly helpful with stubborn or very debilitating illnesses, where it brings in new energy and a new impetus to the healing process.

For all these crystals, wear as a necklace or pendant. It is also possible to take gem essence (3-5 drops, twice daily, and more often if required) or gem water (taken in small sips during the course of the day).

See also: Lymphatic System Health

Impotence

The term impotence covers in men the apparent impairment of sexual activity. It is usually applied to any general lack of ability to practise sex because of an insufficient, or lack of erection of the penis. But it sometimes also covers an inability to ejaculate, failure to achieve orgasm, or climaxing too soon (premature ejaculation). Its causes can be physical or emotional.

From a physical point of view, sexual problems of this nature may occur because of congenital or accidental damage to the penis and the testicles, as well as from problems with the blood vessels (arterial blockage), the metabolism (diabetes mellitus), the nerves (disease or damage to the spinal column) or hormonal balance. General states of weakness, chronic poisoning (e. g. by lead, arsenic or hydrocarbons), and the adverse side effects of some medication, drugs and alcohol, may all contribute toward lowering potency. In all these cases and wherever possible, treatment on a causal level is necessary. Sometimes, in temporary states of impotence, all one has to do is to avoid the impairing factor, such as an excess of "Dutch courage"!

More often, however, the problems have an emotional cause. Competitive pressure, fear of high expectations in sexual performance, the dread of a resulting sense of failure and negative attitudes toward one's partner may all play their part. In addition, an "anti-sex" upbringing (with associated feelings of guilt), fear of venereal disease, possibilities of an unwanted pregnancy and sheer, normal stress and bad moods can all contribute to the scenarios of "nothing works", or to "it was all over too quickly". In such cases, only an open dialogue between the partners can help, communicating one's wishes, fears and difficulties in order to secure the mutual support provided through openness and trust. Should this not be possible, or it produces no apparent success, therapeutic help may be necessary.

The following crystals will only be able to help overcome minor problems; the bigger ones must be treated at a causal level.

Fire Opal helps with impotence and failure to achieve orgasm, but should not be considered in cases of premature ejaculation! It encourages erotic feelings and sexual attraction, removing inhibitions of acting out one's lust. Quite simply, it helps to make sex fun again, so that it becomes spontaneous and impulsive, with an accompanying elimination of any negative thoughts, bad moods, feelings of guilt and other types of inhibition.

Ruby helps with the types of impotence that arise from emotional causes and general feelings of weakness. It encourages an active sex life and brings a renewed passion into what seems to have become boring and every day. Furthermore, it makes it easier to forget any imagined pressure from sexual competition, removes the fear arising from over-expectations or possible failure and – overall – makes one comfortable and joyful about sex.

Thulite encourages lust, sensuality and sexual arousal. It encourages the fulfilment of sexual wishes and fantasies. It also helps to overcome any deep-rooted blockages caused by negative experiences, an upbringing that was off-putting towards sex, feelings of guilt, pressure from competition, fear and bad moods. Thulite helps in achieving a relaxed, natural attitude towards sex and makes it possible to give oneself fully to one's partner – enabling men particular to "just let go" for once.

All these crystals can be worn as a bracelet, necklace or pendant for any length of time. As an alternative, for short but regular periods, place an unpolished stone (Fire Opal, Thulite) a crystal (Ruby), or tumbled stones regularly on the pubic bone. Experience indicates that the time to do this for the best results is the early evening, say, from 7 to 9 pm.

Another well-known and recommended technique is to create a permanent circle of Thulite (raw or tumbled) all around the bed.

Indigestion

see Heartburn

Inflammation

An inflammation is a non-specific, locally limited defence reaction to a harmful irritation. This irritation can be caused by any of the following:

- mechanical (rubbing, pressure)
- chemical (acids, strong alkalis, toxins)
- physical (heat, cold, radiation)
- allergic reaction
- the body itself (tumours, dying skin tissue, infectious product of metabolism)
- external attack (parasites, diseases, germs, wounds)

An inflamed area will nearly always display at least one of the following four symptoms:

- redness
- heat
- swelling
- aching

In order to prevent further spread of the inflammation into the skin tissue, lymphatic system and blood stream, the affected limb should be kept as immobile as possible. Then, consult a doctor or an alternative practitioner in order to clarify the causes, to choose the right treatment and to avoid complications!

Crystals can be applied to relieve inflammation because they do not interfere with other treatments and may, in some cases, prevent the need to take more powerful medicines such as cortisone.

Agate crystals which display an "inflammation signature" of pink spots imbedded within shades of grey or brown are especially suited for treatment – especially if the signature resembles the actual inflammation to be treated.

Place, fix, or wear these Agates, in the form of a thin section or a tumbled stone, as closely as possible to the focus of the inflammation.

Emerald can also be applied in cases of stubborn, chronic inflammations.

In cases of an externally visible inflammation, place or fix a tumbled stone or a crystal on the inflamed spot. In cases of internal inflammation, wear as a bracelet, necklace or pendant with skin contact. Take gem essence (3-5 drops, 5-9 times daily) or gem water (100–300 ml taken in sips during the course of the day).

Heliotrope is nevertheless the first choice in cases of inflammation. It encourages and supports a rapid, successful immune reaction, so that the inflammatory condition can quickly be reversed in a natural way. Heliotrope containing yellow spots is particularly suitable.

If the inflammation is clearly visible, place or fix a polished stone or a thin section on the inflamed area. In cases of internal inflammation, wear bracelets, necklaces, or pendants for longer periods. As an additional method, or as an alternative, take gem essence (3-9 drops, every hour), or gem water (100–300 ml taken in sips during the course of the day).

Ocean Jasper is particularly suitable for inflammations that typically proceed unnoticed (without severe pains, swellings etc.) but that have either a weakening effect or run the risk of damage in the long term. It is a great help in particular in cases of internal, hidden inflammations (eyes, liver, intestine etc.).

Place a thin section or a flat polished crystal on the affected spot; or wear as a bracelet, necklace or pendant. Also, take gem essence (3-5 drops, 5-9 times daily) or gem water (100–300 ml taken in sips during the course of the day).

Influenza

see Flu

Insect Bites and Stings

There is a general a distinction between insect bites – such as those from mosquitoes, blackflies, horseflies, lice, fleas or bedbugs, as opposed to the stings of bees, wasps, hornets, bees and scorpions.

It must be noted at the outset that some people are seriously allergic to such bites and stings, and so may react severely and adversely. In such cases, professional medical help f a professional kind MUST be obtained as soon as possible

Other than that, and outside of the designated and advised malaria-prone regions of the world, mosquito and other insect bites are usually not truly dangerous, even when appearing in larger numbers. They appear as small red spots or swellings that itch a lot and can be painful. However, they can be cured relatively quickly by placing slices of raw onion (or the crystals listed below) on the affected areas.

As indicated above, bites of this kind are only a problem if infections are transmitted at the same time and cause a feverish illness (e. g. malaria, elephantitis or sleeping sickness in the tropics) these should ALWAYS be treated immediately by a doctor.

Stings from bees, wasps, hornets or scorpions cause severe reddening and the formation of painful swellings. However, there is only an acute danger if one has suffered many such stings (about 30 for children and 60 for adults) or in the oral cavity (danger of suffocation in case of throat oedemas) or in the lymph and blood flow of the head.

However, as already alluded to, bee and other stings are at their most dangerous in connection with insect poison allergies, which can trigger extreme swelling, nettle rash, throat oedemas, real allergic reactions and even anaphylactic shock. In such cases, it must be stressed once again that one should call the emergency physician immediately! Until such help is on the scene, the affected person should be made to lie down and keep calm; the upper part of the body should be raised slightly. A moist, cold compress and draining (see below) can sometimes decrease or postpone the effect of the poison.

The same applies to scorpion stings. In the European Mediterranean region, scorpion stings are comparable to bees when it comes to their toxicity. However, they are much more dangerous in the North African Mediterranean lands and in tropical countries. When in any doubt at all, a doctor should be called for safety reasons. (And always shake out your shoes in the morning before wearing them!)

An active draining technique is the most efficient first aid method if stung. It should be carried out immediately, the sooner the better. This is how it works.

Someone assisting the patient places his/her left index and middle finger on the sting and the victim drinks, preferably without interruption, up to one litre of water (and at least half a litre). In this way, the insect poison is neutralised energetically. Even if it still remains in the tissue, it no longer has any effect. If the technique is applied immediately, there will be no pain or swelling at all. Although this remedy seems almost incredible, it really does work – and, above all, is a boon when helping children who have been stung.

Apart from this, the juice from the leaves of lancet plantain (fresh leaves that are chewed or crushed) can be applied, or take a homeopathic sting remedy. Both will bring relief.

Crystal remedies for bites and stings include a number of minerals, **Rhodonite** is probably the best. However the others listed below have specific applications too.

Amethyst and **Rock Crystal** have a cooling effect and relieve swelling and itching in all cases of insect bites or stings. Natural crystal forms, rather than polished stones, help best. Allow the points to touch the location gently. If there is no natural crystal handy, polished crystals can also be placed on the bite, or gem essence can be taken (see below).

Chrysoprase helps neutralise and break down the toxin from the insect's sting. It is particularly recommended if some time has elapsed since sustaining the insect attack, but when there is still itching.

Heliotrope helps particularly with mosquitoes, stable horseflies, blackflies lice, fleas and bedbugs bites that result in inflammation.

Prase is particularly helpful for painful and severely swollen insect bites. It relieves the symptoms and helps neutralise and break down the toxin that has been absorbed.

Rhodonite is the best crystal for all kinds of insect bites and stings. It relieves itching and swelling and helps the body neutralise absorbed poison or toxin. If it is applied immediately, there may well be scarcely any reaction at all to the bite or sting.

In every case, place or affix a tumbled stone or a polished section directly on the site of the sting or bite. Dab undiluted gem essence on the bite and take it as a supplement if required (5-7 drops, 3–5 times daily) or as gem water (100–200ml taken in small sips over the course of the day).

Intestinal Problems

Intestinal problems are very common and can produce a wide range of symptoms. In fact, often only an examination by a medical professional can distinguish between problems of the stomach, pancreas, gall bladder, liver and other associated organs.

Pains and nausea in the stomach area, recurring diarrhoea and constipation, even a permanent sensation of bloatedness, or itching in the anus, should all make anyone consult either their doctor or an alternative practitioner of choice. As an organ of digestion and excretion, the intestine is extremely important for ones physical health as a whole. Nearly all naturopaths agree that a healthy intestine makes a healthy person – and, indeed, an infected or malfunctioning intestine can poison the whole body system.

The intestine consists of two parts: the first being the approximately 4- metre long small intestine, which serves digestion and absorption, and the second the 1.2 - 1.4 metre long colon, which, first and foremost, reabsorbs water and other important substances (e. g. bile) and excretes everything else that is indigestible. In the intestine, pre-digested food from the stomach is brought together [mixed] with digestive secretions from the pancreas and with bile, which serves to digest fats. Furthermore, about 400 species of bacteria and some species of yeasts, the so-called intestinal flora, participate in the process of digestion. Transportation of food and the whole digestive process are driven forward through peristalsis, the contraction of the intestinal musculature, which proceeds in a wave-like motion. The body's immune system is also active within the intestine in order to fend off any pathogens that have entered the body with the food. Thousands of lymph nodes are the bases for the immune cells, which guard the intestine wall and provide us with immune protection. The mucous membranes of the intestine also play an important part in the absorption of nutrients and reabsorption of important substances. In the folds, villi and inversions of these mucous membranes, an active transportation mechanism ensures that – ideally – we will only absorb what our body needs, while everything else is moved on to the colon and transported to the "exit".

However, the human organism is complex and surprisingly interconnected. As a result, emotional influences can often affect physical well being, especially when considering the digestive process. Indeed, they can impair our body's ability to distinguish between what our overall organism needs and what should be eliminated. Emotional strain, fear, stress, conflicts and difficulties in making decisions can sometimes also lead to "wrong decisions" in the absorption processes –seemingly unconnected with our physical self. Emotional burdens, depression, a bad conscience, feelings of guilt or any feelings of being generally ill at easy with life can often accompany colonic problems.

A complicated connection and natural "cooperation" between a whole range of things is necessary in order to ensure that our intestine functions optimally.

It all begins with the composition of our food, whether what we eat is healthily varied or one-sided, well balanced or otherwise, healthy and organic or ready-made, etc. Whatever our diet, its composition and quality will affect directly the efficiency and quality of the digestive secretions and of bile. It also affects the composition of the intestinal flora – meaning, whether or not the right or wrong intestinal bacteria are present – as well as the active or slackened quality of peristalsis, the adequacy of the immune system and, finally, the optimal function of the mucous membranes. If everything is in order – and the intestine is supplying us with the optimum amount of nutrients – the result will be high-quality blood. It is no surprise then that good blood quality means decent health and a subsequently satisfactory quality of life!

However, if things are not in order, such as the diet having insufficient amounts of the necessary vitamins and minerals, nutrient deficiency problems can arise. In turn, this may then interfere with many of our internal functions and may even lead to poisoning. This latter condition is caused by intestinal flora that has become inefficient due to fermentation and putrefaction. Such "poisoning" seriously damages many organs, especially the liver, and may lead directly to several diseases. So, it is more than a truism to say that: a healthy intestine makes for a healthy human!

Intestinal problems that can be alleviated by the use of healing crystals include the following conditions: wind, constipation and diarrhoea (see also main entry), inflammation and infection, disturbances of the intestinal flora, fungal infections, internal bleeding, ulcers, reduced nutrient absorption, the side effects of drugs such as antibiotics, and sluggish intestine. They may also assist in treating the effects of conditions such as irritable bowel syndrome and others that are emotionally triggered by fear, stress or conflict. Nevertheless, all such conditions and problems should be subject to professional medical diagnosis as well, in order to exclude any serious complications such as appendicitis, tumours, intestinal blockage, dangerous infectious diseases or parasites.

Furthermore, it is only worthwhile using crystals within and as a part of a wider framework of comprehensive medical treatment. Depending on any given situation, it may be necessary to include herbal, biological or homeopathic remedies, along with enzyme and nutrient supplements and colonic irrigation. Algae can also prove useful in binding and thereby isolating toxic substances and inappropriate intestinal bacteria. In addition, do not forget exercise, especially for cases of a sluggish intestine or constipation. Finally, there is the obvious need for a suitable diet (without cow's milk) with plenty of fresh water. All of these measures should be coordinated with the help of naturopath or alternative practitioner.

As individual crystals can be applied in different ways and for different intestinal problems, these are summarised in the following table.

Crystal	Effect	Practical applications
Agate	Disturbance of the intestinal flora, with wind and diarrhoea (grey to yellow-brown natural colour), inflammation (pink natural colour), strain, feeling generally run down	A crystal with appropriate signature is placed on the affected area.Wear bracelets, necklaces, or pendants.Take gem water or gem essence.
Amethyst	Diarrhoea, slight nausea, wind and itching anus. Effects of grief, confusion, guilty conscience and feelings of guilt.	Place a crystal on the stomach or wear it on the body.Take gem essence (2-5 drops, 3 times daily) or maximum of one liqueur glass daily of Hildegard von Bingen's Amethyst Water (page 25)
Amber	Digestive disturbances, nausea, inflammation, abscesses, gall bladder problems. Grief and fear	Place the crystals on the affected areas. Wear a crystal with skin contact.Take gem essence or gem water.
Biotite-lenses	Feeling of pressure on the stomach, constipation, sluggish intestine. Stress when making difficult decisions	Place crystals on the affected areas. Wear a crystal with direct skin contact.
Calcite	Digestive problems, reduced absorption of nutrients, sluggish intestine, disturbance of the intestinal flora, wind, constipation, diarrhoea. Lack of exercise, insecurity and difficulty in making decisions.	Place crystals on the affected areas. Wear a crystal with direct skin contact. A long-term treatment is to use Calcite water (up to 1 litre daily) made of crystals with different colours.
Carnelian	Reduced absorption of nutrients, bleeding, sluggish intestine. Effects of unsolved conflicts and problems.	Place crystals on the affected areas Wear a crystal with direct skin contact Take gem essence or gem water
Chrysoprase	Disturbance of the intestinal flora, fungal infections (where it is used in combination with Smoky Quartz), itching anus. Effects of liver and gall bladder problems or antibiotics, supports detoxification of the intestine. Effect of a guilty conscience, loss of security, jealousy and love worries	Place crystals on the affected areas. Or wear a crystal with direct skin contact. Low doses of gem essence (3-5 drops, 3 tines daily) or gem water (20 – 50 ml). For fungal infections, after two or three days, wear Smoky Quartz.

➤→

Crystal	Effect	Practical applications
Dumortierite	Nausea, vomiting and diarrhoea, effects of a bad diet and of chemical additives in food, food allergy, travel sickness. Effects of grief, fear, insecurity, depression, despair and stress.	Place crystals on the affected areas.Wear a crystal with direct skin contact.Take gem essence or gem water
Emerald	Wind, constipation, infections, inflammation (acute and chronic), abscesses, cramps, disturbances of the intestinal flora, side effect of drugs, diarrhoea, and gall bladder problems. Effects of confusion, conflicts, strain and injustice.	Place crystals on the affected areas or wear them on the body. Take gem essence or gem water.
Fluorite	Abscesses, infected mucous membranes, fungal infections, itching of the anus, sometimes also because of food allergy. Effects of stress, strain, or suppressed feelings.	Place crystals on the affected areas. Wear a crystal with direct skin contact. Take gem essence or gem water.
Hematite	Bleeding, sluggish intestine, reduced absorption of nutrients in the intestine. Do not use for infections! Stress and strain, in difficult life situations	Place crystals (preferably a Hematite with kidney signature-red glass head) on the affected areas
Heliotrope	Intestinal infections, nausea, vomiting (only effective under specific circumstances), infection, abscesses. Feelings of lack of control of one's own life.	Place crystals on the affected areas. Wear a crystal with direct skin contact.Take gem essence or gem water.
Jet	Diarrhoea with or without nausea, digestive disturbances, disturbances of intestinal flora, abscesses, difficult life situations, the effects of grief and depression.	Place one crystal on the stomach and one in the mouth at the same time.Take gem essence or gem water.

➤→

Crystal	Effect	Practical applications
Landscape-Jasper	Digestive disturbances, food allergy, nausea, disturbances of the intestinal flora (supports detoxification), sluggish intestine. Effects of environmental pollution, difficult and long-lasting life style changes	Place crystals on the affected areas Wear a crystal with direct skin contact Take gem essence or gem water
Magnesite	Nausea (migraine), tensions in the intestinal musculature, cramps, digestion problems, reduced absorption of nutrients. Effects of great inner tension, nervousness and stress	Place crystals on the affected areas Take gem essence or gem water Wear a necklace or a bracelet for a long period of time
Mookaite	Digestive disturbances, food allergies, reduced nutrient absorption, disturbances of intestinal flora, sluggish intestine, constipation, and bleeding. Effects of overwork, monotony, problems and any stressful emotional experiences.	Place a crystal on the stomach, or wear it on the body. Take gem essence or gem water
Moss Agate, pink	Nausea, sluggish intestine, constipation, intestinal inflammation. Effects of feelings of guilt or feelings of disgust, anger, or revenge.	Place a crystal on the stomach, or wear it on the body. Take gem essence or gem water
Ocean Jasper	Nausea, unexpected infections, gall bladder problems, effects of drugs, sluggish intestine, constipation, food allergies, fungal infections, itching anus. Stress, strain, unsolved conflicts, non-recovery, sleep disturbances.	Place crystals on the affected areas or wear them on the body.Take gem essence or gem water.
Peridot	Digestive disturbances (in connection with gall bladder problems), fungal infections, parasite attacks. Helps detoxification of the intestine, and with a bad conscience and feelings of guilt.	Place a crystal on the body. Place a crystal in salad oil, then take the oil with food later on.

➤➤

Crystal	Effect	Practical applications
Rhodonite	Abscesses, bleeding, wounds, itching anus. Also effects of emotional wounds.	Place crystals on the affected areas. Take gem essence or gem water.
Sardonyx	Digestive disturbances, reduced absorption of nutrients, food allergy, late effects of infections or drugs, disturbance of the intestinal flora, sluggish intestine. Effects of severe exhaustion and of feelings of despondency and meaninglessness.	Place crystals on the affected areas or wear them on the body. Take gem essence or gem water.
Serpentine	Tension in the intestinal musculature, alternating diarrhoea and constipation. Effects of severe inner strain, nervousness or stress.	Place crystals on the affected areas. Take gem essence or gem water. Wear crystals in the form of necklaces or bracelets for long periods of time.
Smoky Quartz	Sluggish intestine, digestive disturbances, fungal infections (in connection with Chrysoprase). Effects of strain, stress, and tension.	Place or wear a crystal on the body. For fungal infections, use Chrysoprase by first taking in the form of gem essence or gem water (see above). After two days, also wear Smoky Quartz all the time in the form of bracelets, necklaces or pendants.
Golden topaz	Nausea, lack of appetite, digestive problems, reduced absorption of nutrients. Effects of exhaustion, depression, insecurity, nervousness and last-minute-nerves	Place crystals on the upper part of the stomach or wear them on the body. Take gem essence or gem water.
Dravite Tourmaline	Digestive problems, food allergies, nausea, disturbance of the intestinal flora, sluggish intestine, constipation, wind, diarrhoea. Effects of self-reproach, loneliness, rejection, and social problems	Place crystals on the stomach or wear them on the body. Take gem essence or gem water.
Black Tourmaline	Wind, constipation, disturbance of the intestinal flora, feelings of distension Effects of inner tensions and negative attitude towards life, feeling of lack of protection.	Place a crystal in the left trouser-pocket or place it on the body. Place it on the colon. Take gem essence or gem water.

162

For most intestinal problems, gem essences should tend to be taken in relatively high doses (5-9 drops, 3-7 times daily, except for Chrysoprase). In contrast, gem water should be taken in **lower** doses (50 – 200 ml taken in sips during the course of the day), especially when absorption is impeded by nausea. Apart from that, the appropriate crystals can be placed on the stomach area in the form of individual crystals, or as raw and tumbled stones. For problems of the colon in particular, follow the physical course of the colon, when placing the crystals on the body (see Fig. 10). Wearing bracelets, necklaces and pendants of the crystal will also have a supportive effect.

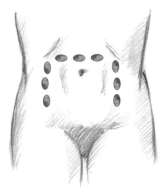

Fig. 10: Arrangement of healing crystals following the course of the colon.

For other healing crystals and references to intestinal problems, see also Stomach Ache; Wind; Diarrhoea; Vomiting; Haemorrhoids; Cancer; Fungal Infections; Travel Sickness; Nausea; Constipation.

Iron Deficiency

Lack of iron in the body is typically characterised by weakness, paleness, tiredness and headaches. It occurs either because of bleeding (e. g. hidden bleeding in the stomach and the intestine region, heavy menstrual bleeding etc), or when there are high requirements of iron, such as during pregnancy, in cases of inflammations, where there is insufficient absorption of iron (unbalanced or one-sided nutrition), a deficient iron metabolism (e. g. in the liver) and disturbances of iron absorption in the intestine.

This latter condition, in particular, plays an important role in regulating the overall iron metabolism, as the intestine is a very sensitive organ. Its absorption mechanisms are easily, and negatively, affected by stress, tensions and any overall feelings of a diminishing quality of life.

With this problem, an increased supply of iron in the food will help only minimally (for example, by eating beetroot and taking herbal juice extracts), as the iron passes through the intestine "unabsorbed". On the other hand, crystals with high iron content stimulate the intestine to absorb iron and will therefore go perfectly well with food that is rich in iron.

Haematite and **Tiger Iron** are crystals with a high content of iron. They improve iron absorption and the role of iron in the metabolism. In this way, they energise and vitalise and improve the supply of oxygen to the organism. Headaches, which typically occur together with a feeling of weakness, will also disappear.

Wear a necklace or a pendant with body contact; or take gem essence (3-9 drops, 3 times daily, when required).

For pronounced weakness, both wearing the crystals and taking gem essence is a very good idea.

As Hematite and Tiger Iron both stimulate inflammation, a doctor or an alternative practitioner should clarify the causes of the lack of iron. However, neither of the crystals should be applied in cases of inner inflammation.

Heliotrope helps with lack of iron caused by internal inflammatory conditions (e. g. when diagnosed as such by a doctor or an alternative practitioner as being caused by low blood pressure). In this case, neither Hematite nor Tiger Iron should be applied until the inflammation has definitely been eliminated.

Wear a necklace or a pendant on the body and/or take gem essence (5-7 drops, 3 times daily).

Itching

Itching is a slight burning sensation or prickling feeling on skin or mucous membranes. It nearly always induces an invol-untarily – or, sometimes, even compelling – desire to scratch oneself. However, when one does this, the result is nearly always that the itching feeling actually increases.

Itches can be caused mechanically, chemically (e. g. insect stings or bites) or physically (burning, radiation), inflammation, skin diseases, hormonal disturbances, and diseases of the blood or metabolism. On a causal level, treatment is more important than on the symptomatic level. However, there is a risk of scratched skin leading to inflammation. Further, because severe itching can almost drive one crazy, it sometimes makes sense to relieve the sensation immediately and directly. If the old saying "don't scratch, wash" proves ineffective, try applying the following two crystals.

Amethyst relieves itching caused by infections and skin diseases when placed on the itch.

However, with large areas of itching, apply Hildegard von Bingen's Amethyst Water (see page 25). In extreme cases, also take gem essence (5-7 drops, if required)

Amber relieves itching caused by mechanical (injury), or by physical (burnings, radiation), hormonal disturbances and diseases of the blood and metabolism.

Place a raw or a tumbled stone directly on the itching areas or wear a necklace or a pendant with body contact for a long period. In extreme cases, also take gem essence (5-7 drops, when required).

Joint Pains and Problems

Usually, joint problems first become obvious as bending and stretching pains. They are caused either by mechanical action (see also Sprains), inflammation (see also: Arthritis), or some degenerative phenomena (see Arthrosis).

Arthritis can be caused by an inflammation of the mucous membrane fold around a bone joint, but the presence of too much uric acid and the concurrent complications (see Rheumatism and Gout) also play an important role. Arthrosis, on the other hand, can be an indirect consequence of arthritis, either through emotional stress, or directly through deposits of toxins. Joint problems should only be treated in conjunction with a doctor or an alternative practitioner, in order to avoid further damage and worsening pain.

Joint problems can result in severe restriction of physical mobility. Whilst such immobility can also be connected with mental immobility, problems resulting from enforced lifestyle change, this is, of course, not always the case. Yet, whenever there is such a connection, it is important to be aware and to highlight such issues.

Thereafter, two things are important for a successful cure: regular detoxification and unrestricted circulation to the body's extremities. In this way, any inflammation can be healed and joints regenerated. The following crystals will to support both these requirements.

Apatite, especially in its blue and green forms, helps with arthrosis and regenerates damaged cartilage. (Interestingly, its chemical composition is close to that of human bone and cartilage.) It also relieves the inflammation associated with arthritis. Emotionally, it encourages a happier mood, flexibility of attitude and the positive aspects of a varied life.

Place (or fix with a bandage) a tumbled stone on the joint. Also, take gem essence (5-9 drops, 3-5 times daily) or gem water (200–300 ml taken in small sips during the course of the day)

Rock Crystal cleanses the joints and helps with both arthritis and arthrosis. It relieves pain and swelling and can supply both the energy needed for the healing process or drain any excess energy. Depending on the specific requirements in each case, an unpolished crystal can be placed on the body in two different ways. If a supply of energy is needed, the crystal should be placed on that side of the joint closest to the torso, but pointing towards the joint (see Fig. 11). However, if there is a need to draw away superfluous energy, place the crystal on that side of the joint, which faces the arm or leg, but pointing away from the joint. When in doubt as to which is needed, try a brief test of about a minute, using each method, one after the other.

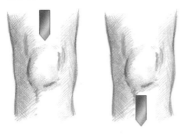

conducting
energy in

conducting
energy out

*Fig. 11: Application of Rock Crystal
for joint problems.*

Garnet Pyrope helps supply the joints with energy and blood, relieving pressure pains in particular and also helps both with arthritis and arthrosis.

Wear as a necklace or pendant with body contact – although it is not necessary to place it near the joint to obtain the beneficial effect. Also, take as gem essence (3-5 drops, 5 times daily) or gem water (200–300 ml taken in small sips over the course of the day.)

Garnet Pyrope crystals primarily help relieve pain in connection with joint problems. But they also cleanse the joint and, in this way, improve the effects of other crystals. They are placed either directly on the painful joint or put into a small cotton bag, which then is fixed on the joint with a bandage. Direct contact of the Pyrite with perspiration should not be allowed for too long, in order to avoid skin irritations caused by iron sulphide compounds.

Green Tourmaline is the most effective crystal for arthritis. Place a crystal along the body axis or on the joints or alongside the extremities. This stimulates the energy flow that is needed for healing through the joint. Furthermore it relieves inflammation and prevents the formation of degenerative damage (arthrosis). If you have no crystal handy, a tumbled stone can be put on the joint. Or take gem essence (5-7 drops, 3-5 times daily) or gem water (200–300 ml taken in small sips over the course of the day). Emotionally, Green Tourmaline also assists in creating open-mindedness, with a flexible and cheerful outlook.

Other types of joint pain manifest themselves as accompanying symptoms of colds, flu and other types of feverish illnesses. They are the result of the interaction with the body's own defence mechanism with the metabolic products and residues from bacteria. The interaction causes a reduced supply of nourishment with a resulting irritation of tissues and nerve endings, disturbances in blood circulation and an accumulation of lymph fluid in the joints.

Whilst joint pains are not a threatening symptom in themselves and are normally only temporary, nevertheless, they can be very uncomfortable.

Blue Chalcedony, **Magnesite** and **Amber** worn as ankle and wrist bracelets are effective in relieving joint pains well. Blue Chalcedony stimulates the lymph flow; Magnesite stimulates relaxation and pain relief; and Amber stimulates the metabolism and the tissues' supply of energy.

Moss Agate, Ocean Jasper or **Sardonyx**, worn as ankle and wrist bracelets have also yielded good results. All three of them belong to the Chalcedony family and, therefore, help bring total healing from disease, stimulate detoxification, regenerate the body and prevent relapses.

See also: Carpal Tunnel Syndrome; Meniscus Problems; Tenosynovitis (TSV); Tennis Elbow

Knee Problems

Just like other joint problems, those with the knee can be mechanical (dislocation and sprain), inflammation (arthritis) or degenerative phenomena (arthrosis). In cases of inflammatory processes such as arthritis, infections in the synovial membranes play a major role. In addition, the presence and consequences in the joint of too much uric acid are rheumatism and gout. Arthrosis, on the other hand, occurs as a consequence of inflammation, toxic waste deposition and overstraining.

Because of the connection between mental and physical attitudes, many knee problems can be associated with factors such as ambition, assertiveness, perseverance, pride, devotion and humility. Even if the problem appears to be pathological, such underlying causes should at least be investigated.

In order to cushion and protect itself against certain types of strain or injury, the knee joint consists of two fibrous cartilage discs between the femur (thigh bone) and the tibia (shin bone). These discs are called the inner and outer meniscus. Sudden movements or twists of the bent knee (e. g. during sport or similar activity) or occupational pressure on the knee over many years (e. g. with floor layers and miners – and, of course, the traditionally eponymous "housemaid's knee"), cause damage and even tearing of these cartilage discs and may also lead, as a consequence, to severe knee problems.

When knee problems occur, the joint should immediately upon the advice and instructions from a doctor or an alternative practitioner. This is essential in order to avoid any permanent damage and additional, even stronger, pain. Once the cause has been clarified, crystals can provide an excellent help together with medically prescribed measures. As with general joint problems, two things are important here: regular detoxification; and a good energetic care of the legs, so that inflammation is rapidly cured and the knees or the menisci, respectively, can be regenerated. (See also: Detoxification; Joint Problems)

Apatite helps with arthrosis in the knee joints. It assists in the regeneration of damaged cartilage substance, as its chemical composition is identical to that of human bone and cartilage. Thus, Apatite can even help cure damage in the menisci. The blue and green varieties of Apatite also relieve arthritis. Emotionally, Apatite helps to make us lively and flexible.

Place or bind a tumbled stone on the knee joint. Alternatively, or as a supplement, take gem essence (5-9 drops, 3-5 times daily) or gem water (200–300 ml taken in small sips over the course of the day).

Aragonite is particularly helpful for damage to the menisci. It relieves pain and stimulates the regeneration of the affected cartilage disc. Aragonite-Calcite stones sold commercially as "Onyx-marble" are also very suitable as they contain about 80% Aragonite. Emotionally, Aragonite helps with stress and strain, particularly when feelings of not being able to cope crop up with certain tasks or situations.

Place a tumbled stone on the knee joint or fix it with a bandage; or take gem essence (5-9 drops, 3-5 times daily); or gem water (200–300 ml taken in small sips over the course of the day).

Biotite-lenses help with sprains, arthrosis, gout and rheumatic knee problems. They help dissolve deposits in the knees and regenerate cartilage and the menisci. For the latter, it is best to combine Biotite with Apatite and Aragonite. Emotionally, Biotite-lenses also furthers flexibility and adaptability without compromising beliefs. Place them on the knee, or bind them there with a bandage.

Dioptase placed over the liver also supports healing of the menisci, as it has an energetic connection with the liver.

Pyrites relieve pain in connection with knee problems. Additionally, they also cleanse the joint and improve the effect of the other crystals. Place them either directly on the tender knee or fix them to the knee after wrapping them cotton cloth. Note, however, that it is best to avoid contact between Pyrites and perspiration over long periods, as iron sulphide compounds that make up Pyrites can irritate the skin.

Pink Tourmaline helps with knee problems, as it stimulates the energy flow through the joint that is needed for healing. It relieves inflammation in cases of arthritis and prevents the formation of arthrosis. Pink Tourmaline furthers commitment to something, desire for enterprise and flexibility. So, it better than Green Tourmaline, which would otherwise be a first choice for joint problems.

Place or bind a crystal or polished stone lengthwise on the knee. As an alternatively, take gem essence (5-7 drops, 3-5 times daily) or gem water (200–300 ml taken in small sips over the course of the day).

Kidney Health

The kidneys are the most important excretory organ in the human body. They perform essential functions for the well being of our whole organism, maintaining our whole fluid balance of minerals, acids/ bases, nutrients, vitamins and hormones. They have to excrete toxic substances and waste products (e. g. uric acid) but, at the same time, retain water and other vital substances.

In essence, the kidneys are large filtering organs, where complicated secretion and reabsorption processes take place. Disturbances in the kidney function that are a consequence of pain-relieving drugs or other kinds of strong medicines, can lead either to a large loss of water, minerals and nutrients, or to an accumulation of toxins and waste products in the body. Both can have serious consequences – or may even become lethal – if they are either not treated, or are treated in the wrong way.

Because of their serious nature, it is not appropriate for this book to deal with true kidney diseases. Any pains in or near the kidneys (which are sometimes accompanied by a raised temperature, shivering and cloudy urine) should be examined and treated immediately by a doctor or an alternative practitioner. Indeed, never instigate any arbitrary treatment without the necessary professional knowledge!

In Traditional Chinese Medicine, our central energy reserve, our life force, or *chi*, is regarded as being linked directly with the kidneys. So, put more conventionally, the health of the kidneys is connected directly to the well being of the whole, thus it makes great sense to strengthen and support the kidney functions. In so doing, the kidneys' efficiency is maintained in their process of detoxification during general diseases (flu, colds and mild infections) or in cases of low or high urine excretion. The most important thing one can do is to drink good, clean water, without any additives such as sugar, flavouring or stimulants!

There can also be an emotional basis to kidney problems – although the overall causes vary from person to person. It can often be that difficulties in communication, within a partnership, career or general living – along with the suppression of emotions, feeling that one is a victim, general fear or desperation – can all contribute to a weakening of the kidney function. When these types of contributory factors are recognised, their elimination (with the help of a therapist, if required) can spare one from many kidney diseases. Just as the kidneys are responsible for a harmonised fluid balance, they are also connected emotionally and mentally to mental equilibrium and harmony. Consequently, crystal therapy can also help in this context with maintaining healthy kidneys and preventing complications.

Chalcedony, Chrysoprase and **Ocean Jasper** improve the flow of body fluids and their overall quality. This helps alleviate stress on the kidneys, but only after an initial phase of increased secretion. These specific crystals should, therefore, be applied as a precaution rather than for acute situations – and always drink of lots of water!

Wear as a bracelet, necklace or pendant on the body. Alternatively, take gem essence (3-5 drops, 3 times daily) respectively; or gem water (100–200 ml [Chrysoprase only 20-50 ml] taken in small sips over the course of the day.)

Jadeite and Nephrite have been known for many centuries to heal the kidneys and actually were named because of their properties in this context: Spanish: *pietra de ijada* "loin stone"; Latin: *lapis nephriticus* "kidney stone". Both strengthen the kidneys function in a similar manner and, if they are applied regularly, they can also prevent the formation of deposits in the uric channels that can lead to kidney stones. They also help one obtain emotional balance and harmony.

Take as gem essence (3-5 drops, 3 times daily) or gem water (100–200 ml taken in small sips over the course of the day); and place tumbled stones on the area over both kidneys. As Green Jadeite is very rare and expensive, the violet-coloured Lavender Jade is an acceptable and effective alternative.

Peridot strengthens the excretory functions of the kidneys. It assists in the release of toxins and waste substances and so helps with urine flow. Emotionally, Peridot helps one recognise personal aspects in one's life that weaken the kidneys, and helps in confronting them.

Place a small tumbled stone in sunflower oil and use it as part of a salad dressing.

Serpentine, like Jadeite and Nephrite, supports all kidney functions. Place a tumbled stone, sections or slices, on the area over both kidneys – or wear as a bracelet, necklace, or pendant for a long period.

Also, take as gem essence (3-7 drops, 3 times daily) or gem water (100–200 ml taken in small sips over the course of the day).

Lack of Energy

see Tiredness

Lactation Problems

Human milk is generated in the female breast in 15 to 20 different small gland lobes, which are embedded in fatty connective tissue. During pregnancy an increased secretion of sex hormones causes these glands to mature and after childbirth, stimulated by a hormone from the pituitary gland, they begin producing milk. Another hormone, activated by the suckling of the infant, then continues to ensure the further production of milk.

During its production, breast milk is stored in the individual glands and then flows through fine channels, the milk ducts, out into the nipple. At the beginning, breastfeeding can be difficult due to a low milk flow; but this can be eased through appropriate massage.

Milk generation at too low a flow rate is often connected to stress and readjustment problems after childbirth. A protected environment and secure atmosphere for mother and child can reduce the external problems, whilst relaxation and meditation help from within.

See also Breastfeeding

Chalcedony, in several varieties, stimulates the lactation process as well as bringing the necessary calmness needed when breastfeeding. Light Blue, White and Pink Chalcedony, without bands, are the types best suited here. They consist of silicic acid, which has flown through fine channels into cavities, where they have crystallised as Chalcedony.

The crystals were therefore generated in a similar process to the production of human milk. Perhaps, then, it is no surprise that White Chalcedony, commonly called "Milk Stone", has been recognised for several hundred years as an aid to lactation at the start of the breastfeeding.

It is most effective in this context when worn as a necklace or pendant on the breast.

Learning Difficulties

Learning is the human ability to absorb, sort, evaluate and apply information. Learning is a part of our daily life. "You never stop learning", is possibly a trite saying, but an accurate one. Learning is decisive in achieving new skills and improving one's life. A failure to understand or fully comprehend – e.g. repeatedly forgetting or ignoring important connections, or feeling that learning something new is "a pain" or source of frustration – can lead directly to a sense of foolishness, feeling stupid and even of being treated unfairly. Psychologically and emotionally, there is almost nothing worse than the feeling that there is something important we do not know, something we cannot do or knowledge and information that we cannot acquire. Therefore, the ability to learn, and to carry on learning, is the key to success, competence and self-respect.

Our ability to learn depends on our intelligence and our so-called "ability to think". Thinking can also be defined as the "ability to recognise and to evaluate"; and our increased intelligence is in direct proportion to our ability to recognise and evaluate similarities, connections and differences.

Intelligence is not innate and unchangeable throughout one's whole life. On the contrary, it can be improved all the time! Further, intelligence has nothing to do with education or the amount of accumulated information. Rather, it is the ability to gain new knowledge – learn from experience, observe life's changes, assimilate information – and then to apply it.

In the first place, the above processes mean that any obstructing issues must be recognised and removed. Typical of such things are: distraction, alcohol, drugs, lack of interest, psychological pressure, hunger, lack of concentration, misunderstandings, tiredness, pain, worries, stress, concern about unfinished projects and plans, constant brooding, despair, all kinds of emotional "downs", as well as physical diseases.

See also: Memory Problems; Concentration Problems; Nervousness; Stress

In addition, three other factors also play an important role – overestimating one's abilities, bad habits and suppression of ideas. This has long been recognised: "Knowing that you do not know anything" was how Socrates put it. Such an attitude remains the starting point of any learning process, just as the idea that you know everything in advance is the biggest impediment.

Further, whilst there are still many arguments about all aspects of education, surely another factor in blocking the learning process arises, ironically, from techniques that have been (and still are) used in the very process of institutional education and learning. One example is simple learning by rote. Whist this method makes it possible to store information, word for word, it does so without any proper understanding of the meaning – accumulating knowledge without any intrinsic value. It creates some very bad habits in connection with the learning process, often leading directly to a form of closed circuit "thinking", when empty ideas or phrases are repeated, parrot-fashion, instead of voicing one's own real thoughts. This is something employed ruthlessly by advertising and some aspects of manipulative popular culture. Yet, better learning techniques often reveal an unknown potential and prove that nobody is actually born stupid. One merely requires a valid means of learning in order to "make it" – through whatever circumstances! Every human being is basically intelligent and, therefore, is able to acquire the knowledge and the experience that he or she needs.

Crystals can be a real support in all of this – although no crystal will ever do our thinking for us! Nevertheless, the application of crystal therapy can help overcome many limitations and thereby further our natural abilities. Specifically, crystals can be of great service in overcoming problems associated with concentration, confusion, and lack of imagination or poor memory skills.

Amazonite is helpful wherever learning is inhibited by serious inner unrest. It is especially efficient when feeling under-challenged, a condition where boredom and lack of interest drown any true motivation and often then open the floodgates to all kinds of distractions. Amazonite helps the mind to remain fully aware and focussed.

Blue Chalcedony stimulates a mental openness to new ideas. It assists in understanding what has to be learned and to then convert acquired knowledge into valid and practical applications. As it simultaneously also furthers articulation, it helps with the application of newly learned skills or acquired knowledge. In this way, it tends to be the crystal of choice for helping with any kind of test.

Chrysoberyl helps with learning problems whenever learning programmes are suppressing rather than encouraging one's potential and where a fear of failure predominates. It also helps with learning discipline, consistently and systematically. It is particularly recommended whenever pressure and stress seem to place a limit upon one's learning ability.

Fluorite helps eliminate any stubborn adherence to limited thinking and poor learning habits. In this, it furthers a positive mental attitude that makes sorting and evaluating information much easier. It furthers the ability to think, improves perception and is, therefore, an excellent learning aid when substantial amounts of new knowledge have to be processed.

Lapis lazuli enhances the ongoing willingness to learn something new, an acceptance that one does not know everything and the ability to absorb evaluate and understand information. It stimulates our ability to think more clearly, so that many insights and recognitions are possible within a short time. Lapis lazuli also furthers the ability to discriminate intelligently, and aids in honesty and sincerity. Finally, since time immemorial, it has rightly been called the "crystal of wisdom".

All of the aforementioned can be worn as a necklace or pendant with body contact for longer periods. You can also make an arrangement of unpolished or polished stones (spheres, pyramids, sections/slices, etc.) at your place of work.

Leg Ulcers

Ulcers develop on the legs and feet when the body tissue there lacks its normal supply of nutrients. As many as 85% of all leg ulcers are a direct result of this and the associated over-accumulation of blood in the veins. More rarely, thy can also be caused by a reduced blood flow in the arteries. In both types, the cells and tissues die without the vital nutrition they require, so ulcers generally tend to occur in the lower leg. Further, they can only really be cured if the underlying, true causes are identified and then treated. Even then, they are very slow to cure, causing considerable distress to those who suffer from the problem.

As far as general precautions go by way of prevention, the most important is thorough removal of toxins (see Detoxification). This usually improves the nutrient supply to the cells and tissues and eliminates the damaging accumulation of toxic substances. A further help is adopting a healthy diet that is rich in vitamins and minerals (if necessary, with appropriate vitamin and nutritional supplements) and reducing one's consumption of animal protein. The latter is deposited in the human body as an important building block of tissue. However, as modern Westernised lifestyle is oversupplied as never before by food high in animal protein, too much of it is nowadays being stored in our bodies. The effect is akin to that of the ever-greater pollution of our environment by toxic waste. This means that the body prepares itself for a poor supply of oxygen and of other nutrients.

So, to summarise, a diet without animal protein is strongly recommended as part of the treatment of leg ulcers – and avoiding pork and any kind of sausage meat, in particular, contributes greatly to a faster cure.

On the emotional and psychological side of things, it is important also to recognise that frustration, stress, anxiety and an overall feeling of being run down may also contribute to blockages or impaired circulation. It can be a vicious circle, in fact, if concerns of this type are then exacerbated by the formation of leg ulcers. Conse-

quently, it is just as important to reduce overall levels of worry and stress (if possible), as it is to eat properly, etc. If necessary, seek the help of a therapist in order to confront ongoing and persistent worry, serious issues, obligation, a fear of failure and identifying sensible life goals.

Physically, when treating a leg ulcer, it is important to clean the area thoroughly and regularly. This can be done using a camomile infusion, or a 0.9% solution of common salt. Such thorough cleansing is very important and should – initially, at least – be performed by a medical professional, doctor, alternative practitioner or nurse. Then, once they have shown you the correct procedures, it is something you should be able to tackle by yourself – though not **too** often, as the wound secretes enzymes, which are beneficial to the cure. As a consequence, bandages should only be changed every two days at the earliest, unless there is a burning sensation or a smell which signifies the presence of bacteria. This latter condition should be discussed with the doctor treating the leg, and the area surrounding the wounds cleansed with oil and healing ointments (from alternative or natural medicine practice).

Physical exercise is also necessary in order to neutralise the underlying accumulated toxins and disruption of the circulation. When seated, raising the feet also provides immediate relief. However, when standing again, slackened blood vessels immediately expand again. It is, therefore, important to wear support stockings or compression bandages when first walking.

Crystals can assist and support the healing of wounds (Mookaite, Rhodonite), as well as boosting nutrient supply to the tissues (Lace Agate, Hematite, Carnelian, Ocean Jasper).

Rhodonite and **Mookaite** can be added to the cleansing fluid used in the form of gem essence (10 drops for 100 ml), be worn in the form of ankle bracelets or be placed inside a bandage close to the wound (but only using a very flat crystal). Mookaite itself also supports a better supply of tissue nutrients, while Rhodonite helps the very slow healing process. Additionally, if worn on the body in the form of a necklace or pendant, they will also stimulate an awareness of any emotional causes and thus also encourage psychological healing.

Lace Agate (with a vessel signature) and **Carnelian** have a supportive effect on the blood vessels in the surrounding tissue and on the blood flow within them. Apart from that, they aid the supply of nutrients and limitation of toxic substances. They also help to cope with frustration, stress and feelings of weakness.

Haematite enhances blood flow and blood quality. Thus, it helps both speed up the circulation and improves the supply. In addition, Haematite also boost the willpower needed to speed the cure and provides the inner strength to cope with it all.

Ocean Jasper also improves the supply of nutrition and the elimination of toxins. It also stimulates the body's immune system and self-healing forces, thereby speeding up the healing process. It is especially effective if it contains cell, vessel or wound signatures. Emotionally, Ocean Jasper also promotes a new sense of new optimism and *joie-de-vivre*, which is also important during the long healing process.

For Lace Agate, Hematite, Carnelian and Ocean Jasper, wear as ankle bracelets (if possible).

Alternatively, take as gem water (200–300 ml taken in small sips during the course of the day), or gem essence (3-5 drops, 5-10 times daily). The dosage should be rather low to begin with, but then can be increased rapidly over the next three days, maintained for several weeks, and finally be reduced gradually once again.

Libido

see Sexual Problems

Liver Health

The liver, together with its function of cleansing, construction and storage, is the organ of regeneration in our organism. It contributes considerably to the detoxification process and it produces our essential proteins. It also acts as a store of many vital substances, such as the red blood corpuscles and the starch-like, energy-storing substance glycogen. The consequence of a weakened liver is a weakened total organism ("tiredness is the pain of the liver") with lowered resistance to infection and other symptoms indicative of insufficient detoxification and regeneration.

It is clear therefore, that maintaining a healthy liver not only leads to better physical harmony, but also to improved emotional states and general equilibrium. The following crystals can have a positive influence on this process.

Amazonite helps with specific metabolic disturbances in the liver, when specific substances can neither be built up nor broken down. Above all, it should be applied when liver efficiency decreases suddenly without apparent cause, or becomes irregular (a possible sign being a drop in performance in the early afternoon).

Chrysoprase is the number-one choice in connection with the liver. It stimulates all liver functions and furthers the cleansing and regeneration of the organ itself. Apart from that, it has also proved to be especially good for detoxification.

Dioptase has a refreshing effect on the liver. This copper silicate is most effective if placed directly over the liver. It stimulates the cleansing function of the liver, aiding the organ itself, as well as processes that are driven by the liver metabolism and by the liver energy in other parts of the body (e.g.

in the eyes, the spinal discs and the menisci).

Emerald furthers the healing and regeneration in cases of liver disease. It has an anti-inflammatory effect and, at the same time, a cleansing and strengthening effect on basic liver function.

Epidote stimulates and supports the building and storage processes in the liver. It is, therefore, mainly a recuperation and regeneration crystal to be used after illnesses or after a long and difficult period.

Malachite stimulates the liver and, in particular, helps with nausea that can be traced back to disturbances in liver function. It has a detoxifying effect and helps with afflictions caused by problems with uric acid metabolism (see Rheumatism, Gout).

Ocean Jasper strengthens the building and storage, as well as detoxifying functions of the liver. It helps with liver diseases (also with inflammatory states), and stimulates the organ's own cleansing processes. It is especially helpful when the liver has been under strain for some time because of malnutrition, alcohol abuse or impaired digestion in the intestine.

Zircon furthers the detoxifying functions of the liver and cell regeneration in connection with liver diseases. It can be applied in particular when there is pain in and swelling of the liver.

Place a crystal, a tumbled stone or a flat slice/section of any of the above on the liver every night; or, if easier use sticking plaster to affix it to the area for a longer period of time. The crystals can be applied in this way every time a process of physical or an emotional regeneration seems to be needed. It is also possible to take gem essence (3-5 drops, 3 times daily) or gem water (50–100 ml taken in small sips over the course of the day).

Long Sight

see Ametropia

Loss of Voice

Loss of voice can be caused by hoarseness, by straining the vocal cords, inflammation of the larynx and disturbances in the actual nerves within the vocal cords. Emotional causes, such as loss of speech associated with sudden, unexpected, shocking and/or traumatic incidents, may also play a part. Always seek the advice of a doctor in order to clarify the causes and avoid serious or even incurable results such as persistent muteness.

See also: Hearing Loss; Hoarseness

Chalcedony can help with loss of voice caused by infections and inflammation of the airways or larynx. Hildegard von Bingen referred to it as the "speaker's crystal" it still remains effective with all problems in the larynx and vocal cords.

Chrysoberyl helps in cases of voice loss caused by brain or nerve disturbance. As a crystal containing the metallic element beryllium, it helps remove many kinds of nerve blockages and thereby re-activates corresponding areas of the brain.

Unlike similar crystals, it should **not** be worn at the neck, but only placed on the forehead, 2 – 3 times daily for about 15 minutes.

Lapis lazuli and **Sodalite** have proved to be very useful when loss of voice is caused by hoarseness, nerve disturbances caused by pent-up anger, shocking experience or problems that are connected with the difficulty in talking about of something disagreeable.

Lapis lazuli, in particular, brings back the voice very quickly. It also helps physically in raising the voice and emotionally in speaking one's mind – the latter especially where there seems to be a need to be heard in order to avoid an injustice or to disclose the truth.

Sodalite helps raise consciousness and awareness of the moment when something really has to be said immediately and ensuring there are no further "blockages" or inhibitions in speaking out.

The best sequence, therefore for these two crystals is Lapis Lazuli for acute cases, followed by Sodalite in order to prevent a relapse.

Larimar helps with a weakened voice that rapidly loses strength and energy; and it also prevents any recurring loss of voice.

Apart from that, Larimar makes it easier to communicate something that has not yet been said, but needs to be.

However, it has a gentler and more "cautious" effect than Lapis lazuli and is also proving to be particularly helpful with feelings of being overwhelmed by a situation in which the throat "tightens up" and that seems to paralyse all speech, thought or activity.

For all of these, except Chrysoberyl, place a slice/section, tumbled or a raw stone on the throat or were in the form of a necklace or pendant.

Lumbago

Lumbago is a pain that occurs suddenly in the spine or in the back's lumbar region. Immediately, it causes a tension within the muscles, a hardening of the spinal musculature and a crooked spinal posture. The associated pains are generally so severe that one can hardly move at all. The causes may be overall "wear and tear" of the spinal column, a slipped disk or a blockage in the flexibility of the small vertebrae. Lumbago is mostly triggered by unaccustomed or excessive strain of the back, as well as by draughts or damp conditions.

In self-treatment of lumbago, pain relief comes as one's first priority, as treatment on a causal level cannot begin before the tensed muscles have been relieved. So, it is very important to take care and, if necessary, stay in bed and keep warm. When the pain decreases, seeing a doctor or qualified physiotherapist, or having a recommended massage can help.

As a support, crystals have turned out to be particularly valuable for relieving the pain of lumbago and for rapidly re-establishing mobility.

Pyrites are the first choice of crystal for pain relief. They should be placed on the affected area in a cotton bag and be wrapped warm pieces of cloth – or, even better, in warmed fur. The cotton bag is necessary in order to avoid direct contact between the Pyrites and skin and sweat, as the latter dissolves iron sulphide (the chemical component of pyrites), which could otherwise lead to skin irritation.

Kunzite and **Sugilite** also have a pain relieving effect, but usually work more slowly than Pyrites. Both crystals can be placed directly on the affected area in the form of a crystal (Kunzite) or a tumbled stone. Take gem essence at the same time (5-7 drops, every half hour).

Tourmaline, particularly Pink Tourmaline and Watermelon Tourmaline, stimulate a re-establishment of mobility. Apply the crystals as polished sections or Tourmaline crystals on the affected area. Alternatively, fix them there with adhesive plasters when the pain is decreasing. The best method is to affix the crystals parallel to the spinal column.

Lyme Disease

see Tick Bites

Lymphatic Health

Lymph is the fluid that drains from the body and is absorbed by a fine system of vessels and, in turn, is conducted back to the blood circulation via larger lymph vessels. The lymphatic system thus consists of these vessels, which contain so-called lymph nodes, and ensures that no toxic substances, harmful bacteria, or damaged or dead white blood corpuscles can return to the blood supply. It is the specific function of the lymph nodes to carry out this process of filtering and detoxification. At the same time, they form the operational base for the human immune system. As a result, the whole lymphatic system is vital for the cleansing and the drainage of the tissues, as well as for the immune defence mechanism. This double function makes it obvious why detoxification and care of the immune defence system are so closely connected. When our tissues are overloaded with deposited toxins and waste substances, the quality and free-flowing nature of lymph are both decreased. The fluid becomes more viscous and the immune reactions are delayed and weakened.

Stimulation and maintenance of a healthy lymphatic system facilitates the drainage of fluid and toxic substances. It cleanses the tissues and the lymph fluid itself, improving both flow and the effectiveness of the immune function of the system. Therefore, any swelling of the lymph nodes that occurs as a result of inflammation and infections, reduces more rapidly. In addition, hypersensitivity to specific foods, acidification, allergy and any predisposition towards infections are alleviated – along with any disturbances of the metabolism, of circulation or heart. Above all, maintaining a healthy and functioning lymph systems remains especially important in supporting the detoxification processes, and in connection with colds, infections and inflammations.

The following have been found to assist in this overall process.

Chalcedony stimulates lymph flow and the removal of fluid accumulations in the tissues (the oedemas). In this way, it supports detoxification and speeds up the shrinking of swollen lymph nodes after infections and inflammation. As a result it also helps with alleviating the effects of most types of feverish diseases (see also Colds; Fevers; Flu).

Moss Agate furthers the cleansing of the tissues and lymph and helps particularly with very stubborn or persistent infections and diseases.

Noble Opal also stimulates the lymph flow. However, it has a stronger stimulating effect on the functions of the immune system, and so, in some cases, is preferable to

179

use instead of Chalcedony – especially in cases of swollen lymph nodes, infections and inflammations.

Ocean Jasper stimulates the lymph flow and helps oedemas shrink back to a normal state. It is especially helpful with accumulations of lymph and stimulates the contraction of the lymph nodes – even in cases of chronic infections and inflammation. It has a stronger cleansing effect than Moss Agate and has a greater strengthening effect on the immune system than has Noble Opal. Its use should certainly be considered in all cases where there is a persistent condition and slow, difficult healing.

For all the above, wear a bracelet, a necklace or a pendant with body contact for a longer period. With oedemas place a slice/section, or a raw or tumbled stone directly on the affected spot. Alternatively, take gem essence (5-7 drops, 3-5 times daily), or gem water (200–300 ml) taken in small sips during the course of the day).

Melancholia

Feelings of constant sadness, worry; misery; general mild depression or even despair – if persistent – can be best summarised under this heading.

Sadness is a vague term, but if we include the above in various forms and combinations, it is nearly always caused by suffering, difficulties and circumstances that make one feel unhappy and that do not seem changeable in the foreseeable future. It is distinguishable from acute personal loss (see Grief), which, as a rule, is due to a specific incident, e.g. a death, a broken relationship, rejection etc. Constant sadness develops over a longer period; sometimes because of a couple of consecutive incidents, – so called "chronic sadness".

Another typical sign of constant sadness is a clinging to the past, which is seen either as the "good old days", "everything was better in the past" or as the time when all the bad things started. However, the past cannot be changed now, despite feelings that maybe one's parents, a former partner, an employer, the War, etc. are to be blamed for everything!

Sadness is characterised by emotional difficulties, unhappy life circumstances and a persistent dwelling in the past. Indeed, all three components are usually present. In contrast to direct grief – where talking about events and associated feelings, and then allowing tears to flow brings relief – talking about sadness and worries, often in a rambling way, merely tends to make the situation worse. Because the suffering has been going on for such a long time, many explanations tend to have arisen or been created in the mind of the sufferer, and which cover up the really painful memories. Furthermore, if you believe that you cannot change anything about the causes of your current situation, the future can look black indeed.

You can only relieve such constant emotions when you recognise that you can actually change your life! This will need to involve looking more closely at painful and sad incidents from the past – if necessary, with the help of a therapist. However, the goal must be to refrain from blaming anyone (and this also includes oneself) for past incidents and to begin to be an active co-creator of one's own life, by assuming total responsibility for oneself. If this change can be made, there will definitely be hope for the future.

See also Depression

Consciously working on oneself possibly with the help from a therapist may be necessary. Nevertheless, crystals can, however, support and ease this work in many areas.

Amethyst relieves sadness and helps one confront the relevant incidents from the past. Amethyst makes the consciousness-raising about key incidents easier and helps one to stop blaming other people. In this way the process of clarification is sustained and inner peace is attained.

Chrysoprase helps with feelings of loneliness, hopelessness and of being lost. It supports the search for ones own truth and brings about self-confidence and security. In this way, Chrysoprase relieves even jealousy and lovesickness. Chrysoprase makes it

possible to look at one's own life with all its blows dealt by fate from a "higher perspective". Thus, it helps create the broader view, which puts many things into a new context and reveals the deeper meaning or the causes of painful or unhappy experiences.

Citrine helps one to release one's attention from previous incidents and to direct it, instead, towards the future. This offers better control over one's life in the "here and now", along with security and self-confidence. Through such positive changes, one can then forget and let go of many incidents that were previously believed (spuriously) to be important and be rid of their persistent influence. Citrine relieves despair by encouraging a growing optimism.

Dumortierite helps one to take things less seriously (hence it being called the "take-it-easy" crystal). Dumortierite makes it possible to look at unpleasant incidents from the past in a new way, to confront them with self-confidence and to talk about them more easily. It is therefore a good support in conversation therapies. It furthers a positive attitude towards life.

Noble Opal quickly draws one's attention to the present and guides it to the positive and brighter sides of life. Boulder-Opals in particular have turned out to be effective as they contain veins of Noble Opal in a mother rock rich in iron, with its associated additional strengthening effect. Noble Opal changes powers of observation, so that attention is increasingly drawn to personal strengths and talents as well as to happy incidents – with a new and better perception of life.

Wear a necklace or a pendant of the above, with direct body contact, for a longer period and/or carry a tumbled stone or a crystal in your pocket.

Memory Problems

A bad memory, or a gradually decreasing ability to remember, is often accepted as being an inevitable process or something that is inherent. With increasing age, in particular, it seems to be impossible to improve the memory. Quite simply, this is wrong!

Totally independent of one's age, there are a number of ways of refreshing the memory function. Foremost among these self-administered methods is memory training. This can be done by such exercises as learning poems by heart, playing memory games, deleting programmed numbers in the telephone or fax machine, going shopping without a list, etc. These exercises should begin with a low degree of difficulty and then gradually be stepped up. Furthermore, any kind of ordering activity is helpful – even tidying up at home and at work, systematic sorting and filing papers, etc. All unfinished activities that are properly brought to an end 100% then help release

mental storage capacity and improve one's memory. Just and try it!

In addition, specific crystals can be applied in order to fortify one's memory. However, they are much more effective when the above training exercises are also carried out.

Amazonite improves the memory when internal unrest and distraction cause lack of concentration. Amazonite is, therefore, particularly helpful with children, who have difficulties with structure at school, such as large classes, ex-cathedra teaching, sitting still, etc. Consequently, they have a very selective memory, recording interesting (to them!) things perfectly, and other things not at all.

Chrysoberyl strengthens one's memory and is especially helpful in stressful situations, or when one feels too stressed to remain in control and think clearly. It is especially good when there is a tendency constantly to forget the most important things.

Diamond helps to reconstruct incidents and, in this way to create, a coherent memory. You can always apply it when you have the feeling that you know something – but just cannot quite retrieve it from your memory.

Fluorite helps to create internal and external order. It strengthens mainly the short- and middle-term memory and so is great help when studying.

Kunzite improves memory and helps

one to recall events or something learned a long time ago that is deeply buried.

Wear a necklace or pendant (if available), or place or fix a rough stone, a crystal or a tumbled stone regularly on the forehead. Also take gem essence (2-4 drops, twice daily) or gem water (50–100 ml taken in small sips during the course of the day).

Menopausal Problems

The menopause tends to take up some 10 to 15 years of a woman's life, during which hormone production within the ovaries declines significantly. These hormonal changes, caused by a decreased generation of oestrogen, can cause problems that are almost always very specific and directly personal.

Irregular bleeding often occurs just before the menopause, along with the infamous "hot flushes" and reddening of the skin. There may also be heavy perspiration, followed by shivering, a disturbed heart rhythm, dizziness and prickling sensations in the upper limbs (a result of disrupted circulation).

Beside that, there may be lack of sleep; nervousness; increased irritability; reduced levels of performance; states of fear and depression. Sometimes there may be metabolic disturbances; weight gain; increase in blood pressure; and osteoporosis (see relevant chapters).

All these problems are all the more pronounced, the faster the oestrogen levels fall. Doctors, therefore, usually administer oestrogen. Alternative practitioners go the opposite way. They ensure that the consequences of the hormonal change are offset by a conscious, natural way of life: balanced diet; avoidance of alcohol, nicotine, and caffeine; regular physical exercise, gym, swimming; and contrast baths. All of these measures may offset the above-mentioned problems.

Moonstone can be an additional help. It delays and harmonises the oestrogen drop, so that the change – over takes place with considerably fewer problems.

Practical application:

Wear as a bracelet, necklace or pendant for longer periods (necklaces are best)

Blue Chalcedony or **Ocean Jasper** is especially useful in acute occurrences such as hot flushes, dizziness, irritability and sleeplessness.

Wear them as a bracelet, necklace or pendant. As an alternative, take gem essence (5-7 drops, 3-5 times daily), or gem water (100–200ml taken in small sips over the course of the day).

Meniscus Problems
see Knee Problems

Menstruation Problems
see Period Pains

Middle Ear Inflammation

Middle ear inflammation is often caused by a cold or flu that has not been totally cured. As a result of the persisting infection, bacteria pass through the connection between the throat and the middle ear. Apart from inappropriate treatment of the disease (working instead of staying in bed) it can be caused by heavily polluted tissue. If this is the case, neither the immune nor the lymph system can fully cope with the disease germs, they are neither able to drain off toxic substances, generated as a consequence of inflammation and infections, nor to excrete them by via the normal route through the kidneys. This can be caused by heavy consumption of dairy produce, especially cow's milk. Modern mass rearing methods of milk cows involves a considerable use of antibiotics to the extent that such milk can only be digested with difficulty so building up antibiotic resistance in the body leading to the pollution and infection of body tissues.

If the body's normal healing process is impeded in this way, it tends to find some form of "emergency exit" through the ear. In this process, pus and toxic substances are excreted via the middle ear, building up until the eardrum splits and the resulting fluid escapes by running out through the ear. This is not only highly unpleasant for the infected person, it is also dangerous as the middle ear then provides an open and relatively easy access to the brain for disease bacteria, germs and other infections. The result can then be life-threatening cerebrospinal meningitis or encephalitis.

It is my earnest recommendation that dairy products from cow's milk ought to be avoided if at all possible. In addition, there should also be a regular programme of detoxifying and any of case of heavy colds and flu treated being seriously (see the relevant chapters), e. g. by staying in bed, the standard advice of the family doctor in the old days. (See also Colds; Flu).

Rinsing the mouth and teeth with organically produced, cold-pressed sunflower oil for some 10 to 20 minutes every day can provide further protection against such infection. This oil absorbs from the tissues any toxic and poisonous substances that might obstruct the function of the immune system. **But do not swallow the oil under any circumstances**; spit it out afterwards and rinse thoroughly with tepid water!

However, if the middle ear has indeed become infected and inflammation has already developed, with accompanying pain, fever and reduction of hearing, seek advice from a doctor or an alternative practitioner as soon as possible in order to avoid any further complications.

If the infection causes severe earache – which, annoyingly and frustratingly, often seems to occur late at night when it almost impossible or impractical to seek any immediate professional help – an effective but quaint "folk remedy" for relief involves placing small bags of raw onion on the ear.

You can also apply an ointment made up of 10 drops of gem essence mixed with 10 drops of Bach "Rescue Remedy" and 10 grams of a basis that consists of 1 part beeswax and 4-5 parts jojoba oil. The ointment is applied around the ear and it helps relieve pains quickly.

As ever, crystal therapy can complement and supplement the above treatments and precautions.

Heliotrope is the most effective crystal for dealing with middle ear inflammation. Small polished pieces of the crystal that have been drilled through with a small eyehole and a thread attached securely are known as "ear olives" These can be introduced into the outer ear carefully and left there until relief is obtained before drawing them out slowly by the attached thread. Great care should always be taken in this application and ear olives placed only in the outer ear.

A related method is to place a tumbled stone or a section/slice of Heliotrope over the ear itself.

Alternatively, take gem essence (initially, some 3-5 drops every 15 minutes, then every 30 minutes and finally around once an hour and at least 3-5 times daily); or drink gem water (up to 1 litre taken in small sips over the course of the day.)

Ocean Jasper can be used if Heliotrope is found to have no effect, or if it has not been applied in time to take effect. Ocean Jasper has a very strong detoxifying effect and apart from that also stimulates the lymph flow and strengthens the immune system. In this way the organism quickly succeeds in curing a middle ear inflammation.

If worn in the form of a bracelet, necklace, or pendant for a reasonable period, it ought not then need to be complemented by any proprietary "cures" for colds or other infections and it will also protect the wearer who shows any tendency towards recurring middle ear infection

For acute problems it can also be taken in the form of gem essence or gem water (the dosage being as above for Heliotrope).

Sardonyx also helps the healing process, especially in cases resulting in such effects as a reduced hearing.

Place an uncut or tumbled stone upon the ear; or wear as a necklace or pendant. Alternatively, take gem essence (5-7 drops, 3 times daily) or gem water (200–300 ml taken in small sips over the course of the day)

Emerald helps with chronic middle ear inflammation, which, while seeming less painful, is identified by period heavy fluid secretion and the onset of hearing difficulties.

In such cases, place an Emerald crystal or a tumbled stone over the ear; or wear as a necklace or pendant.

Alternatively, take gem essence (5-7 drops, 3 times daily or gem water (200–300 ml taken in small sips over the course of the day).

Migraine

Migraine is a very strong headache, most of the time, it affects only one side of the head and starts with a flickering before the eyes and sight disturbances, often accompanied by nausea and vomiting.

The pain itself is often rhythmic, throbbing and beating and is intensified by noise and light. A sufferer might also start sweating heavily, have palpitations, cramp, stomach ache, diarrhoea, sense disturbance and paralysis phenomenon.

Migraine results mainly from disturbances of the brain's blood circulation and blood vessels. These undergo rapid contraction and expansion, affecting the brain's hypersensitive nerves. This is experienced as the aforementioned unbearable pain and associated phenomena.

However, migraine can also be caused by the Earth's natural radiation or by electromagnetic pollution (e. g. microwave communication, power lines, radio clocks), metabolism problems in the liver, the gall bladder or the pancreas, and accumulated lymph or hormonal disturbances. Food, drink and tobacco (red wine, chocolate, cheese), climatic or hormonal changes

(e. g. during the menstrual cycle) can also trigger migraine fits.

In addition to all of the above, migraine is one of those afflictions that occur when one is totally stressed, unhappy, worn out, restricted by a strong sense of duty but with a crying need for relaxation. Migraines of this type often occur at exactly the moment when relaxation ought to be possible (often called "weekend migraine").

In order to reduce the number of migraine attacks, it is advisable to make relaxation, meditation and exercise a regular feature and part of one's life – and once in a while to detach oneself from ones duties. In this way, one does not necessarily have to pay the price of a strong headache for the right to peace and recreation.

Rhodocrosite is the first choice for acute migraine. Firstly, locate the medulla oblongata, the place under the back of the head where the spinal column passes through into the brain through an opening in the skull. It is relatively easy to find, as the spot is pressure sensitive. Then, place the Rhodocrosite crystal there and the migraine will ease off after a short time.

Emotionally, Rhodocrosite also helps one to recognise personal needs and to assert them. Wear as a necklace or pendant for this purpose.

Magnesite and **Amethyst** relieve migraine and reduce the tendency towards attacks if they are applied for lengthy periods. Amethyst helps first and foremost with migraines that occur in connection with climatic changes and during times of great personal changes. Magnesite is more helpful with migraines that are nutrition-induced or which recur regularly.

For both crystals, wear as a bracelet, necklace (the most effective) or pendant.

Ocean Jasper helps with migraine connected to metabolic disturbance, accumulations of lymph or detoxification. There is also a connection in this context with migraine that occurs shortly before menstruation. This is a result of the body releasing poisons and toxic substances at an increased rate in order to exploit the menstrual flow for the excretion of these substances.

Strangely, it is not necessary to wear Ocean Jasper especially close to the head or the neck in order to make it help with migraine. Crystals kept in a trouser pocket or around the bed have proved helpful help in many cases.

Minor Bleeding

Minor bleeding that is caused by cuts, scratches, scrapes, grazes or other similar kinds of injuries, can easily be healed with crystals. Obviously, standard first-aid measures should be applied as an initial priority and any further loss of blood needs to be prevented after more severe injuries.

Carnelian, Mookaite, Snowflake Obsidian, and Rhodonite all help stop minor bleeding. In addition, Mookaite and Rhodonite also support further recovery, with Rhodonite being regarded as by far the best. With the help of Rhodonite, small cuts and scratches are healed within a few seconds, so that an adhesive plaster is often not even needed.

The crystals mentioned above can be pressed directly on the wound in the case of minor lesions. Apply either uncut or tumbled stones, or slices/sections. Of course, in all cases, they should be cleansed and washed thoroughly beforehand. As a rule, bleeding will cease after a couple of minutes. Apply diluted gem essence (10 drops dissolved in 100 ml of water) or gem water for scrapes or grazes.

Mouth Problems

Problems in the mouth – such as furring, mouth ulcers, blisters on the tongue, inflammations of the mucous membranes, bad breath, plaque on the teeth and bleeding gums – are usually connected with diseases or infection of the airways, problems of digestion, metabolic disturbances, lack of oral hygiene or toxin-affected tissues (see also Detoxification).

The most effective treatment is gargling or rinsing the mouth and teeth with organic, cold-pressed sunflower oil for 10 to 20 minutes every day. This oil draws out from the body tissue the toxins and poisons which obstruct the work of the immune system. **Under no circumstances should the oil be swallowed**; spit it out afterwards and rinse the mouth thoroughly with lukewarm water! A definite, noticeable improvement of the above mentioned symptoms should be apparent after doing this just a couple of times.

Jet helps especially with oral furring, blisters, ulcers, general mouth inflammation, bad breath or bleeding gums.

Emotionally, Jet helps one to overcome any withdrawal and the reserve that may have arisen as a result of bad luck or suffering, enabling one to "open up" once more. This is connected with the mouth because the mouth features so strongly in human expressions of openness and interaction – such as eating, speaking, kissing, etc.

Chrysoprase and Smoky Quartz in combination, will, however, be more effective than Jet in cases of oral fungal infections (see also Fungal Infections).

Ocean Jasper is another important crystal in this context. It aids open-mindedness and conflict resolution. Besides that, it is also very effective with infected airways, inflammation and metabolic upsets. It has a detoxifying effect and stimulates the lymph flow, to the extent that mouth problems disappear rapidly.

For both Ocean Jasper and Jet, place a tumbled stone in the mouth; or wear as a necklace or pendant for a reasonable period of time. Alternatively, take gem essence (3-5 drops, 3-5 times daily) or gem water (200–300 ml taken in small sips during the course of the day).

Muscle Tension

Muscle tension can be caused physically by bad body posture, pain, inflammation, overwork (especially if not part of a daily norm). Emotionally, any involuntary tension resulting from mental pressure or anxiety can also produce tenseness in muscles, as will intense concentration over unusually long periods, for example, driving a car at high speed for several hours may also lead to muscle tension.

In fact, such emotional and psychological states are not for nothing described as one being "tense", or "strung out", in appropriate circumstances or when anticipating an event or a need to take important steps to change something.

See also: Cramp; Joint Pains; Muscle Injuries; Muscle Weakness

Crystals that are of help with tension not only have a relaxing effect on the muscles, they also promote emotional relaxation. Believe it or not, their effect on the muscles is so profound that even displaced vertebrae sometimes fall into place, or at least can be repositioned correctly much more easily, via the crystals' relaxing properties.

Amethyst relieves tension, especially if

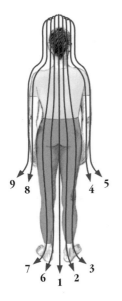

Fig. 12: Treatment with Amethyst
to relieve muscle tension.

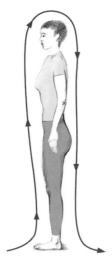

Fig. 13: Compensating movement
to stabilise the blood pressure.

used in the form of a druse the size of a saucer to stroke the body, as if using a brush, but without touching the body. The druse should be moved from the forehead, over the scalp, neck, back and the legs; then over the arms and downward to the floor (see Fig 12). Areas of the body, which are regarded as especially tense, can be treated in this way several times.

If the blood pressure falls very quickly because of the treatment, creating feeling of dizziness, then this has too be stabilised by means of a "compensating" movement of the crystal over the body. In other words, the stroking should be applied to the body's axis, starting at the front, passing over the head and downward along the back (see Fig. 13).

If Amethyst is worn in the form of a necklace, it will also relieve muscle tension and will help with the identification and negation of the emotional and mental causes of tension.

Magnesite has a relaxing effect on the whole muscle system. It helps overcome fear and grief and thus also brings about the required relaxation.

Place a tumbled stone on the affected areas or wear as a bracelet, necklace or pendant. Alternatively, take gem essence (3-7 drops, 3 times daily), or gem water (200–300 ml taken in small sips over the course of the day).

Smoky Quartz relaxes the whole body. Hold two crystals or tumbled stones in the

189

hands and allow yourself a couple of minutes rest. Alternatively or as a complementary treatment, place a crystal or a tumbled stone on affected muscles. If used in crystal form, ensure they point downward toward the feet or the hands.

Smoky Quartz also helps one to remain relaxed in trying times and reduces any innate tendency to become stressed. For this purpose, it can be worn as a bracelet, necklace or pendant.

Tourmaline crystals (in particular the small, narrow ones) of any kind help with tension. Emotionally, Tourmaline enhances a sense of mental flexibility and agility.

Place the crystals along the body axis or along the joints, pointing downwards. In this way, the energy flow is stimulated in the affected areas. In instances where the joints have also become stiffened by stress, wear the crystals as a bracelet, necklace or pendant.

Muscle Injuries

Muscular problems can range from aching and pulled muscles to actual tears in muscle fibre. All can be caused by undue strain on the muscles, or – in cases of severe injury – by sudden, excessive demands on an already taut muscle (e. g. stretching, squeezing and twisting).

Aching muscles can be best defined as being experienced as only temporary pain and/or stiffness. Such aches are caused by metabolic products of the muscles working without sufficient oxygen (with a resulting production of lactic acid) and inflammation and swellings on any small tears in the muscle fibres after extreme exertion. A hot bath (alkaline based) and physical exercise offer the best treatment for this type of pain relief.

Pulled muscles are caused by strain on individual muscle fibres. The symptoms are experienced as localised pressure and pain when moving the limb, very occasionally accompanied by slight bleeding. Truly severe pain may mean that there are major tears in muscle fibres. The application of a cold arnica poultice or compress should alleviate the pain.

The most serious form of muscular injury is full muscle rupture. Here, a substantial mass of fibres, or even whole muscles, are torn apart. This leads to stabbing pains, along with severe bruising, swelling and a substantial reduction of use or movement in the affected area. Treatment requires that the affected limb remains motionless along with the application of a cold arnica poultice. If necessary, in very severe cases, the torn muscles may even require stitches.

With the exception of merely aching muscles, any other form of muscular injury should be examined by a doctor – especially if a pulled muscle is suspected.

The application of crystal therapy is

helpful in all the above types of tears in the muscle fibres, as muscular injury nearly always results from such lesions.

Rhodonite is probably the best crystal to use. It relieves pain, swelling, and bruising and speeds up the healing process.

Place or tape a tumbled stone or a slice/section on the affected muscle; or keep it in place with a bandage.

As a supplement, take gem essence (to begin with, once an hour; later some 5-9 drops, 3-4 times daily) or plenty of gem water (up to 1 litre, taken during the course of the whole day).

Muscle Weakness

The signs of muscle weakness are that the muscles perform less well, become tired much too fast, and that there is an increasing lack of energy during strenuous work. These problems can be caused by overburdening, infections, bad nutrition or lacking *joie-de-vivre* and, more seldomly, through autoimmune diseases. In order to exclude these possibilities in connection with a continuous weakness of the muscles, one should be examined by a doctor or alternative practitioner. Any emotional cause, or lack of *joie-de-vivre*, should also be checked out by a therapist. When treating weak muscles the greatest natural therapy successes are obtained if one can rediscover the aims and goals, which previously awoke one's enthusiasm which have been gradually forgotten, and one begins to enjoy them anew. Enthusiasm is always the factor which helps best, when weakness has to be overcome, and new strength is to be found.

Garnet Pyrope and **Rhodonite** in combination is helpful in connection with weak muscles. Garnet Pyrope mobilises the energy reserves and stimulates the metabolism, circulation and muscle regeneration. Rhodonite is particularly helpful with infections and autoimmune diseases, as it regulates and normalises the immune system.

Emotionally, Rhodonite helps one to let go of lingering, hurtful feelings and pain, while Garnet Pyrope supports one's focus on new goals that arouse one's enthusiasm.

Hold Garnet Pyrope in each hand (as a tumbled stone or a crystal) and place Rhodonite on the thymus gland. The best time to do this is late morning. A Garnet necklace with a Rhodonite pendant, which hangs over the thymus gland, is also suitable, or you can wear as a bracelet, necklace or a pendant with body contact for a longer period.

Take gem essence (3-5 drops, 3 times daily) or gem water (200–300 taken in small sips during the course of the day).

Myopia

see Ametropia

Nausea

Nausea is not an illness, but a sensation that is itself a symptom of several different illnesses or functional disturbances of the internal organs. For example, it can be caused by the following: over-eating and irritation of the stomach (e.g. alcohol); stomach or intestinal diseases; various kinds of inflammation; poisoning; nerve and brain diseases; travel sickness; sun stroke; migraine.

Apart from the above, nausea can also be caused by unpleasant experiences, smells, disgust, grief etc. – in principle, therefore, by anything, the mere thought of which makes one feel bad.

See also: Stomach Problems; Vomiting

As nausea is an extremely non-specific symptom, it is best left to a doctor or an alternative practitioner to clarify its causes – as long as it is not caused by self-evident excessive consumption of alcohol or bad food.

Treatment at causal level is, of course, the first priority. Nevertheless, finding some initial relief in order to avoid any unnecessary discomfort is perfectly sensible and advisable.

Here are some crystals suitable for alleviating nausea.

Antimonite is good for all stomach problems with nausea and vomiting.

Aquamarine works best for nausea, which is a consequence of problems with the pancreas or general stress and anxiety.

Amber eases nausea arising from stomach, pancreas and gall problems.

Dumortierite relieves all types of nausea and the feeling of wanting to be sick. Make it your first port of call, if ever in doubt.

Heliotrope and **Pink Moss Agate** are the crystals to use with nausea arising from intestinal infections.

Magnesite for nausea caused by migraine or gall bladder problems.

Ocean Jasper for problems with the liver, gall bladder, intestine and pancreas or for nausea caused by worries, stress, anxiety or unresolved conflicts.

Turquoise can be applied for nausea caused by a wide range of stomach problems, including, vomiting or heartburn.

For all of the above, hold a tumbled stone, or place a flat slice/section, on the stomach. Or wear as a necklace or pendant, with direct body contact for the best results. Alternatively, take gem essence (8-12 drops in 100 ml water) or gem water.

Neck Pain

Neck pain nearly always results from tension due to a range of causes; for example incorrect posture, dislocated vertebrae, unfamiliar/new working postures and any involuntary strain of the neck muscles in connection with strain, emotional tension or stress. Even such activities as concentrating hard for rather long periods – for example, driving a car rather fast and/or for long distances – may cause neck tension.

Emotionally, the same effect can be the result of worries about any business, or anything causing worry that makes one feel uncomfortable and that gradually seems to become becomes ever more pressing or urgent.

Crystals are helpful with neck tension and have a relaxing effect on both muscles and emotions. They can be so effective that even dislocated vertebrae may sometimes slip back into place all by themselves – or, at least, prove easier to manipulate (only by a professional!) back into place.

Amethyst releases neck tension by means of a few calm stroking movements, from the back of the head and downwards over the neck, with a druse the size of a

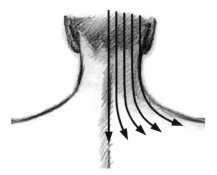

both sides, 3-4 times, repeating

Fig. 14: Amethyst treatment in cases of neck tension.

saucer. Use the druse as if it were a brush, but without actually touching the skin (see Fig. 14).

Make four or five parallel strokes from the centre of the head to the ear, and the neck tension will often disappear very quickly, especially if the treatment is repeated 3-4 times on both sides.

Amethyst worn in the form of a necklace will also help with easing the tension and it is also useful in enabling one to recognise and eliminate any emotional causes of the tension.

Amber, **Magnesite** and **Smoky Quartz**, especially if worn in the form of necklaces, can also relieve neck tension. They have a relaxing effect, physically and emotionally, so that it becomes possible to remain relaxed and calm, even in stressful situations.

Rhodonite, together with Magnesite and Bach's Rescue Remedy, are another great help in cases of neck tension.

Place the gem essence from the two crystals, together with the Bach remedy, (3-5 drops of each) into a glass of water, and drink this during the course of the day. Apart from that, one should take copious quantities of liquid. This combination will help the sufferer to let go of any fears and worries and so bring about a complementary emotional release.

Tourmaline in all forms helps relieve neck tension, especially in the form of small crystals rods. Place or affix them in some way onto the back of the head, pointing downwards. In this way, the energy flow in the rear of the head is stimulated, which, in turn, furthers relaxation and flexibility. Emotionally, the crystal enhances openness and mobility.

Nerve Pains

see Neuralgia

Nervousness

Nervousness is best described as any form of emotional tension. In other words, feelings of unrest, haste, clumsiness, hypersensitivity, irritability, disharmony, hyper-activity and impatience. As a rule, insecurity, pressure, fear, stress, excessive demands or unresolved conflicts are hidden behind such "nervousness". Any commonly ascribed state-of-nerves – such as stage fright – is often easier to overcome than true, basic nervousness. The latter lasts for a long time, and its true causes can remain unknown – often only be solved permanently with the help of a professional therapist.

Meditation is excellent in assisting the calming process, as are physical activities and exercises such as Tai Chi, yoga or forms of autogenic training.

Many crystals – indeed, too many to list here – have an alleviating effect, calming nervousness and encouraging a relaxed

attitude. Consequently, only the most effective and specific crystals are listed here.

Aventurine furthers inner peace, patience and relaxation in connection with stress and insecurity. It also helps particularly with irritability, over-sensitivity and a sense of emotional disharmony.

Amber brings freedom from cares and encourages a relaxed attitude, strengthens confidence and self-confidence – particularly when nervousness causes stomach ache.

Chrysoberyl relieves any form of nervousness that causes excessive haste and clumsiness. It is also very helpful in overcoming fears, and when one feels that too high a demand is being made and when one is under any kind of pressure.

Dumortierite helps one take things much more easily and relieves feelings of fear and insecurity. It is helpful in coping with heavy emotional burdens, obsessive behaviour and with problem solving.

Larimar is effective in cases of mood-induced nervousness or when one might sense that a "disaster" is approaching (one that other people have no inkling of). Larimar can enhance sensitivity to such subtle perceptions, but enables one to preserve a sense of inner peace and to deal more easily with the situation.

Magnesite eases nervousness that occurs alongside severe restlessness and hectic behaviour such as hyperactivity. It induces relaxation, calmness and helps in coping with anxiety, hypersensitivity and irritability.

Golden Topaz is the best crystal for last-minute nerves such as stage fright or before an important interview, examination, etc. It helps one feel secure and self-confident, strengthens the ability to express oneself and helps in facing up to public appearances in a relaxed way.

Hold a crystal (Chrysoberyl or Golden Topaz), or a raw or tumbled stone (Amber or Magnesite) in the hand for immediate effect; or wear as a bracelet, necklace or pendant for a longer period.

Alternatively, take gem essence (3-7 drops, 3 times daily), or gem water (100–200 ml taken in small sips during the course of the day).

Neuralgia

Nerve pains can occur as a consequence of a trapped nerve, pressure on or a squeezing of the nerves (e. g. as a result of conditions such as a slipped disc), by infection, poor circulation, poisoning and as a consequence of other diseases. Overall, nerve pains are categorised as neuralgia, neuritis and nerve degeneration

The chief symptoms of true neuralgia are sudden attacks of drawing, cutting, stabbing or boring pains – although the nerves themselves display neither anatomical changes nor functional failure.

The more serious inflammatory state of neuritis, depending on which nerves are directly affected, occurs together with pain, disturbances of sensation, paralysis phenomena and other functional disturbances.

In contrast, degeneration phenomena are often painless, although they are generally accompanied by signs of functional disturbance or failure. They are often responsible for numbness or partial paralysis.

Injuries of many kinds can also cause severe pains (e. g. in case of trapped nerves) and irritation. In the most extreme cases of fully severed nerves, there can be complete functional failure of a limb or specific areas.

In all cases of nerve pain, one should always consult a doctor or an alternative practitioner, in order to clarify the exact cause and to initiate relevant measures. Injured or inflamed nerves may, under certain circumstances, continue to react sensitively and painfully to the smallest irritations for a long time. However, it is something of a myth that nerve cells cannot be regenerated. On the contrary, nerves can indeed be regenerated, and can even be totally healed – and crystal therapy is a great help in this process.

Nerve problems can also be connected directly to emotional problems, inner conflicts, and any form of stress. Therefore, it makes sense to think seriously about what is "getting on one's nerves", and to identify any worries or problems that are preying on one's mind. Of course, such issues have to be tackled on an emotional level and, if necessary, with the help of a therapist. However, as with nerve pain from direct physical causes actual crystals can also be helpful.

Larimar is very helpful with neuralgia that occurs suddenly and unexpectedly, or where no recognizable pattern of attacks can be established. In addition, it helps organically sound but previously trapped nerves to regain their function after the actual cause has been eliminated but where function remains impaired.

Emotionally, Larimar helps to overcome over-sensitivity and panic attacks, particularly at times of dramatic change.

It is best to place a slice/section or a tumbled stone on the affected areas or on the areas where the nerves emerge. As an alternative, take gem essence (3-7 drops, 3 times daily) or gem water (100–200 ml taken in small sips during the course of the day).

Lavender Jade relieves recurring nerve inflammation and neuralgia after previous inflammatory states. Emotionally, it enhances a sense of harmony and inner peace.

Place a tumbled stone on the affected spot, or wear as a necklace or pendant for a longer period. Alternatively, take gem essence (5-9 drops, 3-5 times daily) or gem water (100–200 ml taken in small sips during the course of the day).

Kunzite and **Sugilite** also help with nerve pain of any kind, be it neuralgia or as a result of injury and its efficacy is only surpassed by Lavender-Jade in cases of an inflammatory state.

Emotionally, Kunzite and Sugilite help neutralise tension and improve one's mood. Kunzite helps primarily when compliance, humility and acceptance are necessary (e. g. in order to accept things that cannot be changed, without resistance), while Sugilite backs one up so that one can stick to one's point of view and initiate the necessary changes.

Their use and application are as described above for Lavender Jade.

Tourmaline assists in the regeneration of injured and degenerated nerves. Green Tourmaline in particular is most effective in cases of degenerative phenomena, whilst Pink Tourmaline is better for treating actual nerve injuries. Water Melon Tourmaline, which contains a core of pink and a coating of Green Tourmaline, is also a good choice – though if none of these specific varieties of Tourmaline are to hand, other forms can also be substituted to good effect.

Tourmaline is a dynamic, vibrant and vitalising crystal, helping to harmonise the body, soul, spirit and intellect as a whole.

Place or affix Tourmaline crystals (or small crystal rods) along the body axis or along the axes of the individual joints. The crystals should always point away from the head and towards the hands and feet. In this way, pain can be relieved and any disturbing sensation, numbness – and, sometimes, even paralysis – can be healed.

If no crystals or small rods are available, slices/sections and tumbled stones can also be placed on the affected spot, or bracelets, a necklace or pendant can be worn.

Also, take gem essence (3-7 drops, several times a day) or gem water (100–200 ml taken in small sips during the course of the day).

Neurodermitis

see Dermatitis

Nightmares

Nightmares are dreams that cause fear and are often accompanied by tossing back and forth whilst asleep, severe tension and heavy perspiration – when you wake up bathed in sweat. They are caused either by the unconscious processing of unresolved conflicts, emotions or impressions from previous experience; or by stories, literature, radio or TV, etc.

A remedy for nightmares, on a causal level, may be the clarification of any such conflicts and past experiences – and maybe an avoidance of further stimulating images! In addition, therapeutic help may

be needed – especially when the specific contents of dreams remain a worry when awake.

In addition, crystal therapy can help in dealing with nightmares.

Agate in the form of a section/slice beneath the pillow makes sleep deeper, calmer and more recuperative. Dream content also becomes more pleasant. If the Agate contains Rock Crystal, dreams can be remembered more easily, enabling one to relate more directly and cogently to their contents.

Amazonite relieves nightmares that occur in stressful periods of life and where there is a very clear and obvious connection to immediate daily situations. Extreme moodiness during the day and very troubled sleep at night are further indications for the use of this crystal.

First wear Amazonite around the clock, in the form of a bracelet, necklace or pendant. Later, when matters seem improved, wear it only during the daytime!

Chrysoprase helps with almost all types of nightmares, in particular with any including repeated themes or content. It is particularly effective with children, who may wake up at night, seeming disturbed and unable to orient themselves – even in familiar home surroundings and unable on occasions even to recognise either their parents, sisters and brothers. Chrysoprase liberates the brain from worrying and threatening images and lessens the fear of falling asleep again and having the same dream after waking up.

Place a tumbled stone of Chrysoprase under the pillow; or wear it as a pendant, necklace or pendant.

Ocean Jasper brings calming sleep with renewed energy and pleasant dreams. However, there may be a temporary worsening during the first few nights of its application and is caused by the processing off the inner conflict. If you can withstand this effect, it may be advantageous to go through the phase, as Ocean Jasper strengthens the ability to manage conflicts.

It is best to wear it as a bracelet, necklace, or pendant during the day and arrange it as a circle of raw or tumbled stones around the bed at night.

Nosebleeds

Nosebleeds occur because of lesions in the mucous membranes of the nose. The most common cause is a blow on the nose, or even blowing one's nose too vigorously. Dry inflammatory states or adenoids can also cause nosebleeds. Apart from that, nosebleeds can be a symptom of problems such as high blood pressure, arteriosclerosis, blood coagulation problems, infectious diseases (such as diphtheria, measles, or typhoid fever) and lack of vitamins K and C.

(It is worth noting that during puberty and adolescence, nosebleeds can also occur spontaneously, although the medial cause is still unknown.)

If nosebleeds are a result of one of the specific problems identified above, they should always be treated professionally. However, bleeding can normally be stopped by lying down and placing a cold compress on the nose and another at the back of the neck.

The following crystals can also be applied to ease nosebleeds.

Carnelian is recommended for regularly occurring nosebleeds and should be applied according to Hildegard von Bingen's advice, where a crystal (raw or polished) is placed into heated (if required, simmering) white wine. This is then taken during the course of the day. The tendency towards nosebleeds will dissipate after a short time with this treatment.

Rhodonite will stop acute nosebleeds, no matter what the cause. Simply place a section/slice, or a tumbled stone, on each side of the nose.

Taking gem essence (5-9 drops) or gem water (100–200 ml) will also staunch the flow of blood.

Numbness

Numbness can occur in specific areas of the body because of inefficient or lack of blood circulation, damaged nerves, or a general lack of energy supply. To be safe, one should, therefore, have the condition examined by a doctor, or by an alternative practitioner, in order to identify the exact causes and take suitable measures to alleviate the problem.

Crystals may also be of service here.

Rock Crystal helps with general numbness. Place naturally grown crystals on the body in such a way that they point towards the numb area. In this way, the affected spot and tissue receive energy, stimulating its transformation in the cells and in the metabolic process.

Pyrope Garnet helps with localised circulation problems and improves the distribution of energy in the whole organism.

Wear as a necklace or pendant, or place a raw or a polished crystal on the affected areas at regular intervals.

Tourmalines, particularly the pink variety or Watermelon Tourmaline, are the best of all crystals to apply in cases of numbness. They enhance the energy supply and the blood circulation of the affected are and even help regenerate trapped or damaged nerves.

Place a Tourmaline crystal, or pieces of crystal, along the axis of the body or the joints (they can also be fixed there with sticking plaster). They should always point away from the head and towards the affected area. If no crystals are available of the type mentioned above, other kinds of tourmaline can also be applied.

Also, wear as a bracelet, necklace or pendant; or take gem essence as a supplement (3-7 drops, 3 times daily), or gem water (200–300 ml taken in small sips over the course of the day).

Nystagmus

Nystagmus is an involuntary movement or quivering of the eye, usually horizontally. As a symptom of a disease, however, it can be accompanied by severely impaired sight, disturbance of the eye muscles, poor circulation, damage to the cerebellum and affected balance.

Extended periods of eyestrain, due to inadequate lighting conditions, can also cause nystagmus (one recognised as an occupational disease such as "miner's nystagmus"). However, this form is curable – so with any of the above symptoms immediate professional medical clarification is recommended.

Ideally, a holistic cure should be sought and in this connection, all the obvious factors come into play, i. e. plenty of fresh pure drinking water, getting plenty of sleep, reducing stress levels and muscle tension. Then in this context, the appropriate treatment for the specific complaint can begin (see Eye Problems; Cataracts; etc.).

Amethyst relieves nystagmus that is accompanied by severe muscle tension or nervous problems. A special treatment using pieces of Amethyst druse and tumbled stones is the best form of crystal therapy (see Eye Problems.)

Aquamarine helps particularly with nystagmus associated with severely impaired vision and with nerve and eye muscle problems.

Smoky Quartz helps particularly with nystagmus connected with stress, worry and anxiety – or when an existing condition is being made significantly worse by these types of concern.

Sardonyx is the most suitable crystal overall for nystagmus, however, as it has an alleviating effect on all the causes already described. It will also be an additional help if the sense of balance is also affected.

All of the above can be placed on the eyelids in the form of small crystals, or raw or tumbled stones.

Alternatively, they can be taken as gem essence (5-7 drops, 3 daily), or gem water (100–200 ml taken in small sips during the course of the day).

A combined treatment using several of the crystals has also been shown to have good results.

Start first with the Amethyst treatment (see Eye Problem). Next, hold two pieces of Smoky Quartz in the hands. Finally, place small pieces of Sardonyx or Aquamarine directly over the closed eyes. Ideally, this should be repeated every day preferably – or at least twice a week.

Obesity

see Weight Problems

Oedemas

Oedemas are accumulations of fluid in tissue, skin, mucous membranes, lymphatic vessels, or in organs such as the lungs or brain. They occur when the flow of lymphatic fluid from the blood into the tissues is a greater than the reverse process. As well as resulting directly from disturbances in the outflow from the lymphatic vessels, oedemas can also occur as a result of the deposition of toxins in the tissues, high blood pressure associated with a weak heart, weakened kidneys, general metabolic problems and any damage to the blood vessels resulting from allergies, inflammation or poisoning. The occurrence of oedemas shows the possibility of heart or kidney disease and so should always be checked by a doctor or an alternative practitioner. (See also Lymphatic Health.)

In addition to treatment at causal level (in consultation with the doctor or alternative practitioner), it is beneficial to stimulate the lymph flow in order to drain the tissues and ensure an adequate diet. As well as good lymph drainage, two crystals are recommended to support such treatment.

Blue Lace Agate stimulates the lymph flow and thus furthers draining and redirection of the tissue fluids back into the blood circulation. It also helps dissolve toxins deposited in tissues and accumulations in the lymphatic system, thus eases the draining of oedemas.

Ocean Jasper is a Chalcedony variety, which, because of imbedded iron compounds, also stimulates detoxification and enhances the immune system. It has a similar effect to Blue Lace Agate and so is even more effective at a causal level.

Place a tumbled stone or a section/slice of Ocean Jasper on the affected area, where there is an obvious indication of fluid accumulation. For prolonged treatment, lymph flow can be improved and stimulated by wearing Ocean Jasper as a bracelet, necklace or pendant.

As a supplement, take gem essence (5-9 drops, 3 times 5 daily) or gem water (200–300 ml taken in sips over the course of the day).

Operations

Whilst a vital part of medical practice, in the context of crystal healing and associated therapies, operations should be regarded as injuries to the body (see also Wounds).

However, unless undertaken in a total emergency, most operations are something we know about in advance and so there are other considerations to bear in mind. For example, extraction of teeth, removal of adenoids and warts, as well as surgery of the inner organs, are all forms of operation. Consequently, it is not the nature of the intervention that matters in itself, rather it is the very fact that an intervention of or in the body is being carried out which has an injurious effect – so it is very important that the body is prepared for any form of operation or surgery.

Before the operation: Basically, it all starts with the right mental attitude. Prepare your body; well in advance of the time that the operation is to take place. Find a quiet, comfortable spot and imagine that you are able, in your thoughts, to talk with your body, as if it were a person, Greet it and thank it for its good services. After all, you really do have a lot to thank your body for and it is part of your overall being. Tell it what actual operation is going to be performed and why. Do this in simple terms, as if you were talking to a sensible child. You can even ask its opinion.

The outcome will become self-evident during this inner conversation. Of course, such things as fear, worries and concern will crop up, and under no circumstances should you ignore or even devalue such trepidation. Rather than trying to pass off fears by saying, for example, "it's not that bad!", just acknowledge and accept them and confirm that you now know all about these reservations. Simply go ahead and ask your body how best you can support it, so that it can accept the operation and overcome it successfully. Moreover, do not be surprised by the apparent answers, for they can often be very specific – "get plenty of sleep", "take vitamin C", " eat a steak", etc. – and are definitely worth taking very seriously. Even if you feel truly ridiculous about such a conversation, it is still worthwhile – and more than once. It never hurts to have a few more similar conversations. You may even find out what is truly good for you but has hitherto remained hidden inside. In summary, you only need to ask.

Apart from this mental preparation – which has already been proved medically to contribute to vastly improved benefits and the success of operations and their outcome – there are still a couple of other precautions that can help. The timing of any surgery is very important. If at all possible (notwithstanding the ongoing pressures and difficult scheduling experienced by health services), use a lunar calendar and try to ensure that this is the time that the operation to will take place. Why? Because the Moon's precise position is very important for quicker and easier healing. In addition, wound healing is improved by a reduced consumption of animal protein (in particular dairy products) about four weeks before the operation, particularly if accompanied by a gentle programme of cleansing (see also Detoxification).

Chrysoprase can be used for this purpose, as it also relieves worries and fears about the operation.

Dumortierite, Rhodonite or **Sugilite** can also be applied to lessen any sense of fear – Rhodonite or Sugilite especially if the fear becomes very intense.

All four of the above can be worn as bracelets, necklaces or pendants during the weeks preceding the operation. It is almost certain that they will need to be removed during the operation (including dental treatment) and this request should be complied with readily. Indeed, they should not be worn under any surgical procedures as they may cause any anaesthetic to be much less effective – or not work at all!

After the operation: In the first instance, it is best to apply all the alternative rescue remedies such as Arnica (as a homeopathic treatment, and if at all possible and reasonable, as a poultice), then Bach Rescue Remedy.

Obsidian then provides additional help, if a tumbled Obsidian is held in the hand, or placed close to the operation wound, in order to dissolve shock from the injury on a cellular level.

Rhodonite or **Mookaite** can then be applied by placing a tumbled stone or section/slice of on the spot. Bracelets, necklaces or pendants, of Rhodonite or Mookaite will support the wound healing.

Beside that, if possible, take gem essence (5-9 drops dissolved in some water, every hour).

However, do NOT use Rhodonite or Mookaite if post-operational wounds are draining pus or are of a type that may not heal immediately. Instead, continue with Obsidian, which relieves and improves the healing process, but does not speed it up detrimentally.

Apatite can be used in a similar way after bones have been re-set, or after any type of bone operations, as it speeds up the re-fusion of the bones quite remarkably.

After any operation, it is a good idea to continue with a diet of reduced animal protein, until the wounds have healed well and before undergoing any reinstitution of detoxification measures.

Sardonyx is then suitable as it continues any part of the healing processes that may be incomplete and starts detoxification slowly and gently.

Chrysoprase may follow, but only after a week, in order to neutralise the medication and residues of the anaesthetic.

Both Sardonyx and Chrysopase are applied either externally to the body, or are taken in the form of gem essence (3-5 drops, 3 times daily) or gem water (Sardonyx about 100 ml, Chrysoprase about 20 ml daily).

Sugilite is also recommended for pain relief after operations. It is either placed of fixed on the painful or tender areas, or worn in the form of a bracelet, necklace or pendant.

Osteoporosis

Osteoporosis is caused by a reduction of bone mass and bone structure, causing bones to break more easily and even resulting in spontaneous fractures, under certain circumstances. Basically, it results from a disruption or cessation of the normal regeneration of bone so that the amount of newly generated bone mass does not correspond to the amount already broken down or degenerated. Although the basic mineral composition of the bones does not change, there is an overall loss of substance and strength.

The loss of substance is often connected with changes in metabolism or in hormonal balance. Women are especially prone to the condition as it is usually the hormonal changes, which occur during the menopause, along with reduced activity in the sexual glands and higher thyroid activity that result in osteoporosis. A lack or deficiency of calcium and vitamin D, plus certain types of medication (such as cortisone), can also be major factors, when body tissue has an excess of toxic deposits. Overall metabolism is thus impeded, and together with insufficient physical exercise, this also can contribute to osteoporosis.

Detoxification, which includes a diet without animal protein but rich in calcium and vitamin D, and appropriate physical exercise, are therefore the crucial factors in avoiding the onset of osteoporosis. Crystals too can be especially effective; especially those with significant calcium content such as Apatite, Aragonite, Calcite and Fluorite, all stimulate the body's calcium metabolism and encourage bone growth and health.

Apatite, as calcium phosphate is therefore the chief one of the four to be recommended, its chemical composition being similar to that of bone fibre. Its healing effect is particularly evident with fractures, where it stimulates the regeneration of new bone.

Fluorite is calcium fluoride and also enhances generation of new bone substance.

Calcite and **Aragonite** are forms of calcium carbonates and encourage absorption of calcium in the intestine. In turn, the metabolism then supplies the calcium to the body and so encourages the strengthening of the skeleton

All four crystals complement each other perfectly well and can also be applied together. Wear them as a necklace or pendant for a longer period, with direct body contact. In addition, take gem essence (3-5 drops, 3 times daily)

Pain

Injuries, inflammations, and damaged nerves can cause physical pain. The purpose of pain is twofold; firstly, to direct the mind's attention towards the affected area of the body in order to avoid further damage; and secondly (especially) to initiate measures that lead to healing and improvement.

Thus, simply taking pain-killing drugs is akin to removing the brake lights or internal warnings on one's car. However, if one understands the signal and solves the problems on causal level – with the help of a doctor or an alternative practitioner when necessary – pain-relieving measures can be a definite help of course. Nevertheless, it is best to employ remedies, which have no adverse side effects – healing crystals therapy, for example.

Beside that, there is another immediate treatment that does not involve crystals, but which relieves pain caused by external injuries such as cuts, scratches, abrasions, blows, strains, dislocations, sprains etc. This method involves "re-enacting" the whole incident of the injury's cause and is a consciousness-raising method that directs our attention, and consequently our life energy, towards the affected area and thus furthers the healing process. One repeats the injury exactly as it took place, where it took place and as quickly as possible after the incident. Of course, all this is done without hurting oneself again and sometimes requires repeating a couple of times. The pain suddenly increases, after which it decreases or even vanishes; this is the point at which one should stop.

See also: Gout; Joint Pain, Lumbago, etc.

Depending on the circumstances under

which a pain occurs, and where it is felt, there is a selection of crystals for use largely in connection with specific pains.

Rock Crystal can relieve pain very quickly. Take two crystals the length of a finger and place them pointing towards the aching spot, but so that their tips are also pointing diametrically opposite each other (see Fig. 15). In most cases, there is a spontaneous and initial increase in the pain, which then diminishes and gradually stops.

Pain is an accumulation of energy, so this method supplies even more energy, until the blockage is dissipated – explaining why, at first, the pain becomes worse before it fades away. This method is most efficient with pains that are caused by injuries, tension, nerves, muscle cramp, etc. In cases of stomach pain, however, avoid this treatment as the initial increase in pain can become too extreme.

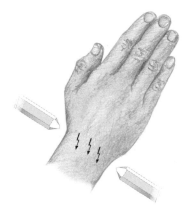

Fig. 15: Application of Rock Crystal in case of pain.

Double-pointed Rock Crystals, especially the bright "Herkimer Diamonds", can also be used, when arranged in a triangle around the tender spot they have a similar pain relieving effect.

Kunzite helps particularly with easing nerve pain, whether actual neuralgia or from a pinched or injured nerves. Typical signs are drawing, dragging gnawing and radiating pains (e. g. as in cases of sciatica).

Malachite relieves cramp and pains in the inner organs, in particular in the female reproductive system. As a result, it also applied in cases of menstruation problems and during the birth process (see also: **Childbirth; Period Pains**), Typical symptoms for applying Malachite are, therefore, cramp-like pains.

Pyrites relieve all types of pains in principle, except certain types of headache, and are particularly effective in cases of severe pain, such as lumbago or severe joint pain.

Rhodonite helps particularly with pain caused by external injuries such a cuts, abrasions, blows, dislocations, sprains, and during the healing of wounds. Typical of these are burning, sharp, stabbing and gnawing pains.

Sugilite relieves severe nerve pain and toothache. Its effect is somewhat slower than Kunzite but, on the other hand, it is stronger. Typical indications for the application of Sugilite are severe twinges, acute and throbbing pains.

Black Tourmaline, together with

205

Obsidian, helps to relieve sharp, acute and pressure pains – and especially with easily detectable tension pain.

Place a little tumbled Obsidian (its "Apache's Tear" form is the best) directly on to the tender spot and place four Tourmaline rods, pointing outwards, around it. The Obsidian dissolves the pain whilst the Tourmaline drains away the excess energy.

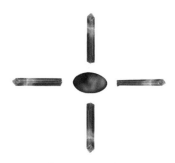

Fig. 16: Treatment of pain with Black Tourmaline and "Apache's Tear".

Zircon helps particularly with cramp and diffuse pain in larger areas, in particularly for pains of the inner organs (see Period Pains). Otherwise, dull, twinges, cramp-like and gnawing pains are typical indications for the beneficial use of Zircon.

For all of the above, except Rock Crystal placed or tape them on the aching area. They can be in the form of actual crystals (Kunzite, Zircon), raw stones (Pyrites), tumbled stones (Kunzite, Malachite, Rhodonite, Sugilite) or sections/slices (Malachite, Rhodonite). For safety reasons, place the Pyrites inside a cotton bag before

it is placed on the skin as iron sulphide in the Pyrites can react with perspiration and cause skin irritation.

Periodontosis

see Gum Disease

Period Pains

For many females, menstruation is often accompanied by pains, weakness, charged emotional states or other forms of discomforts. These problems can be caused by hormonal disturbances such as irregularities in the individual hormonal cycles, problems associated with the mucous membrane of the uterus, heavy bleeding and so forth

Of course, there are also emotional problems and reasons. Among these can be a general psychological "rejection" of the menstruation process and cycle itself. Women have even been known, on occasions, to refer to it all as "uncomfortable, annoying and unclean". The truth and expertise varies as widely as the actual number of females in the world, one can be sure of problems. But to some degree or other there can also be problems with a partner or family, with sex, feelings about overall femininity and womanliness, religious and ideological attitudes, etc.

Therefore, strong and repeated menstruation problems – so called "period pains" along with their emotional causes should be discussed with therapists, midwives or experienced women. As mentioned already, each case is always an individual one, needing an individual solution.

So, there can be many causes – including a possible association with the lunar cycle and consequent interaction between the Moon and menstruation cycles. Whatever the causes, symptoms and effects can all be relieved with the following crystals.

Agates containing a "uterus signature" relieve unusually heavy bleeding and provide emotional strength and stability. Agate also supports the desire for rest and withdrawal; and it helps create the space necessary for this need.

Place Agate sections or slices containing an appropriate signature directly on the body over uterus.

Biotite-Lenses help from the point at which discomfort first appears, all the way through to feelings of strong pain. Such pain may be experienced some time before the menstruation, often becoming worse, before subsiding with the actual onset of a period. Biotit-lenses relieve such problems and cause a faster and easier commencement of menstruation.

Lapis lazuli extends the menstruation cycle if it regularly starts too early. Emotionally, it also helps the sufferer to cope with any problems occurring with a partner or in the family. In so doing, it assists in open discussions of the problems.

It is best to wear Lapis lazuli as a necklace or a pendant.

Malachite relieves cramp pains, precipitates the start of any delayed bleeding and regulates the emotions. It can be used with both extended but light bleeding and for short, heavy bleeding.

Emotionally, Malachite assists in any problems associated with one's sexuality or femininity. It can bring out into the open many repressed feelings and experiences with which one has not yet come to terms. In so doing, it helps identify those issues that are best talked over with a person in whom one has full confidence.

In practical applications, one can place a tumbled or polished stone on the area over the uterus – or take gem essence (7-9 drops when necessary)

Moonstone helps bring the menstruation cycle into line with the lunar cycle, so that the ovulation takes place at full Moon and the menstruation starts at new Moon (unless personal predispositions conflict with this). Through this harmony of exterior and interior rhythms, tensions are broken down and menstruation is greatly eased. (It is also worth noting in this context that Moonstone also aids fertility.)

Emotionally, Moonstone helps a woman accept her femininity and to live with it with enjoyment.

You can place a tumbled stone in your bed or wear as a necklace or pendant for several lunar cycles.

Tiger Iron helps with feelings of weakness and lack of energy during menstruation. Emotionally, it also enhances strength, perseverance and resoluteness.

Place a triangle of Tiger Iron pointing downwards on the sacrum. However, in extreme cases, supplement this with gem essence (5-7 drops, 5 times daily) or gem water (200–300 ml taken in small sips over the course of the day).

Zircon helps with strong cramps and pains, and in particular when menstruation seems delayed and for stimulation if expected menstruation does not occur. Emotionally, it helps one to "let go" and overcome personal loss or dependence.

Place a Zircon crystal (preferably a double terminated form) on the area over the uterus, where it has a very strong effect. In view of its effectiveness, applications should not really exceed half-an-hour.

Piles

see Haemorrhoids

Pregnancy

In pregnancy, the initial hormonal changes, and later physical changes, may cause a number of problems and areas of discomfort. However, for the most part, these should not be regarded as any kind of "illness".

Sometimes, though, there is a need for support or relief and crystal therapy can be very helpful. In order to summarise all the conditions and applications during pregnancy, the information is presented here in the form of a table:

(See also: Childbirth)

Crystal	Effect	Practical applications
Kunzite	Acceptance of pregnancy and the mother role	Wear as a necklace or pendant. Take gem essence (5 drops)
Amber	In cases of worries and existential fear	Wear as a necklace or pendant. Take gem essence (7 drops)
Chrysocolla	In case of emotional crises	Wear as a necklace or pendant. Take gem essence (7 drops)
Dumortierite	Against nausea and vomiting and for patience and ease.	Wear as a necklace or pendant. Take gem essence (7 drops)
Moon Stone	In order to ease the hormonal changes	Take gem essence (5 drops)
Garnet Pyrope	In order to ease the metabolic changes	Wear as a necklace or pendant

➤→

Crystal	Effect	Practical applications
Agate (Water Agate or Uterus Agate)	Furthers the growth and the function of the uterus and protects the unborn child	Carry a tumbled stone, which can be placed on the stomach in the evening
Pink Tourmaline	For stability and contact with the unborn child	Wear as a necklace or pendant
Hematite, Tiger Iron	Against lethargy, tiredness and lack of iron	Wear as a necklace or pendant at first. Take as a supplement gem essence (5 drops) later
Rhodo-crosite	Stimulates the blood circulation in cases of exhaustion	Wear as a necklace or pendant for a short time
Blue Lace Agate	Drains oedemas (accumula-tions of fluid) in the body	Place a tumbled stone on the affected areas and take gem essence (5-7 drops). Wear if necessary as a necklace or pendant
Agate (Eye Agate or Lace Agate)	Prevents varicose veins and helps the blood vessels to regenerate	Place a tumbled stone on the affected areas. If necessary, wear as a necklace or pendant

Prostate Problems

The prostate is the male sexual gland about the size of a walnut and located near the urethra and underneath the bladder. The two sperm ducts leading from the testicles to the urethra pass by the prostate, the function of which is primarily to release an alkaline secretion during ejaculation. This is needed in order to neutralise any acidic urine residue and, in this way, to secure the mobility of the sperm-containing semen.

With increasing age, enlargement of the prostate may occur because of hormonal changes and can often lead to considerable problems, particularly if the urethra becomes increasingly narrow.

In the first stages, it often causes diffi-culties in emptying of the bladder (stimula-tion stage). Then, in the second stage, the resulting enlarged bladder cannot be emp-tied sufficiently, which can lead to the risk of inflammation from urine residue. Finally, in the third stage, the elasticity of the bladder is totally lost. This leads to a condition termed overflow incontinence, where urine is released constantly, drop by drop – but with accumulated urine remain-ing within the urethra that can damage the kidneys – an extremely dangerous situa-tion.

Screening is now available for reduced prostate function where a doctor or practi-tioner is able to motor blood and urine levels of PSA (prostate specific antigen) and it recommended for all men over the age of 50 even where there are no immediate symptoms.

In some cases the emotional factor of sexual insecurity also contributes to prostate problems. For example, in the second half of a man's life, changes in partnerships, feelings of, or actual, reduced ability to achieve things or deep discussions about subjects such as the meaning of life and death often cause changes in self-image. In turn, such readjustments can have an influence on one's sexuality and so the function of the sexual organs, including the prostate, may well be affected. Thus, in addition to screening, trying to identify any such psychological and emotional background – if necessary, with the help of a therapist – can be of great assistance. Of course, having one's sexual needs fulfilled, as one gets older, also seems to be one of the best remedies against an enlarged prostate!

Agates or **Ocean Jasper** with an eye signature (concentric rings), as well as tubular crystals of Agates, can be applied at the early stages of the enlargement process. Placing a section/slice or a tumbled stone over the base of the penis has been shown to prevent further enlargement, or even to reverse the process.

Zoisite can be applied at all stages of the condition and may contribute to the reversal of the process. It is also helpful for clarifying emotional problems, as it also sup-

ports the retention and sense of one's own value and self-confidence during any aged-based changes in one's sex life.

Ruby helps one to overcome sexual insecurity, especially in combination with Zoisite.

For Zoisite and Ruby, place a tumbled stone regularly on the base of the penis – although it is also helpful to wear them as a necklace or a pendant. In addition, take gem essence (5-7 drops, 3 times daily).

Psoriasis

Psoriasis is a non-contagious skin disease that is characterised by flat, irregularly shaped, sharply delimited and partially itchy, reddish areas. These are covered with flakes of silver coloured dry skin cells that are easily scratched away. However the exposed, fresh skin is subject to spot-like bleeding. The elbows and the knee joints, the chest and the back, the hairy scalp and the fingernails are all especially susceptible areas.

Psoriasis tends to follow a chronic, phase-based pattern of spreading and in about 4-5% of cases is accompanied by chronic inflammation (*Arthritis psoriaca*), which causes very painful swellings of the joints, particularly in the fingers and toes.

Infections, damage to the skin, metabolic disturbances and hormonal changes (e. g. at the beginning of menstruation or during and after pregnancy) appear to encourage or intensify the outbreak or spread of the disease.

The reddish patches occur because there is a high level of renewal and detachment of the skin in its upper layer. All this points to a disturbed cell metabolism, which, in turn, is caused by tissue that is impaired by an accumulation of toxic waste deposits and that is under-supplied with nutrients (see Detoxification).

However, this alone does not explain the stubborn persistence of the disease, which resists both conventional and alternative treatments. It seems as if emotional causes also play a role here, something about which there has been much speculation.

When we take into account that skin is the largest human organ in direct contact with our environment, along with the fact that many internal processes are mirrored in the health of skin, it seems unlikely that there is any one single cause for psoriasis. Therefore, it has to be assumed that the emotional element of the cause of psoriasis is different in each case and from one individual to the other. Nonetheless, its one common characteristic remains its stubborn persistence!

So, the question arises as to whether there may be a particular and high degree of stubbornness in our lives, thoughts, feelings and actions? Or, to put it another way, which changes do we resist most stubbornly? As the maintenance of a healthy state equates with the ability to change oneself, the onset of disease can often mean resistance to change – and, in this case, a particularly stubborn resistance.

Obviously, questioning oneself in this way can lead to some totally different areas of one's life. Yet, interestingly enough, this type of insight (e. g. into overall therapeutic methods and practices) have been shown to clarify and identify such areas of resistance and have already led to real improvement in many cases of psoriasis.

A holistic, alternative treatment of psoriasis should, therefore, also include already identified and as yet undiscovered emotional or psychological causes. On the physical level, detoxification is the most important procedure, and this is where crystal therapy can play its part.

Chrysoprase has turned out to be one of the most effective crystals in this respect

Aventurine and **Green Zoisite** are the next best choice, as both are especially suitable because of inclusions within the crystals of a silvery platelet signature.

Antimonite, however, is *the* most important treatment for psoriasis. It is a chemical compound the two interesting elements antimony and sulphur.

The latter is known to be cleansing element with profound effects and is applied both in traditional medicine, in order to bind toxic substances, and in homeopathy for the holistic cleansing and solution of stubborn processes. (The traditional dosing with brimstone and treacle is a case in point, where 'brimstone' is the old name for sulphur.) Its further strength is evident in its ability to combine with antimony, an element, which usually displays considerable "unwillingness" to form compounds.

Antimony is diamagnetic, i. e. it does not orientate itself to the Earth's magnetic field, but, instead, always takes up a position at right angles to the field. As already noted, it is only very 'reluctantly' bound – except with sulphur. It even has explosive modified forms and expands physically upon solidification from its liquid sate (rather like ice from water). As Antimonite, its most common natural form is that of needle-shaped, radial aggregates. These seem to point in all directions, as if it were trying to express a need to escape from everything. It is as though it represents a stubborn reluctance to be bound in any sort of conventional framework. This is a characteristic which one often meets in connection with psoriasis – for where else should this display of resistance against a framework or restrictive shell show up than in the skin. After all, our skin is indeed our 'shell'!

Antimonite is applied primarily in the form of gem essence (5-7 drops, 3 times daily), or as gem water (100–200 ml taken in small sips over the course of the day).

It can also be applied externally, where a piece of Antimonite is immersed in clean water for a whole day before 20 drops of sulphur essence are added per litre of this water. The affected spots should be moistened with this liquid several times a day.

Psychic Protection

Feeling the need for protection arises when conflicts, arguments, negative situations, apparent coercion, contrary influence and the actions of others or unfortunate experiences have such an overwhelming effect that one's own energies do to not appear adequate to handle it all. Problems of personal space in large crowds, as well as technological, radiation or electromagnetic influences and pollution may also result in feelings of an increased need for protection.

So, whilst protection may be necessary at certain moments or specific times, it is by no means a long-term solution. Instead, it is more important to find a solution to problems or conflicts at a causal level. This involves working on increasing personal stability; resolution of conflicts and of negative external influences and can be achieved by staying calm whilst still expressing one's own point of view in an open-minded manner. At the same time, it also means acquiring knowledge of any physical or spiritual connections, in order that one has a greater control over areas of conflict and no longer feels like a victim of external circumstances.

This "internal protection" can only be gained through personal, individual energy and abilities. However, under certain circumstances, this may have to be developed through instruction and with the help of a therapist. Until it has been developed, crystal therapy can also help protect against external influences, although used as the sole remedy, they tend to have rather a weakening effect in the long term.

Crystals in therapy are never intended to create dependence. In this context especially, a distinction has to be made between the "shielding crystals" – those that protect against external influence – and the ones that have a strengthening effect, and help one obtain stability and develop one's own skills. The real, overall goal is always to end the need for any kind of remedy once therapy is completed – and this includes the use crystals as much as any another form of help.

Agate encourages the development of one's own abilities and strengths. In particular, Agates with concentric rings (so-called Eye Agate) further inner concentration and centring. This leads to a higher degree of stability in dealing with external influence and helps maintain a point of view during arguments. So, Agates help build internal protection using one's own energies.

Obsidian used in the form of a tumbled or polished stone, acting as a mirror to reflect negative mental and technological pollution or influences of all kinds. Place it close to windows and locations where the influence is felt or suspected to be. Point in the direction of the source of the power

(according to one's feelings or after taking actual scientific measurements). However, do **not** wear Obsidian on the body as it can have the effect of creating feelings of inner turmoil and disquiet!

Serpentine has a protective effect in situations where you might feel uncomfortable, in crowds and in cases of verbal aggression or psychic attacks. It creates external protection – but should not be worn for too long, as it sometimes makes one *too* compliant and ready to compromise ("for the sake of a quiet time"). It is best worn as a pendant or necklace or, if required, held in the hand as a tumbled stone. Alternatively, place it on the solar plexus, the throat or the kidneys, depending upon where the external threat is felt.

Turquoise also provides an initial external protection. However, it then provides inner protection as it dissipates any tendencies to "give in" and enhances strength and courage to take matters into one's own hands. In this way it is has a more comprehensive effect than Serpentine.

Turquoise works best as a pendant or a necklace worn on the solar plexus, though not for too long in order to avoid it becoming too much of a habit.

Black Tourmaline helps in making a person less susceptible to negative external influences, whether physical, emotional or psychological, thus avoiding direct resistance and simply allowing energetic and spiritual effects to flow through. It removes obstacles in the body's energy pathways and also creates internal protection by inducing a state of unassailability

Wear it either as a necklace or pendant. If in an actual crystalline form, ensure that the pendant points downwards, or carry it in a pocket, again with the point downwards.

Revitalisation/Regeneration

Revitalisation – or "regeneration" (Latin: *regenerati* "rebirth") – is a return to an original, healthy and harmonious state of well being. Physically, regeneration means renewal or rejuvenation of our cells, tissue and organs. Emotionally, it means a return of strength and abilities and an improvement of the general mood.

Regeneration is an ongoing, daily necessity, for both mind and body, after the hardships, trials and tribulations of the day. Of course, sleep provides us with our most important period of such regeneration It is the mental equivalent of food digestion, whereby the daily input into our senses and brain – and the subsequent processing of daily impressions, experiences and information that remain incomplete or unresolved whilst awake – can be finished, sometimes in the form of a dream.

If this form of essential regeneration and emotional relaxation is there every day, one can remain vital, healthy and rejuvenated and not feel "worn out". (See also Sleep

Disturbance.)

Second only to this is any form of valid and positive emotional recreation. If we neglect the daily renewal process or carry it out only inadequately, then the mind and body will, sooner or later, demand longer breaks and periods of rest. Thus, taking a break or a holiday can be the real alternative to becoming ill and feeling worse and worse. During such holidays, sport and physical exercise can have a real recreational effect – as long as there is no serious competitive pressure and personal enjoyment and limitations are respected.

If getting away is impractical or there is financial difficult, one should at the very least rest and relax, concentrating on personal well being and avoiding excessive physical and emotional strain.

Everyone has periods in his or her life of heavy stress and pressure. There may be conflicts that are hard to resolve, serious physical illness or injuries, problems in personal relationships, study or at work, etc. Naturally, all these demand extra amounts of time for recreation if they are to be held in check and not to have a detrimental effect.

Yet, all this cannot be taken for granted. For example, the resumption of old habits at the end of an illness will often cause an immediate relapse. During or after an illness, avoid any emotional stress, severe pressure or activities that cause lasting tiredness or exhaustion, always give in to the feelings and need for physical and emotional regeneration. Healthy food that is rich in vitamins, daily walks, relaxing baths, sufficient sleep and time on one's own are all very important in this revitalisation process.

Crystals that speed up the regeneration and revitalisation processes can be very supportive – although without the application of the above programmes of self-healing, they cannot by themselves bring about a full recovery and their use alone will only have a short-term effect.

Epidote helps revitalisation after times of great strain and/or severe illnesses. It is a particularly good choice for feelings of total exhaustion or an inability for even the simplest activity. Emotionally, it helps one to regain a sense of a healthy and happy existence and to revitalise forgotten ambitions, goals and ideals. In this way, feelings of courage, strength and confidence for the future will return.

Ocean Jasper detoxifies and (through stimulation of lymph flow) boosts the nutrient supply to the body tissue along with the removal of toxic waste. In this way, it contributes to basic cell renewal and physical revival. In addition, it fortifies liver function and so provides both physical and energetic improvement. In parallel, it also strengthens emotional renewal and brings new hope and courage and has even been described as the "crystal bringing with it the energy of waking up on a spring day".

Rutile Quartz furthers cellular renewal and thus also the regeneration power in the all cells and organs. In addition, it brings hope during very difficult periods, when everything seems dark and hard to take. It helps one to "think big" and to view the true situation from a more subjective point of view. A resulting, but simple, change in attitude often serves to bring about a new sense of strength and confidence in the future.

Zoisite, especially forms containing Ruby, encourages regeneration during sleep of cells and tissue after an inflammation or severe illness. It enhances recovery from any exhausting, strength-draining efforts or experiences.

For all of the above wear as a bracelet, necklace or pendant. They may all be used to complement and enhance the effect of other relevant crystals during the overall healing process. Additionally, or alternatively, take as gem essence (5-9 drops, 3 times daily) or gem water (200–300 ml taken in small sips over the course of the day).

Rheumatism

Rheumatism is a broad term that covers painful changes and/or functional disturbances in the joints and sinews, muscles or in the connective tissue. In the former, it is more correctly termed rheumatoid arthritis and in the latter, soft-tissue rheumatism. However, both types involve a chronic inflammatory processes connected with deterioration of the autoimmune processes, excessive protein intake and acidification (uric acid accumulation). Consequently, a diet free of or low in animal protein and regular detoxifying measures are preconditions for a cure. (See also: Detoxification)

Rheumatoid arthritis often develops intermittently with joints on the hands and feet being particularly affected. It begins with painful inflammations in the inner part of the joint, with synovitis and inflammation of the joint's mucous membranes, leading to severe stiffness and pain. Following this, there may even be direct damage to cartilage and bones, which further limits and hinders movement. Then, as the disease progresses, other joints and even the spine may also be affected.

The fact that the condition first affects peripheral parts of the body indicates that our organism is trying to keep the causes as far as possible away from central, vital organs such as the liver, spleen, lymph nodes and the heart. In order to prevent such a spread, one should undergo professional medical treatment where further measures can be initiated to de-acidify and cleanse the affected tissues.

Emotionally, rheumatism often goes hand in hand with feelings of frustration, bearing a grudge, suppressed annoyance or anger or any sort of thing that can lead to a sense of bitterness – the psychological equivalent of physical acidification. Long, unhappy periods, particularly if one's mobility and freedom are limited, seem to increase the physical symptoms of rheumatism. In such circumstances, any way of removing such mental barriers is a positive step, if necessary, with the help of a therapist.

In applying crystal therapy as a part of the treatment of rheumatic illnesses, it has been shown that those which have turned out to be particularly effective have both a detoxifying, de-acidifying effect and the beneficial property of creating harmony, emotional balance and freedom. So, they should, be employed not only during the acute phase of a rheumatic attack, but also as part of the long-term treatment, in order to change the basic physical and emotional environment of rheumatism.

Amber relieves both the pain and the underlying inflammation of stiff joints and limits the subsequent damage. Furthermore, it encourages a calm and cheerful disposition, brings about a sense of freedom from care and helps in letting go any frustrations and anger.

Place a raw or a tumbled piece of Amber on the tender areas; or wear a necklace or pendant with direct body contact. Also, take gem essence (in acute cases, 3-7 drops every half hour; then later 3 times daily).

Chrysoprase stimulates detoxification of tissue and is the best choice for a long-term treatment that can eliminate the causes of rheumatic disease. Emotionally, it brings worries and suppressed annoyance into the open and so helps in their elimination.

Place a tumbled crystal on the tender or painful spots or wear as a necklace or pendant during periods when there are no rheumatic problems. Alternatively, take gem essence (3-5 drops, 3 times daily).

Malachite relieves pain arising from acute rheumatism, as it detoxifies and de-acidifies the affected areas very rapidly. Emotional causes, such as annoyance, anger and frustration are often brought into the open very dramatically with Malachite. Nevertheless, such spontaneous outpourings can help to vent one's anger in a fundamental and complete way, so that, afterwards, there are only feelings of relief and freedom.

Place a tumbled stone or a section/slice on the tender areas. A short, intense pain may be experienced to begin with, but it will considerably shorten the total time that pain is experienced.

As Malachite is particularly suitable in the treatment of an acute attack, it combines well with the use of Turquoise.

Turquoise also has a pain-relieving and detoxifying effect. It helps rheumatic problems to dissipate gradually and contributes to a complete and long-term cure from the disease. Turquoise neutralises acidification and thus changes the body's own long-term environment. Used in combination with Malachite, it has a stronger effect in reducing inflammation.

Turquoise also helps in dealing with frustration, bitterness and extreme emotional ups and downs by inducing a sense of balance and inner, as well as outer, harmony.

Place a tumbled crystal on the tender areas in cases of acute problems or wear as a necklace or pendant during periods when there are no rheumatic problems. Alternatively, take gem essence (3-5 drops, 3 times daily).

Green Tourmaline is helpful, both in the early and progressive stages of rheumatism. It detoxifies, de-acidifies, adjusts the metabolism, impedes inflammations, relieves pain and furthers the regeneration of affected joints, muscles, or organs.

Emotionally, Green Tourmaline is helpful in dealing with sadness, frustration, long-lasting unhappiness, impatience and bitterness. It encourages us to find new perspectives, to see life from new angles and to develop a new interest in others and in our surroundings and our own life.

It has a swift, pain-relieving and revitalising effect, especially if a crystal or section is placed in front of a torch and the resulting green-coloured beam is directed on to the affected areas. Depending on requirements, this treatment can be carried out 3-7 times per day for 5-15 minutes.

In addition, it can be worn as a bracelet, necklace or pendant. Also, take gem essence

(5-7 drops, 3-5 times daily), or gem water (100–300 ml taken in small sips over the course of the day).

Rocky Mountain Fever

see Tick Bites

RSI

see Tennis Elbow

Sadness

see Melancholia

Scars

Scars are formed as a natural process of the skin in order to substitute for lost or damaged tissue after injuries or inflammations. They consist of coarse, white connective tissue with many fibres, but with few cells and blood vessels. Scar tissue has much lesser elasticity and overall resilience than normal connective skin tissue. Furthermore, it often has a very deleterious effect on the blood circulation and supply of natural energy to neighbouring tissues and organs. This is especially the case with scars that lie transversely to the body's basic axis and four limbs. If nerve pathways have also been interrupted, this may cause problems with the sense of touch, and numbness can occur.

Scars and resulting skin malformations are often accepted as being unchangeable visible features. However, this is not necessarily so. Even with quite old scars, the actual scar tissue can be partly changed into a version that is much more efficiently supplied with blood, nutrients and the body's energy.

Any scar, even if involving severed nerves, can be healed with the help of crystals.

Chrysocolla is very effective in cases of large, lumpy scars, even if they are relatively old. As a mineral rich in copper and silicic acid, it stimulates the regeneration of skin and tissue, so that they can be transformed into a healthy form.

Place a polished section/slice on the scar, fixing it with sticking plaster if required. Then, take either gem essence (3-5 drops, 3 times daily) or gem water (100–200 ml taken in sips during the course of the day) at the same time.

Rhodonite helps particularly with transforming the tissue of deep scars and fresh wounds. It improves blood circulation and encourages the formation of new cells – sometimes to the point that no scar forms at all.

Its application and use are as detailed above for Chrysocolla – but it can also be worn in the form of a bracelet, necklace or pendant.

Tourmaline in particular can be applied in order to stimulate the flow of energy through scars that have a blocking effect, to improve the formation of nerves in the tissue and to heal cut nerves. The crystals or rods should always point away from the head and towards the hands or the feet, in order to stimulate the nerves (in cases of numbness etc.). In cases of a blocked flow of energy the point should point upwards on the front of the body– but downwards on the back (Fig. 17). All types of Tourmaline can be applied for this kind of treatment. The most suitable ones, however, are watermelon tourmalines.

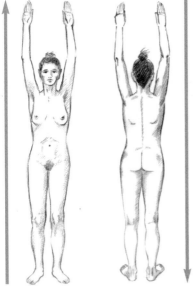

Front: Back:
Energy flow upwards   Energy flow downwards

Fig. 17: Energy flow patterns in the body.

Sea Sickness

see Travel Sickness

Sexual Problems

Sexuality is one of the basic human needs and a sexual relationship that is harmonious and satisfying contributes substantially to a happy loving relationship. If the needs and desires of both partners can be lived openly and with sensitivity there is hardly anything that creates more joy in life.

Unfortunately, for many reasons, sex is often burdened with more problems than with actually creating happiness – and there are a host of phenomena that are involved in causing such a contradictory situation. An upbringing which is hostile towards desire and the body, seemingly meaningless moral principles, unpleasant experiences, abuse, fears (including those of unwanted pregnancy), communication problems within relationships, conflicts between the two people in the partnership, inhibitions, pressure to perform, fear of sexual failure, withholding fantasies and wishes, feelings of guilt and perpetual myths ("men are only interested in one thing", "women never feel desire", etc.) all impede the joy of sex and turn it into a battleground or arena of conflict.

Therefore, the real solution to overcoming sexual problems is the need for clarification of the causes, which can be

219

achieved through having an open dialogue with one's partner or with the assistance of a therapist.

See also: Impotence

The crystals listed below can, however, serve in raising a desire for and a delight in sex. As well as improving sexual activity, increasing pleasure and enjoyment, they also improve the physical and emotional preconditions for a truly fulfilled sexual life.

Fire Opal furthers erotic attraction, it encourages the unrestrained acting out of one's desires and brings pleasure in sex. It makes one spontaneous and impulsive and quickly dispels disturbing thoughts, bad moods, feelings of guilt and other inhibitions. It is also helpful with impotence and lack of orgasm – however, it should not be used if there is a tendency towards premature ejaculation!

Garnet Pyrope helps one to overcome inhibitions and taboos, in particular when obsolete or seemingly meaningless moral views lie at the root of the problem. It furthers an active, harmonious sexuality and is helpful with potency problems, frigidity, any sense of disgust and an antipathy towards sex.

Malachite is helpful with sexual problems that are based on any unfortunate or negative previous experiences. It will identify any lingering fears and injurious images, bringing them to the light and helping one to talk about them. In this way, it also supports therapeutic processes and

eliminates feelings of shyness and bashfulness, helping to express and to act out sexual wishes and needs.

Rose Quartz furthers sensuality, romance and tenderness – and helps to overcome sexual problems by enhancing empathy and openness with a partner. It also improves circulation in the genitals and thereby increases a sense of sexual desire.

Ruby can bring a new passion into the greyness of every day life making it easier to let go of pressure to perform and alleviate false expectations and fears about failure. It stimulates an active sexuality and brings about a comfortable well being and pleasurable feeling about sex.

Rutile Quartz encourages a fulfilled sexuality, where fear and feelings of guilt create problems. It helps particularly with sexual problems that are the consequence of extreme tension, e.g., problems with potency or premature ejaculation.

Serpentine furthers gentle, tender sexual activity and relieves stress, fear and nervousness. It also helps women who could not previously achieve orgasm because of their feelings of tension during sex.

Thulite improves desire, sensuality and sexuality. It furthers the acting out of one's own wishes and fantasies and helps one to overcome any deeply-rooted blockages resulting from previous negative experiences, an upbringing that is hostile towards sex, feelings of guilt, the pressure to perform, outright fear and the detrimental effect of bad moods. It helps in attaining a more relaxed and natural attitude towards sex, and makes it possible for men in particular, to "let themselves go" for once.

For all of these crystals, wear as a bracelet, necklace or pendant; or place a tumbled stone under the pillow. Besides that, a well-known and much appreciated ploy is to spend time in a circle of Thulite crystals (raw or tumbled) arranged around the bed!

Shock

In medical terms, "shock' is used to describe two different processes.

Firstly, there is shock to the circulation – an acute, life-threatening breakdown of the blood circulation. This can occur because of actual loss of blood or body fluids, a breakdown or collapse of the kidneys or the heart, chronic infections, severe lack of blood sugar, extreme allergic reactions (anaphalactic shock) or severe injuries. The obvious signs in cases of this type of a shock are skin pallor, cold sweats, nausea, a fast but weak pulse, shivering and feelings of cold, fear, restlessness and confusion. After immediate first aid precautions – the staunching of bleeding, for example – place the affected person in a supine position with the legs raised and **call the emergency services as soon as possible.** Avoid any panic or excitement and try to speak calmly and quietly to the patient.

Secondly, there is psychological shock. This leads to an emotional disturbance, probably without severe physical injury, but with symptoms similar to physically-induced shock. This is because it too leads to disturbances of the circulation, with a subsequent lack of oxygen to the brain, shivering, fainting, hot flushes, confusion, disorientation, excitability or rigor. One should take the same first aid precautions as with physical shock, but there are additional methods that can be applied to rapidly relieve the effects of the shock. The first of these precautions, after first aid, is to bring the person back to normal consciousness. The fact is that emotional shocks can lead to a situation where the affected person is still "stuck" in the frame of mind in which the incident of shock occurred. Their consciousness has therefore to be disassociated from the incident and be directed towards the present. This can best be done gently but by asking them to repeat what you have just said to them

The procedure may have to be repeated a couple of times, until the affected person is – often suddenly – able to repeat your last words, indicating a return to normal consciousness and the present and can then be spoken to calmly and answer coherently. It is often then useful to continue with gentle instructions such as: "Put your hands down and feel the ground"; and when this has been competed successfully adding something like: "Press the ground firmly!"

Again, this must also be repeated a couple of times, until one can tell that the person has fully "come to". Bringing a shocked person "back to the present" and helping then to be "grounded" can often dissipate the effects of psychological shock almost completely. In other words, by restoring the patient's outer order, the inner order can then be restored further – for example, by collecting objects that are lying about after an accident. Whatever else, though, always listen attentively when they are talking about the shocking experience.

There are a couple of crystals that can also be employed in order to alleviate states of shock.

Obsidian will assist in the process of restoring a normal conscious or state of mind if a tumbled stone is placed in the hand of the affected person. The most effective form is actually Rainbow or Black Obsidian. In addition, if used as described the temporary state of psychological paralysis will dissolve suddenly and enable a normal conversation to take place.

Rhodonite can then be used in order to further the recovery of normal consciousness. It can be either held it in the hand, taken as gem essence (7-9 drops), or as gem water (100–200 ml taken in sips during the course of the day).

It is always worthwhile being ready for cases of shock by having a pre-prepared mixture of Obsidian and Rhodonite essence together with Bach Rescue Remedy. This mixture can be kept at home, or in the medicine chest, and be taken immediately as required (7-9 drops).

Short Sight

see Ametropia; Sight Problems

Sickness

see Vomiting

Sight Problems

Weak or impaired sight is typified by a very strong reduction in the sharpness of vision. This can be caused either by a blurring of the lenses and by diseases in the retina or choroids (the tissue layer behind the retina that contains many blood vessels). Other causes are a lack of, or impaired formation, of the so-called "yellow spot" (the point upon the retina, where the eye is sharpest) and disturbances in the nerves or the sight centre of the brain. In turn, the latter may be connected with varying or unequal vision in the eyes or squinting.

Weakened sight is not really a disease in itself. Rather it is a symptom of the consequence of many, often complex, causes.

See also: Ametropia; Cataracts; Eye Problems; Squinting

A central issue in all of this is the body's metabolism. Increasing deposits of toxins and waste, together with infections, cause a blurring of the eye or the lens, diseases of the retina or infection and damage to the choroid.

See also: Detoxification; Diabetes, Liver Health; Lymphatic Health, Revitalisation, Thyroid Problems

As there is a close connection between the eyes, efficient vision and a healthy liver function, treatment of the optic nerves, as well as those of the retina, are also possible using homeopathy, along with a sensible diet and drinking lots of clean water in order to regularise the metabolism.

Agate crystal containing an eye signature is particularly helpful in connection with diseases of the retina or choroids and any type of blurred vision. Agate sections/slices or a tumbled stone with central inclusions of Rock Crystal are particularly recommended and should be placed on the eyes regularly for about 15 minutes (evenings are best).

Rock Crystal is particularly helpful in the early stages of blurring. Place a small crystal or a tumbled stone directly on the closed eyelids. The clear, bright so-termed "Herkimer Diamonds" are particularly suitable.

Chalcedony and **Noble Opal** improve the fluid regulation of the eye as well as being beneficial to the body's overall lymphatic system. As a result, they are therefore helpful in cases of blurred vision as well as with some diseases in the retina or choroid.

Chrysoberyl is helpful with weak sight and impaired vision, particularly if the latter is caused by disturbances of the optic nerve or the sight centre of the brain. Place a crystal between the eyebrows (on the "third eye") for about 15 minutes, 3 times a day.

Diamond reduces the accumulation of toxins in the eye, particularly if taken in the form of gem essence (3-7 drops, 3-5 times daily) and gem water (200–300 ml taken in small sips over the course of the day). Diamond likewise affects the optic nerve and the sight centre of the brain, which makes it an important crystal with which to treat impaired vision. A Diamond can be placed directly on the closed eyes or between the eyebrows (on the "third-eye") as a supplementary treatment.

Dioptase has a positive effect on the eyes, primarily through the eyes connection with the liver. In cases of impaired vision, place a small crystal or a small group of crystals, directly onto the liver. Dioptase eye drops applied at the same time heighten the beneficial effect of the body's metabolism on the eyes.

Emerald is also helpful in connection with metabolic problems. It also has a positive effect on disturbances in the nerves, poisoning and chronic as well as acute infections. Place it regularly on the eyes and on the liver, preferably at the same time. Beside that, one can wear a necklace or pendant, or take gem essence (5-9 drops, 3-5 times daily) or gem water (200–300 ml taken in small sips over the course of the day).

Ocean Jasper has a similar effect to Agate in this context, especially when it also contains within its structure an eye signature and/or if acute or previous infections have contributed to the impairment of sight. In such cases, it can also be worn in the form of a necklace or pendant, be placed on the liver, or be taken in form of gem essence (200–300 ml taken in small sips over the course of the day).

Sardonyx, being a tri-coloured Chalcedony and as an Agate-related mineral, is also the best and most important crystal in cases of weak sight and impaired vision. It affects all the affected areas (eye metabolism, the retina, the choroid, the nerves and the brain) and will thus show exceptional results in some cases. It is best applied both internally and externally.

Place a raw or a tumbled stone directly on the eyes and take either gem essence (5-7 drops, 3-5 times daily) or gem water (200–300 ml taken in small sips over the course of the day).

Tourmaline, with its various colour varieties (blue, pink, green and water melon), is especially helpful, when impaired vision is caused by nerve disturbances or damage. Place either a crystal or a tumbled stone directly on the eyes or take gem essence or gem water (dosage as for Emerald).

Sinusitis

In most cases sinusitis, arises in connection with a cold, flu or inflamed dental roots in the upper jaw. Occasionally, it may also arise as a result of injuries or blood infections. Its symptoms consist of pulsing, throbbing pains in the sinus area and in the forehead. The pain is caused by pressure, particularly when bending forward, or by a high temperature and obstructed nasal breathing (often only through one nostril). The resulting, unpleasant mucous from the nose is initially yellowish and pus-like, turning later to a greenish-yellow.

As a precaution, sinusitis should always be treated by a doctor or an alternative practitioner, in order to avoid further complications and inflammation of the eyes, the optic nerve or the cerebral membrane. It is important to prevent sinusitis from developing into a chronic state, which, although showing few direct symptoms, can lead to a heavy build up of mucous in the membranes such as the adenoids.

The emotional causes of sinusitis can sometimes be found in taxing situations that lead to confusion and loss of emotional bearings. As mental clarity disappears, the nose becomes more and more "stuffed up" and exposed to inflammation. Looked at another way, one has only to remember how the ability to think is often diminished in even the mildest cases of the common cold.

Some relief may be obtained by rinsing the mouth and teeth with organic, cold pressed sunflower oil for 10 to 20 minutes every day. This oil absorbs toxic and poisonous substances, which results in a rapid improvement of the situation. **Do not swallow the oil under any circumstances**; spit it out afterwards and rinse thoroughly with lukewarm water!

See also Colds; Flu

Emerald has been shown to be the most effective crystal for use with sinusitis. It relieves inflammation of the mucous membranes very quickly, un-blocks stuffy noses and thus eases breathing through the nose. Furthermore, it also supports clarity of thought and feeling, with a positive effect on the nose and sinuses. As a rule, Emerald prevents the outbreak of chronic sinusitis, but also helps as part of a cure once it has occurred.

Heliotrope, **Blue Chalcedony**, **Moss Agate** and **Ocean Jasper** may also contribute to relief from any cold and flu-like condition and from sinusitis itself. Heliotrope is most effective at the beginning of the inflammation, i. e. with the first signs of yellowish mucous, with the initial pain, or when bending the head forward. Chalcedony can then be used during the course of the disease, in order to support the cleansing process via the lymph system. If the condition is very stubborn and retreats only very slowly, apply Moss Agate and Ocean Jasper.

For all the above, place or affix a polished crystal or a section/slice on the sinuses or on the forehead. Their effect is also enhanced if they are worn as a necklace or pendant

Additionally, take gem essence (depending on the intensity of the disease, 5-7 drops from 3 times daily up to a maximum of once an hour) or gem water (200–300 ml taken in sips during the course of the day).

Heliotrope can also be applied as an ointment with a beneficial and rapid effect. Mix the gem essence with Bach Rescue Remedy (10 drops of each in 10 g of ointment base (1 part beeswax and 4-5 parts of jojoba oil). This ointment can then be rubbed into the area over the sinuses and relief obtained.

Skin Care

The skin may be affected internally or externally by such things as an unhealthy environment, a poor indoor climate, polluted air, radiation, toxic deposits in the tissues, intestinal disturbances or a range of different illnesses. This means that merely treating disorders of the skin makes little sense. Indeed, it can even be harmful as, in certain circumstances, suppressed skin symptoms may often shift their effect to other organs, e. g. the body's mucous membranes or the airways, and thus lead to a general deterioration of health. A regular course of detoxification (see Detoxification) and – if necessary – colonic irrigation, is the most important factor in enabling the skin to heal from inside.

On the other hand, gentle care can support the skin in its natural secreting and cleansing function. As a result, unpleasant symptoms can be relieved and the skin itself remains intact and healthy. Skin care like this has to be positive and not suppressive in nature. It should be based upon furthering its natural functions, leading to normal regeneration and self-healing.

Amethyst has turned out to be especially beneficial for cleansing and healing the skin. As elsewhere (see also: Abscesses; Acne; Blisters; Itching; Dandruff; Sun Stroke), Hildegard von Bingen's Amethyst Water (see page 25) is particularly effective. This gentle, but profoundly effective, water-based preparation should be used as the sole cleansing agent for ones skin, i.e. without additional use of soap, alcohol-based cleansing agents or cosmetics.

It regenerates and cleanses all the skin layers and makes oily skin, couperose (the visible small blood vessels in the face), reddish spots (rosacea), dandruff, eczema, abscesses, and excessive build-up of hard skin and calluses improve or even gradually disappear.

Sleeping Problems

The experience of sleep disturbance may include an inability to fall asleep, or sleeping uninterruptedly yet still feeling unrested on waking; there may also be an increased feeling of tiredness of even a need for sleep during the day. Apart from physical diseases (such as inflammation, cysts and "bad nerves"), activities such as shift work, jet-lag, negative energy fields near the bed or in the bedroom and various types of emotional stress may also cause sleep disturbances.

Whilst physical diseases often cause an increased need for sleep, in order that the body has time for relaxation and regeneration, emotional stress and worries often have the opposite effect. The result can be that of experiencing a really hard time in falling asleep or having a full night's sleep. It might feel, for example, as if one cannot, or does not want to, let go of the day's events and incidents.

As long as sleep disturbances only occur occasionally, or because of clearly understandable and identifiable reasons (excitement over specific incidents), one need not worry. However, if they persist, or occur more frequently, some remedy must be found.

Of course, obvious diseases and emotional problems should be treated at a causal level. However, it is recommended to use meditation as an immediate aid in seeking an improvement in sleeping.

By employing some mentally relaxing exercises or taking an evening walk, whilst still maybe thinking over the day's events, one can then also bring them to a close.

See also: Nightmares

In order to improve one's sleep effectively, it is important to be aware of the natural sleep cycles. From dream research, it is known that light sleep (called rapid eye movement – or REM – sleep and which is filled with dreams) and deep sleep, alternate during the night. Emotional and physical regeneration also follow this same sleep cycle. In this way, toxins and waste products are excreted from the tissue and the processes of renewal take place during periods with deep sleep.

It can be seen therefore that if a phase with deep sleep is interrupted, one feels weary, downcast and unrested. On the other hand, waking easily and normally at the end of a phase of deep sleep, one feels clear and has a feeling of being fully rested. So, wherever possible, one should arrange the length of one's sleep, so that one wakes up after a phase of deep sleep; but how can one do this?

The answer lies in the importance of knowing the length of personal sleep phases – which are also the same as the body's own regeneration periods. This can be done by means of simple observation and recording the times when one awakes feeling rested and then calculating how much time has elapsed since one fell asleep. It is obvious pretty quickly that the periods of waking up feeling rested are of a more or less constant length of time. This is then regarded as a whole number resulting from the multiples of one's sleep cycle.

For example, if one wakes up after 5 hours and 20 minutes, or after exactly 8 hours, the common divisor is 2 hours 40 minutes – this is the time of one regeneration phase after which you feel rested. You find multiples of these phases throughout your sleep: 2 x 2 hours 40 minutes = 5 hours 20 minutes; 3 x 2 hours 40 minutes = 8 hours.

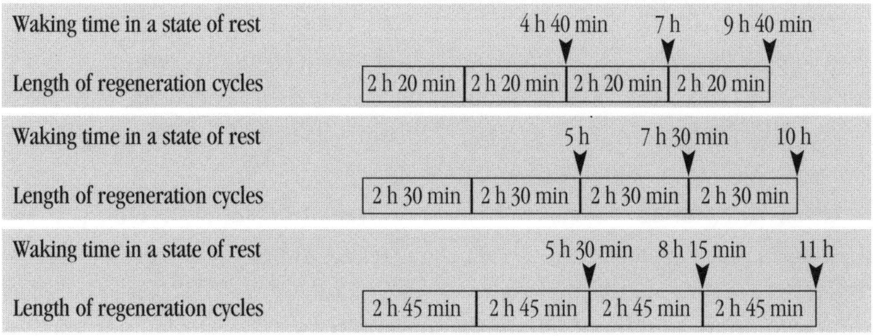

Waking time in a state of rest		4 h 40 min		7 h		9 h 40 min
Length of regeneration cycles	2 h 20 min	2 h 20 min	2 h 20 min	2 h 20 min		

Waking time in a state of rest		5 h		7 h 30 min		10 h
Length of regeneration cycles	2 h 30 min	2 h 30 min	2 h 30 min	2 h 30 min		

Waking time in a state of rest		5 h 30 min		8 h 15 min		11 h
Length of regeneration cycles	2 h 45 min	2 h 45 min	2 h 45 min	2 h 45 min		

Fig 18: Regeneration cycles during sleep.

On the other hand if one wakes up rested after 5 hours or 7 hours 30 minutes, the common divisor is 2 hours 30 minutes: that is 2 x 2 hours 30 minutes = 5 hours; 3 x 2 hours 30 minutes = 7 hours 30 minutes. This common divisor indicates the length of a single regeneration phase during sleep.

As a rule, the regeneration cycles take between two and three hours. If one is emotionally and physically in good shape, they can be somewhat shorter – but with diseases and heavy emotional problems, they may be somewhat longer. Normally, the body needs three of these regeneration cycles in order to "digest the remains of the day". Thus, one generally has to assume an average time of eight hours in order to get enough sleep.

However, if one sleeps for one or two extra cycles, the body will have the time to carry out more regeneration work. This is why an illness often causes a need for more sleep.

When we sleep for longer, say, during holidays, this brings emotional and physical rejuvenation. On the other hand, if we sleep for less than these three phases, or cycles, every night, this will result in increased deposits of toxins and waste. Then one really gets "worn down", lacking the beneficial effects of the body's essential regeneration. Accommodating sleep requirements according to the regeneration cycles is, therefore, a very important support programme for body and soul. It helps not only with sleep disturbances, but also with a host of other problems (see Revitalisation).

To summarize, one can say that it is important to find the length of one's own regeneration cycles, preferably to ensure one has three of these cycles every night during sleep – and especially to set the alarm correctly, so that one wakes up in the morning exactly between two regeneration cycles. (Of course, this is only if a wake-up call is still needed at all. The more precisely one knows personal regeneration cycles, the more exactly one can predict and tell oneself when to wake up.)

This investigation and observation of one's own rhythms is much more important and effective than any sleeping pills, barbiturates or even "natural" alternative sleep inducing agents. If the above methods are combined with others that help one fall asleep – meditation, relaxation, walks, etc. – the result will be sound sleep. In which case, use of the following crystals might only be necessary in exceptional cases, effective though they will prove to be on such occasions, assisting in the mental relaxation necessary in order to meet the physical and emotional needs, when one is rested and ready for therapeutic, healing sleep

Agate is helpful in the form of a section/slice under the pillow. It helps induce a deeper, calmer and revitalising sleep. Furthermore, any dreams will be experienced as being comfortable and unthreatening.

Agate also assists if there is any tendency towards waking up early and not being able to fall asleep again.

Amethyst improves the quality of sleep, in cases where unfinished business cause disturbing or anxious dreams. Such dreams are typical of an increased need for sleep and the simultaneous decreasing quality and value of the sleep. Anything that we feel unable to tackle directly and that is put aside during the day then turns up at night and is processed during sleep. In this way, the sleep is of a type that is simply "clearing out the junk" of the day, with incidents, worries and conflicts repeated several times and often in different variations, until they are "digested" and dealt with. Because dreams like this are just as much mental work as is conscious daytime thought, the brain's resulting activity means that the sleep lacks the necessary depth for the vital physical and other forms of renewal and regeneration.

Initially, a bright, clear Amethyst crystal, or a tumbled stone under the pillow, will actually stimulate such "clearing out junk" dreams and so one may feel an initial deterioration as a result of this increased activity during the dream-time. However, it is in this way that many unfinished matters are dealt with effectively and conclusively after a couple of nights. Then, from this point on, sleep becomes deeper, more recreational and the body's regeneration cycles become shorter.

Wearing an Amethyst during the day, in the form of a necklace or a pendant, raises one's awareness of the fact that many experiences and much information can be best dealt with immediately, freeing sleep for its true purpose of revitalisation

Aventurine makes it particularly easy to fall asleep, because it helps in "letting go" of persistent cycles of disturbing thoughts, images and feelings. It brings with it the necessary calmness and relaxation, so that one can fall asleep peacefully.

Chrysoprase is helpful when it is difficult to sleep through the night, or in dealing with nightmares, in particular with children, who wake up fretful in the middle of the night (see also **Nightmares**). It also frees the mind or worrying images and very unpleasant feelings.

Ocean Jasper makes it easier to fall asleep and to sleep deeper. It also furthers night time renewal, especially if one places several raw or tumbled stones in a circle around the bed.

Black Tourmaline improves sleep, bringing about rapid relaxation. It makes it easier to fall asleep and also to sleep through until morning. It is also helpful when electronic pollution disturbs one's sleep pattern and there is no other way of shielding or neutralisation.

For Aventurine, Chrysoprase and Black Tourmaline, place a tumbled stone under the pillow or wear a necklace or a pendant with body contact.

Slipped Disc

The spine consists of vertebrae, each of which is separated from its upper and lower neighbour by a thin disc of ligament, a ring of connective tissue with a jelly-like core and high water content and whose purpose is to keep the spine flexible. The vertebrae themselves can become worn and the intervening disc can loses fluid from out of this jelly-like tissue and, with it, the intended elasticity. Consequently, the vertebrae become flatter and their flexibility is decreased. This can then cause pain in the back (although not always necessarily).

In extreme cases, the ring of connective tissue expands too much, or is actually torn or damaged. This makes the jelly-like substance flow partly, or totally, into the spinal channel, where the spinal nerves are situated; and it is this that we call a slipped disc – or disc prolapse. Compression of nerves can result in truly severe pain, which then either radiates sideways or into the joints of the body.

It is essential to consult a doctor or an alternative practitioner as soon as possible in order to obtain an accurate diagnosis. In addition, some crystals have turned out to relieve pain extremely effectively and to be helpful during the renewal of the damaged ligaments. Of course, as with so many physical conditions, there can often be a psychological or emotional factor that causes the problem. As ever, this is always something to be taken into account.

Amazonite relieves stiffness and inflexibility as a result of its lead content ("like heals like" as they say). Flexibility and motion is important if the discs are to absorb fluid and maintain their elasticity. In this way any further erosion is prevented. Amazonite also soothes when sudden pains strike.

Aragonite with signature bands, being a calcium carbonate rich in water crystal, is probably the number one choice in treating cases of a slipped disc. It enhances the renewed absorption of water in "worn" ligaments and renews their elasticity. Place or affix either a section/slice or a tumbled stone on the affected spot. An Aragonite-Calcite-crystal, sold commercially under the name, "Onyx-Marble", has also been shown to produce good results.

Dioptase helps with slipped discs. Fix a crystal or a crystal cluster on the liver as discs are energetically connected with the liver's energy meridian. A combination of Dioptase placed over the liver and Aragonite upon the discs also has a good effect.

Kunzite relieves the pain of pinched nerves. For a slipped disc, Kunzite can be placed or fixed on the affected area together with Aragonite, either in the form of a crystal or a tumbled stone.

Pyrites relieve the pain from a slipped disc. However, as they contain sulphur and can react with sweat, and thus cause skin irritation, they should only be applied for a short period. For any longer term uses, they can be worn on the tender area if contained within a small, thinly woven cotton bag

Wear them as a bracelet on each hand; or as a necklace or pendant during sleep for best effect. Alternatively, take gem essence (5-9 drops before going to sleep), or gem water (200 ml).

Snoring

Snoring is the term we use for sounds produced by breathing when asleep, especially those noises which occur when breathing through the mouth while lying on one's back. Snoring is caused by the vibrations of the slackened soft palate and is further exacerbated by the tongue sliding backwards, when the body is supine. Oral breathing is usually a result of impeded breathing through the nose that is caused by adenoid swelling or a cold – and in children by tonsillitis.

Loud snoring is also associated with emotional tensions, which have considerable effect on sleep. Sleeping on one's side, stress reduction and relaxation before falling asleep – and the effective treatment of colds and other diseases of the airways – are some of the most important measures that can be taken to prevent snoring.

Heliotrope, Ocean Jasper and **Emerald** can be applied to relieve snoring. They also help with colds, tonsillitis and other diseases of the airways, and have a relaxing effect on tension.

Sore Throat

see Throat Pains; Tonsillitis

Speech Difficulties

see Hoarseness: Loss of Voice; Stuttering

Sprains

A sprained joint is caused by sudden, violent and excessive movement beyond its normal range of movement (e. g. twisting an ankle). Tendons become overstretched or torn apart. Sometimes, even the joint enclosure itself is damaged as well.

The usual result is very obvious swelling with severe pain – sometimes with bruising.

As with all similar types of injury, it is always valuable to initiate some form of pain-relieving exercise as soon as possible – even if simply to ensure a full awareness of the injury and the circumstances that caused it.

One method involves repeating the motions, circumstances or sequence of events immediately after the incident – but of course, without repeating the actual injury). If, for example, the foot was twisted, the last movement before the injury can be repeated (slowly) once more. It might even be necessary to repeat the whole incident a couple of times until the pain suddenly increases, but then decreases rapidly; and this is the point at which to stop. This form of exercise focuses both attention and life energy on the affected part of the body and thereby furthers the healing process.

Afterwards, the swelling can be relieved by a cooling arnica poultice and (if part of one's normal self-treatment) by taking homeopathic Arnica and Bach Rescue Remedy.

However, to be truly safe and reassured, see a doctor, in order to ascertain whether or not the tendons and ligaments have merely been stretched, or whether they have been torn apart and the whole joint has been affected.

Obsidian can be applied to sprains. Use Obsidian immediately after the accident as it dissolves the pain and the state of shock inflicted on the cells. Place a tumbled stone on the aching spot – particularly important if the above consciousness-raising process cannot be carried out.

Rhodonite can then be used as a follow-up, being applied afterwards in order to heal the sprain and limit any possible bruising.

Place a tumbled stone or a section/slice over the affected area or ensure there is one it inside any supporting bandage.

As an alternative, place a necklace around the joint; or take gem essence (5-9 drops, initially every hour, then later 3 times daily), or gem water (up to 1 litre taken in small sips over the course of the day).

Squinting

Squinting- also sometimes referred to as strabismus or strabism – is a consequence of a positional defect in one or both eyes. This results from the eyes being not quite parallel when observing anything distant and thus one cannot quite focus on a specific spot nearby. The overall condition is often caused by disturbances in the eye muscles and their associated nerves, along with errors of refraction or pronounced differences in the visual power of the eyes.

Deviations in eye position might only be occur during tiredness or strain, etc. – which is termed latent squinting – whilst the problem is present all the time in the cases of a permanent squint.

As squinting produces a double image, the brain suppresses the information from the weaker or squinting eye. This leads to reduced sharpness and acuity of sight and – sometimes – can cause progressively weakened vision. Consequently, squinting should always be treated.

Traditional medicine involves exercises for improving sight (e. g. in cases of unbalanced sight, where the stronger eye is covered), or the correction of refraction errors by means of sight-improving measures. Very pronounced anomalies in the eye muscles are also corrected physically using surgery.

In the field of alternative medicine, it is also recognised that squinting can often occur together with the vertebrae being out of alignment or with bad posture. As a result, body therapeutic measures (e. g. craniosacral therapy; osteopathy; Dorn-Breuss method, etc.) can sometimes cure squinting.

In children, squinting has sometimes been known to occur after vaccinations. Such instances can be treated with appropriate cleansing measures (see Detoxification), or with homeopathic remedies, as there is undoubtedly a close connection between the eyes and the liver

In order to be sure that all of the possible interactions and causes are taken into account, I strongly recommend that a homeopathic or anthroposophic eye doctor, or an alternative practitioner, be consulted alongside any other type of squint therapy.

See also: Ametropia; Eye problems; Sight Problems

Whilst crystal therapy may support such measures within the framework of a holistic therapy, crystals should not be applied alone.

Aquamarine and **Emerald** are without doubt the best crystals to use in connection with squinting they relax the area surrounding the eye, stimulate the nerve activity and have a positive effect on the eye musculature.

Place small crystals or tumbled stones on the eyes, or wear them as a necklace or pendant around the neck. Alternatively, take gem essence (5-9 drops, 3-5 times daily), or gem water (200–300 ml taken in small sips over the course of the day).

Rock Crystal and **Amethyst** can have a positive influence on squinting. Amethyst works in particular in connection with the treatment described in the chapter on "eye diseases", in which one places Rock Crystal, Aquamarine, Emerald or Sardonyx directly on the eyes.

Sardonyx is useful when squinting is caused by a marked difference in the strength of the eyes. It is applied like Aquamarine or Emerald.

Tourmaline, with its different colour varieties (blue, pink, green and water melon) can also improve squinting, especially when it is caused by nerve disturbances or injuries. Again, it is used like Aquamarine or Emerald.

Stings

see Insect Bites and Stings

Stomach Ache

Stomach ache is an immediate symptom of a whole range of problems. Practically any organ in the abdominal cavity – stomach, intestines, pancreas, kidneys, liver, bile, uterus, etc, – can be its cause.

Other causes might include such things as displaced vertebrae, emotional problems, grief, a gall bladder "racked with rage", blows and falls, etc. Consequently, it is far too imprecise to refer simply to "pains in the stomach", if a specific treatment is to be suggested.

It is important to identify exactly where the pain is first noticed (that is, if it can be located specifically at all), at what time of day it occurs, what has been eaten soon before, the actual nature of the pain and what, if any, are its accompanying symptoms (e. g. nausea, vomiting, perspiration attack, diarrhoea, etc.).

All this should be clarified by a doctor or by an alternative practitioner, in order to obtain an accurate diagnosis. As a stomach ache can sometimes also have a dangerous or life-threatening cause, it should not be self-treated without having first had professional help and NEVER if the pain is very strong, manifests suddenly, or continues for a long time!

Once the underlying cause has been determined, crystal therapy can help bring about relief to many kinds of stomach ache and – at the same time – contribute to a cure on causal level. The many different possibilities of symptom and treatment are summarised in the following table.

Crystal	Effect	Practical applications
Agate	Stomach, intestine and uterus problems (grey to yellow-brown natural colour), also inflammation (pink natural colour); feelings of being alone or overburdened	Place a crystal with a suitable signature on the affected spot or wear it on the body
Antimonite	Stomach problems with nausea and vomiting	Place a crystal on the stomach, or take either gem water or gem essence
Aquamarine	Problems with the pancreas, gallstones, bile congestion, nausea in the late morning, allergic reaction to food; consequences of stress, overburdening, or hasty consumption of food.	Place a crystal on the left side of the upper stomach, or take either gem water or gem essence
Amber	Stomach, intestines, pancreas and bile problems. Consequences of grief and fears	Place a crystal on the affected spot, or wear it on the body ➤➤

Crystal	Effect	Practical applications
Biotite-Lens	Unspecific feelings of pressure or bloated ness, menstrual problems; stomach ache when difficult decisions have to be taken	Place a crystal on the affected spot or wear it on the body
Chrysocolla	Liver, gall bladder and menstrual problems; consequences of overburdening, violent outbursts of feeling or suppressed anger	Place a crystal on the upper right part of the stomach, take either gem essence or gem water or wear it on the body
Chrysoprase	Liver and gall bladder problems, cramps; consequences of bad conscience or loss of security	Place a crystal on the affected area or wear it on the body
Citrine	Stomach problems, bloatedness, consequences of having eaten too much, grief, depression or fear of conflict	Place a crystal on the affected area or wear it on the body
Diaspor	Stomach problems, heartburn; dissatisfaction, disappointment	Place a crystal on the affected spot or wear it on the body
Emerald	Liver, gall bladder an intestinal problems, inflammation and cramps consequences of confusion, conflicts, strain and injustice	Place a crystal on the affected spot or wear it on the body
Heliotrope	Intestinal infections, liver, gall bladder and bladder infections; lack of delimitation or control in one's own life.	Place a crystal on the affected spot or take either as gem essence or gem water
Magnesite	Cramp, migraines, gall bladder and stomach problems, heartburn; strong emotional tension, nervousness, stress	Place a crystal on the affected spot or take either as gem essence or gem water; wear as a necklace or bracelet
Malachite	Cramp-like stomach, gall bladder and abdominal pains (also menstrual pain); fear of every day matters, inhibitions, repressed feelings	Place crystals on the affected areas
Moss agate, pink	Nausea, sluggish intestine, constipation, intestinal infection; feelings of guilt, disgust, grudges, anger or revenge	Place or wear a crystal on the area over the intestine or take either as gem essence or gem water

➤➜

235

Crystal	Effect	Practical applications
Ocean Jasper	Liver and gall bladder problems (mostly green crystals), stomach and intestinal problems (mostly brown crystals), spleen and pancreas problems (mostly grey-white crystals). Food allergy, consequences of overburdening, unresolved conflicts, lacking rest, bad sleep	Place a crystal on the affected spot; wear on the body or take as gem water
Rhodonite	Pains following punches, blows or injuries. Consequences of emotional wounds	Place a crystal on the affected spot or take either as gem essence or gem water
Sardonyx	Spleen pain, stitches in the left side, long term consequences after infections, food allergy, despondency, consequences of strong overburdening	Place a crystal on the left side or take either as gem essence or gem water
Serpentine	Kidney and intestinal problems, alternating diarrhoea and constipation; consequences of a strong inner tension, nervousness, and stress	Place a crystal on the affected spots or take either as gem essence or gem water. Wear it in the form of a necklace or bracelet for a longer period
Golden Topaz	Nausea, lack of appetite; depression, nervousness, last-minute-nerves	Place or wear a crystal on the solar plexus, or take either as gem essence or gem water
Turquoise	Nausea, vomiting, heartburn; feeling of lack of protection or helplessness	Place or wear a crystal on the stomach area, or take either as gem essence or gem water
Tourmaline, black	Constipation, feelings of bloatedness; inner tension, negative attitude towards life	Carry a crystal in your left trouser pocket; place it on the intestine, or take either as gem essence or gem water
Zirconium	Strong cramp-like pains from the stomach, gall bladder, liver or the uterus, menstrual pains; fear of personal loss, feelings of pointlessness	Place a crystal on the affected spot

With stomach ache, the dosage of gem essences is typically high (5-9 drops, 3-7 times daily); but for gem water typically low (50–200 ml taken in small sips over the course of the day), in particular when ingestion is impeded by nausea.

Stomach Problems

Symptomatically, most stomach problems are difficult to distinguish symptomatically from diseases in the pancreas, the gall bladder and the gall ways, the liver or the intestine. Nausea and vomiting are not automatically a sign that there is something wrong with the stomach (see also Vomiting).

Professional advice from a doctor or an alternative practitioner should always be sought for clarification of the real cause – especially when symptoms persist for rather a long time or occur at regular intervals. Consequently, the crystals described later in this entry are only effective, when symptoms such as a sore throat, feeling full or bloated, having no appetite, nervous tension – or simply "having the collywobbles" due to worries and problems – are unambiguously linked to the stomach.

Just as our stomach is occupied physically with the digestion of absorbed nutrients, it can, in the same way, also be associated with our psychological and emotional "digestion" of experiences and information. Matters that might be described as

being "emotionally indigestible" can sometimes cause the same problems as items that are physically indigestible. This has long been recognised in both folklore and common experience – to the extent that certain popular sayings illustrate this clearly: "butterflies in the stomach"; having a bad feeling in the "pit of one's stomach"; "that makes me sick", etc, etc.

So, as ever, physical and emotional nutrition are interconnected. Healthy, organic food in a varied diet will provide different results than processed or "fast" food. Furthermore, why not consider staring out with a short meditation in order to make the day different, rather than consuming with breakfast the news of the day with, all too often, its bulletins of human and natural disasters?

Stomach problems should always remind us of the fact that we should review our nutrition from a holistic perspective. As a result, crystals which help in relieving stomach problems also help us find it easier to deal with things emotionally and make us ready and able to digest "big stuff". So, in summary, it makes little sense to use the following crystals if there is no accompanying readiness or willingness to change lifestyle and – where the stomach is concerned specifically, changing dietary habits.

Agate that contains within its crystal form a "stomach signature" helps with all kinds of physical and emotional stomach problems. It strengthens the mucous membrane of the stomach, relieves inflammation and helps with feelings of bloatedness. Gently, it stimulates the stomach and has an emotionally stabilising effect, so that even uncomfortable matters do not "lie too heavily" there.

Amber helps with nausea caused by inflammation such as gastritis, or with stomach ulcers. It also strengthens the mucous membrane of the stomach. However, is much more likely to help with lack of appetite or stomach problems caused by "nerves", as, emotionally, Amber furthers happiness, cheerfulness and freedom from care.

Diaspor helps quickly with cases of sore throat and too much acid in the stomach (acidosis). It relieves the type of nausea that, typically, occurs after heavy or rushed eating.

Emotionally, it has a calming effect on feelings of nervousness and fear – and of guilt without any apparent cause.

Magnesite also helps with sore throats, excessive stomach acid or stomach cramps. It relieves hiccups and is calming in cases of nervousness, anxiety and irritability.

Place a crystal (if Diaspor), or a tumbled stone/section slice (of any of the above) on the stomach. Alternatively, you can wear them as a necklace or pendant. Take as gem essence (5-7 drops, 3-5 times daily) or gem water (100–200 ml taken in small sips during the course of the day).

Stress

Stress is usually caused by the feeling that there are too many loose ends still to be tied up or situations to be resolved. These all contribute to a sense of carrying a real emotional load, accompanied by a deep feeling of dissatisfaction. The resulting stress is a direct result of feeling that personal wishes and actions are being pushed aside constantly by ongoing obligations or influences from other sources (often described as the "parent syndrome"). Added to this can be a wide range of other external factors that have a direct affect on emotional stability or general quality of life – such as noise and other forms of pollution, direct physical danger and illness, emotional or personal conflicts, crises, personal loss, etc.

Stress is intrinsically an "internal" phenomenon. Nevertheless, external signs can be very obvious. For example, in observing two individuals in similar situations, you may often notice that one of them is already totally "stressed" and on the brink of losing control, while the other one is still totally relaxed. The tendency to allow oneself to become stressed is thus connected directly with the ability to face the present and future – as it exist s, and as it may turn out. This does not mean one has to actually like the present or the probable future; but it does mean that we have to able to face up to things as they are. The more one dwells on the past and the unfinished things, or on unfulfilled wishes, then the less one is capable of accepting the status quo. So, already you begin to feel stressed…

Yet, the problem is that we can neither stop nor channel the influences to which we are exposed. Thus, we become so confused that all thoughts, feelings, actions and – soon after – our physical functions also become thoroughly confused. The resulting sense of ineffectiveness and an inability to take any action only serves to make matters even worse – and the vicious circle becomes a downward spiral.

The best remedy is to try to get a handle on all the loose ends and, in so doing, gain more personal freedom – for rest, recreation and wish fulfilment. Sometimes, simply just drawing up a list, where the tasks are arranged according to necessity and chronological order can be a great help. Then, as there emerges a general idea of what has to be done "immediately", "soon" and "later", the burden of unfinished business is greatly reduced. It is no longer feels as though everything is weighing you down at once. Instead, you can now make free time and create some space in which to do one thing after another, systematically and free of stress. When this way of working or living becomes the norm, the freedom, at first merely temporary, becomes a permanent – and there is again much less stress.

In this way, you will notice that not only will internal stress decrease, but that the influence and affect of external stresses will also decrease. Of course, it is always more productive and beneficial to work in peace and quiet than surrounded by in noise ("turn off that radio"), or in clean air instead of the polluted atmosphere of a big city. However, the internal factors, the weight on the mind of anything unfinished can be several times greater than any external stress. For example, one can feel extremely uncomfortable in the most idyllic setting, if one knows that the rent is overdue of that the bailiffs will be calling the next day! Yet, in contrast with a meditative attitude, one can have an enjoyable time even in the hurly-burly of the big city.

There can be no doubt; the solution to stress is to clean up and de-junk – on all levels.

However, in addition, there are a number of other ways to relieve feelings of stress. Together with plenty of sleep, daily walks, meditation exercises, Tai Chi, saline foot baths in the evening, any sensible relaxing or focussing activity will encourage stability, a balanced outlook and a much-reduced susceptibility to problems arising from stress.

In cases of acute stress the following crystals will also help matters.

Aventurine helps when one is distracted and confused by creating a sense of distance from previous and future incidents and assisting in applying oneself fully and effectively to the present. Aventurine also brings about relaxation, regeneration and recreation and thus reduces the influences of external stress factors.

Bronzite promotes liveliness and activity whilst remaining calm internally. This enables one to become swift and effective, which helps in dealing with anything left unfinished quickly and without stress. It strengthens the nervous system and helps in having a relaxed attitude in the face of conflicts and extreme situations. It is also particularly suitable when it proves hard to have any enjoyable time on one's own ("the parent syndrome", see above), even in circumstances when one really does have a great need for peace and recreation.

Chrysocolla helps one keep a cool head when bombarded and overwhelmed by too many simultaneous impressions or stimulations. It is particularly helpful in situations of sudden stress or of rapid change. Chrysocolla helps one to stay neutral, calm and composed in all manner of conflicts and disputes.

Dumortierite enhances the ability to see everything with an easier and more relaxed attitude. It softens harshness and blind ambition, and communicates courage and confidence for future situations. Not for nothing is it often called the "take-it-easy-crystal", for it is applied especially when there is a need to abandon patterns of compulsive behaviour, etc.

Magnesite has a relieving and relaxing effect, when there is a danger of "losing one's nerve". It relieves stress, nervousness, anxiety, and irritation and encourages patience.

Smoky Quartz is quite simply *the* "anti-stress" crystal. Simply hold two crystals or tumbled stones in the hands, and the stress and tension will disappear. If worn for a longer period, it increases the ability to cope with worries. Smoky quartz communicates a sense of level-headedness and perseverance, in order that any steps necessary can be taken consistently after thorough consideration. Beside that, Smoky quartz can also reduce any tendency to be stressed and reduce any susceptibility to external stress factors.

For all of these crystals, wear as a bracelet, necklace or pendant for a lengthy period in order to bring about the best relief from stress. Alternatively, in more immediate circumstances, take a large, polished stone in the hand, when feeling particularly stressed.

Strokes

A stroke or aneurysm (historically called "apoplexy)" is, in effect, a cerebral thrombosis, embolism or haemorrhage, a sudden malfunction in the blood circulation in a part of the brain. This can cause unconsciousness, paralysis, sight disturbances or loss of speech. Weakness, sense disturbances or paralysis in one side of the body, visual disturbances (also double vision), speech disturbances, dizziness, feelings of insecurity when walking and an abrupt onset of a very severe headache are some of the symptoms which can often appear very suddenly and quickly.

These phenomena can last a couple of minutes or be permanent. If the attack is indeed merely a few minutes in duration and the effects last no more than 24 hours with a seeming full recovery, the condition is called a TIA (transient ischaemic attack)

Nevertheless, in these cases, **call for the emergency medical services or a doctor immediately**! The faster a stroke is diagnosed and the faster it is treated, the better. Only a few hours are available for some necessary treatment (i.e. dissolving of blood lots; see below)! Until the ambulance arrives, the affected person should be seated or laid down comfortably and be freed of any clothing that is too tight. The sufferer should not eat or drink anything, as there is a danger of suffocation in cases where the patient slips into unconsciousness!

If the cause is a cerebral embolism, the arteries that supply the brain are blocked by a blood clot and so the affected areas of the brain are under-supplied with blood. With a cerebral haemorrhage, arteries in the brain burst.

In both cases, the origin is defective blood vessels, which are often caused by arteriosclerosis in connection with high blood pressure, diabetes, diseases in the walls of the blood vessels (more rarely) or because of disturbances in the coagulation (blood-clotting) process.

For stroke prophylaxis, see also Blood Pressure (high), Arteriosclerosis and Diabetes.

In this context, traditional medicine tends to refer only to causes such as excess weight, lack of physical exercise, and smoking, too high consumption of alcohol or severe emotional burdens. However, often forgotten are the need for general detoxification, a diet with the correct nutritional value, and (especially) the damaging effect on the blood vessels of a high degree of stored proteins. A balanced diet consisting of healthy organic food, or, if necessary, a diet without animal proteins, physical exercise outdoors, stress reduction and a regular detoxification regime are thus the most important prophylactic precautions in connection with strokes. (See also: Detoxification)

Aventurine, **Diamond** and **Heliotrope** are the appropriate crystals to apply (see Arteriosclerosis).

Diamond in particular has proven its worth after a stroke and traditional medical treatment (but, in some cases, during treatment) and Hildegard von Bingen wrote about it some 850 years ago:

"the person who suffers from gout, or has had a stroke, the disease, which affects one side of the body, so that one can no longer move, should put a diamond into some wine or water for a whole day and drink this. In this way, the gout will leave him, even if it is so strong that his joints feel as if they are threatening to tear apart. The consequences of a stroke can thus be alleviated."

So, Hildegard von Bingen had already recognised the connection between the consequences of toxins and waste products (gout) and strokes. However, wine is not now recommended in the first weeks after a stroke, though the Diamond water advised by Hildegard von Bingen has shown its worth in many cases. As a complement to the above diet and any accompanying rehabilitation measures such as physiotherapy, Diamond enhances the breakdown of blood clots and – at the same time – it also assists in the reorganisation of the brain, whereby healthy parts take over the functions of the damaged sections.

Stuttering

Stuttering is a disturbance in the flow of words caused by a spasmodic inhibition of speech, as well as by multiple repetitions of sounds, syllables and words. It is often caused by very strong tensions, which, in turn, are emotionally based in some way.

Stress, strain and conflicts, in particular, aggravate stuttering, while, in contrast inner stability, harmony and relaxation improves the flow of speech.

Stuttering is much more common in children and young people than in adults. This is especially the case if the sufferers feel stressed at home, under parental and/or other pressure to achieve or to succeed, or subject to forms of strongly controlled social behaviour.

However, these are far from being the only causes. In many cases, these may even be the sufferer's own ambitions or inhibitions, whilst in other cases it is often impossible to identify any cause whatsoever.

Interestingly enough, it is the self same crystals that are helpful with stuttering, which also emphasise one's character, an identity of self, and which eliminate undue external influences. These are crystals that enhance and stimulate courage and confidence. As Hildegard von Bingen expressed it in respect of Blue Chalcedony, they are the crystals "which bring firmness and courage so that one can make a speech and express elegantly what one wishes to say". It is hard to find a better description even today of the connection between our emotional state and trouble-free speech.

Rock Crystal strengthens "what is already present", one's own character and aims. It clarifies one's thoughts, brings firmness and calmness. Thus it is also very successful in connection with stuttering.

Blue Chalcedony is the classic "orator's crystal", according to Hildegard von Bingen. It helps one express one's self well and fluently, as it brings emotional ease and a relaxed attitude. This crystal makes it possible to stay relaxed, so that spasmodic voice inhibitions disappear.

Chrysoberyl is the best crystal for stuttering. It helps one remain completely sober, clear and self-confident (the "military commander crystal"), even in the greatest conflict and stress situations, i.e. especially during tests, fears of going to school, pressure to perform or other burdening factors. Thus it also brings enormous improvement and progress in connection with stuttering.

It is best to wear all of the above in the form of necklaces (if Rock Crystal or Chalcedony), pendants (if Chrysoberyl), or as drilled, tumbled stones (if available) over longer periods of time. When making a speech or giving a talk, or some other presentation, they can also be held in the hand in the form of crystals (Rock Crystal, Chrysoberyl), or as tumbled stones (Chalcedony).

All three are also very effective if taken as gem essence (3-7 drops, 3 times daily).

Sunburn

Sunburn is caused by over exposure of unprotected skin to the sun's short-wave ultra-violet (UV) radiation. This condition can be even worse if there is also additional exposure to these same sun's rays reflected from snow and ice surfaces

In its initial stages, sunburn causes inflamed, reddened skin that is painful and has a sensation of tightness. Later, in the advanced stages, painful blisters occur and then the skin loosens. In cases where larger areas of skin are affected, phenomena very similar to those after burns can be observed. In which case, **seek professional medical assistance immediately.**

Sunburn can be relieved by exposure to orange-coloured light, the application of the fresh, gel- like sap from the leaves of *Aloe* Vera and the oil from St. John's Wort – with added immortelle and lavender essences. It is also very important to drink lots of fluids.

The following crystals also have a relieving effect – and even a prophylactic effect in the case of Prase.

Amethyst helps with the healing of sunburn in its initial stage of reddened skin. It is best applied in the form of Hildegard von Bingen's Amethyst Water (see page 25), treating the affected areas with this water several times daily.

Aventurine is particularly helpful in relieving pain arising from sunburn and speeds up the healing process.

Take gem essence (5-7 drops, 5-7 times daily) or gem water (up to 1 litre taken in sips over the course of the day). Alternatively, for external treatment, arrange a circle of 8-12 tumbled stones around the affected person.

Prase is, however, the best choice of crystal in connection with sunburn. For a reduction of the skin's sensitivity to light and sunburn, place a Prase stone in the mouth like a sweet, or wear as a necklace or pendant on the body.

For the actual healing of sunburn, place a section/slice or tumbled stone on the affected area. Alternatively, take gem essence (5-7 drops, 5-7 times daily) or gem water (up to 1 litre taken in sips over the course of the day).

Sunstroke

Sunstroke is an irritation of the membrane surrounding the brain, arising from long, intense exposure to the rays of the sun on the unprotected head or neck. Its symptoms are severe headache, a red and hot head (though not always), lethargy, dizziness, breaking into a sweat, nausea, vomiting and – in extreme cases – a state of confusion.

In cases of sunstroke, **always call a doctor!**

However, immediate first aid involves moving the affected person into the shade and lying them down with their torso raised. Clothing should be loosened or opened to cool the patient and moist towels should be applying cool the forehead and neck.

In addition, and/or until a doctor arrives, and after the patient has been attended to, crystals can be applied to bring relief.

Aventurine helps relieve sunstroke quickly, when the affected person is able to lie down again.

Arrange 5-9 tumbled stones in an arc around the head for some time or until an initial improvement is noticed. After that, move the stones gradually further and further away from the head, so that the arc becomes ever larger (see Fig. 19). Carry on with this procedure until the headache has decreased significantly. This treatment can be repeated every hour if needed.

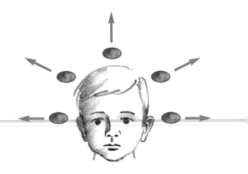

Fig. 19: Treatment of sunstroke with Aventurine.

Apart from that, Aventurine can be worn in the form of a bracelet, necklace or pendant; or take gem essence (5-7 drops,

5-7 times daily), or gem water (200–300 ml taken in small sips over the course of the day).

Prase helps with sunstroke. Place a slice or a tumbled stone on the head or wear as a bracelet, necklace or pendant, but with direct body contact.

Place a crystal in the mouth – but **only** if the person is conscious and monitor constantly! For example, when still in the sun, place a crystal in the mouth like a sweet. It may sound incredible; but this has been effective in many cases. Nonetheless, it is no substitute for a hat or any other kind of sun protection in the long run.

Also, try gem essence (5-7 drops, 5-7 times daily), or gem water (200–300 ml taken in small sips over the course of the day).

Smoky Quartz can be held in the hand or placed on the head (in the form of a crystal or tumbled stone) in cases of sunstroke. It is also possible to wear it as a bracelet, necklace or pendant.

Synovitis

Synovitis is a painful inflammatory state that occurs within the membranes surrounding the sinew of a joint. It is especially prevalent in long sinews such as those in the forearm and is often caused by chronic or acute overuse of a limb (e. g. overstretching or wrenching of the appropriate sinew).

However, it may also be caused by an infection, or as the consequence of rheumatic conditions.

See also: Joint Pain

In order to identify the cause, it is, as ever, important to look into any possible emotional causes of sinew problems. For example, any sense of feeling unfulfilled – partially or totally – can be a reason for such inflammation, especially if there arises any sense of one's deepest wishes becoming drowned in the everyday grind of life.

Recognising this situation and accepting that there is a sense of being unfulfilled, and then turning it into a feeling of fulfilment, has often caused what might seem like "miracles cures" of this condition.

Overall, the symptoms are that the smooth movement and function of the sinew is impeded and creaking sounds can be heard. However, synovitis caused by infection creates accumulations of both fluid and pus, which are associated with the most severe and painful outbreaks of the condition. Consequently, whatever the circumstances, synovitis should always be examined by a doctor or an alternative practitioner so that complications and lasting effects can be avoided.

The affected area should be cooled and kept motionless with a splint or plaster cast during treatment. In traditional medicine, the 'dry' variety is mostly treated with cortisone and the infectious variety with antibiotics or by surgery. However, alternative medicine involves the application of cantharides plaster (which drains the skin area), enzyme supplements, comfrey ointment or homeopathic remedies or ointments.

In addition, posture and its affects upon the spinal column need to be considered, along with any blockages of neighbouring joints. The latter have been shown to play a role in the condition, particularly in cases of chronic, therapy-resistant cases of synovitis.

Luckily, there are crystals with an anti-inflammatory effect that can help relieve the pain and speed up the healing process.

Agates of a natural pink colouring thus containing within their structure an inflammation signature (e.g. a pink band or strand) are especially suited for the treatment of synovitis. Agates also assist in helping with a realisation of personal wishes and ideas and also protect personal free space.

Amazonite is particularly helpful with so-termed "dry synovitis" caused by severe stress and which is therapy-resistant. It should also be applied when associated pains increase or decrease without any apparent reason. Amazonite also supports one's deepest yet suppressed yearnings.

Amber is helpful with "dry synovitis" or the consequences of rheumatic diseases. It relieves pain and should, if necessary, be replaced several times with a fresh, cooler piece, if the first one becomes too hot.

Amber enhances a positive mood, eliminates worries, gives confidence for the future and helps one to await quietly the correct time for the fulfilment and activity needed to fulfil any heart felt wishes.

Chrysocolla helps with all types of synovitis. Its compound of copper (the metal of Venus), and silicia relieve infections and inflammation and contributes to the regeneration of affected tissue. It also stimulates life improvement

Heliotrope is particularly helpful with infectious synovitis that may be accompanied by a raised temperature. It stimulates the ability to feel free from any external influences that are constantly distracting.

Lavender Jade is helpful with suddenly recurring synovitis, especially cases occurring as a consequence of acute stress or strain – as with, for example an overstretched sinew. The sprain itself can be treated immediately with Rhodonite, but Lavender Jade animates inner images and dreams and helps inner protection and the realisation of truth and spontaneity.

Ocean Jasper is helpful with infectious, long-lasting synovitis. It strengthens the immune system, relieves the inflammation, lowers high temperatures and supplements the normal draining of fluid accumulations. Being a crystal that encourages the solution of conflicts, it also helps when obligations and professional necessities appear to be in conflict with any original life goals.

Emerald is helpful with very stubborn chronic cases of synovitis – no matter what the cause – as well as with rheumatic diseases. It has a fast pain-relieving effect and impedes inflammation. It also helps find new directions if or when one's inner desires seem to have been lost.

Green Tourmaline is helpful with acute and chronic synovitis, no matter what the cause. It also has a rapid, pain-relieving effect. In addition, it has a positive effect upon regeneration of any affected tissue. Emotionally, when life seems to consist of nothing but effort and struggles, Green Tourmaline reopens the miraculous and wonderful side of existence, making it easier not only to do things but to allow them simply to happen.

For all of the above, place a section/slice or a tumbled stone on the inflamed area or as close as possible to it. If necessary, hold in place with sticking plaster, or use a bandage; alternatively wear as a bracelet, necklace or pendant around the clock.

In addition, or as an alternative, take gem essence (3-9 drops, every hour), or gem water (100–300 ml taken in small sips over the course of the day).

Teeth Grinding

Grinding one's teeth during sleep is the consequence of some form of emotional tension (stress, anxiety, worries, conflicts, grief, etc.), which persists into one's sleep and dreams. The subconscious concern and worry about the problems causes considerable tension in the jaw muscles. The teeth are clenched and ground against each other – almost as if one were having to chew through a problem. The consequences of the grinding are toothache caused by inflammation in the root area (because of the pressure being applied) and subsequent neuralgia (see Nerve Pains; Neuralgia).

Because of its underlying causes – worry, anxiety, problems, etc, teeth grinding is something that needs attention and ought not to be merely accepted. The basic tension has to be identified and addressed properly and therapeutic help is often necessary

Jet relieves the jaw muscles and helps reduce any inflammation that has occurred as a consequence of grinding one's teeth.

Kunzite and Sugilite help to reduce any emotional tension. Kunzite makes it easier to accept things that cannot be changed whilst Sugilite assists in maintaining a regular relaxed mood, in spite of problems and resistance. Both can alleviate nerve pain that often accompanies teeth grinding.

Magnesite relaxes the jaw muscles and decreases any tendency to grind teeth during the night. It also has an emotionally soothing and relaxing effect, as well as encouraging patience and increasing one's capacity to deal with emotional stress.

Place any of these crystals in the mouth in the evening. But remove well before

247

you go to sleep and place it under the pillow.

When the grinding causes actual pain, wear the crystal as necklace or pendant; and take gem essence (5-9 drops), or gem water (200 ml) before going to bed.

Teething Problems

"They arrive with pain and leave with pain" goes an old saying on the subject of teeth. While we do have at least a chance to do something about avoiding the second part of the saying, we are, to a large extent, unable to influence the teething process in the infant and small child. Teething is often connected with pain, a temporary accumulation of lymph fluid, general discomfort with accompanying sleep disturbance, raised temperature (often with reddened, hot cheeks) and diarrhoea.

Amber is traditionally applied for teething troubles and can be worn as pendant (using a large chunk), or as an amber baby necklace (approximately 30 cm long). Both should be lose fitting and care must be taken to avoid the pendant or necklace being too tight. Overall, Amber relieves pain and discomfort and draws away the heat caused by erupting teeth.

Blue Chalcedony can be used with Amber in the same type of necklace to an even better effect, as the latter dissipates accumulated lymph fluid and brings about faster relief through a feeling of coolness.

Because Amber is petrified resin, it "stores" information and overall atmosphere very well. The mother should, therefore, wear the necklace for a while, before placing around the child's neck. In this way, the mother's "'imprint" is transferred to the child, which increases the mineral's positive effect.

Tennis Elbow

Tennis elbow is a term used to describe an aching and inflamed irritation of the periosteum of the upper arm bone at the elbow joint. The problem is often caused by straining sinews, which are attached there at the bone protrusion. The condition can be caused by unaccustomed or excessive playing of tennis – hence the name – or by any other regular activity of the elbow joint. It can also occur as a result of upper spinal problems in the areas on a level with the chest, neck or the shoulder joint. In the latter case, the condition tends to affect both sides of the body.

See also: Joint Pains

In order to identify its exact cause, all cases of tennis elbow should be examined professionally.

In respect of self-help, the first measures to be taken are rest and quiet. In acute cases, the area should also be kept cool – although, whilst seeming contradictory, cases of really chronic pain, require heat treatment.

Traditional medicine usually treats any serious case of tennis elbow with cortisone – or even surgery, where the sinews attachment to the bones, is "nicked", or even cut away.

However, things do not have to be quite that bad! Alternative medicine recommends the application of cooling herb poultices of herbs as treatment, using preparations of comfrey and rue. Homeopathic remedies and body therapies (such as cranio-sacral therapy, etc.) are also valuable, along with acupuncture and other treatments from traditional Chinese medicine

For complementary crystal therapy, the following minerals are recommended.

Amazonite relieves the inflammation and pain of tennis elbow, having a slow but very strong effect. It can, therefore, be combined with Green Tourmaline (see below) initially, or with other pain-relieving crystals, such as Pyrite (see Pain).

Amazonite is particularly suitable for treating chronic conditions, where it prevents the degeneration of the affected muscle. Being feldspar that is rich in lead, it should be applied particularly when tennis elbow is experienced at time of stress or emotional frustration

Chrysocolla also helps with a persistent condition, especially where there may be affected tissue, caused by stress or strain. As a compound of copper and silicic acid, the crystal relieves inflammation and pain, and supports tissue renewal. Chrysocolla also helps especially when tennis elbow is connected with the repetitive and monotonous activities associated with certain manual jobs or activities – an overall condition sometimes now referred to as RSI (repetitive strain injury) and much associated with computer keyboard working.

Green Tourmaline helps with acute and chronic problems. It has a fast pain-relieving effect, inhibits inflammation and also stimulates the regeneration of affected areas.

Emotionally, Green Tourmaline helps especially when one's life seems full of anxiety, stress and strain we and everything seems like a fight requiring great effort. When things seem this way, we tend to neglect the better things in life far too much. However, treating this state of mind with the crystal also leads to free-flowing physical movements, rather than those of a stressed nature and which cause or exacerbate conditions like tennis elbow.

For all the of above, place a slice/section or a flat, tumbled stone as close as possible to the elbow, fixing it there with sticking plaster or a bandage. If necessary, wear as a bracelet, necklace or pendant around the clock.

As an alternative, take gem essence (3-9 drops, every hour), or gem water (100–300 ml taken in small sips over the course of the day).

Temperature Sensitivity

Sensitivity to changing or certain temperatures can signify a number of things. These include: a personal predisposition or perceived bodily aversion; an excessively emotional attitude to heat or cold; a degree of individual imperviousness to a range of temperatures; or a number of physical causes. The latter range from tiredness, through circulation, nerve or glandular disturbances (thyroid gland, adrenal gland), inflammatory states, infections, fever and fluid imbalance, to a wide variety of diseases.

If an infection or disease is the reason, it is important to determine the real cause. Indeed, any sudden occurrence of unusual and lasting sensitivity to temperature should be examined and treated professionally.

Because of this, I cover here only non-specific sensitivity to temperature, i.e. ones which seem to occur regularly, as a general tendency or which prove worrying or annoying at specific times. Examples of this condition are sensitivity toward heat that becomes extremely irksome and a problem during a hot summer; or sensitivity toward cold, which makes the winter unbearable; or difficulties experienced during the damp-cold transitional months of the year. All these problems have one thing in common: they demonstrate our difficulties in adapting, or a reduced ability to deal with, particular aspects of our surroundings.

The physiological components of the human body that are stressed in such situations are what traditional Chinese medicine calls the "triple warmer". This "triple warmer" is the ability of our organism to regulate its own energy. It controls the distribution of the vital life force in all of our organs and joints. It does this by regulating blood circulation in the different parts of the body. It also controls our overall, basic metabolism, as well as the specific energy metabolism of and within cells. Further, it balances any localised lack or surplus of energy and raises or lowers body temperature, depending on the requirements of our overall organism.

In order to strengthen the "triple-warmer", physical exercise is needed to promote and support good circulation. An intake of plenty of fluids is also a great help in ensuring an efficient and beneficial energy distribution, assisting perspiration and subsequent cooling. Add to this plenty of fresh air, as the body needs a good supply of oxygen as fuel. The body is also strengthened by the means of rapid temperature changes (e.g. alternating hot and cold baths/showers, sleeping with an open window, temperature differences in the house, staying out in the open in all kinds of weather, etc.). Thus, only if we "educate our triple warmer" will it be able to react adequately in future.

Our emotional or psychological attitude toward heat and cold is also very important here. The more we "withdraw" from the traditional and natural influences of the seasons – with indoor heating, air conditioning and so forth – so, gradually, we will come to dislike them. This is an attitude that, for example, most children are not yet able to perceive or appreciate ("Why do I have to put on a pullover, just because mummy or daddy are cold?"). So, spend much time outdoors as you can on a regular basis – in all kinds of weather. This induces a feeling of confidence and creates an ability and propensity to defy heat and cold, – and any previous sensitivity to temperature is enormously reduced!

However, if a tendency toward sensitivity to either heat or cold remains, certain crystals – with their corresponding properties of cooling and regulating heat sensitivity – can be applied to great effect.

The following crystals are best for their cooling properties:

Amethyst has a cooling effect. It lowers the circulation rate and assists with efficient perspiration. It also helps in letting go of any tendency to complain or moan about the weather or 'this unbearable heat or cold'.

Aventurine and **Prase** both reduce sensitivity toward heat and also help overcome any psychological resistance towards heat and direct sunlight (see also: Sunburn; Sunstroke).

Aquamarine regulates the functions of the thyroid gland and thus reduces any heat and energy overproduction in the cells.

Beside that, Aventurine brings about general feelings of ease and a relaxed attitude, which make it easier to cope with heat.

Rock Crystal, applied during hot weather, enhances a feeling coolness and eases perspiration. Stroking the head and the joints with the crystal produces an instant and a distinct cooling effect. To achieve this, take a so-called "generator crystal" and allow its large, pointed surface to touch the skin, while moving it from the top, downwards – or from the centre, outwards – over the face, head and the hands (see Fig. 20). If necessary, also stroke the back, body and legs.

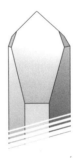

Fig. 20: Generator Crystal

Chalcedony has a cooling effect and improves adaptability to sudden climate changes or those occurring during the transitional seasons of spring or autumn.

Sodalite and **Blue Tourmaline** have a distinctly cooling effect and help in coping with the heat. At the same time, they regulate the circulation and bodily fluid balance and thus dissipate internal heat energy – which is actually what is making the external heat unbearable.

In contrast, the following crystals have a warming and beneficial effect in connection with sensitivity to cold.

Fire Opal stimulates the circulation, makes one warm and active, and is therefore very helpful when one feels chilly and internally cold. Beside that, it stimulates those delightful "hot thoughts"...!

Garnet Pyrope stabilises the blood circulation and generally decreases sensitivity to the cold. Like Ruby, it contributes to overcoming the psychological resistance to frost and cold.

Carnelian stimulates the metabolism and the blood circulation gently but efficiently. As a variety of Chalcedony, it also helps principally during the transitional times of spring and autumn.

Obsidian is one of the best crystals to use in cases of severe sensitivity to cold. It stimulates the energy production of one's cells and improves the blood circulation. In this way, it is very helpful with cold hands and feet. For best effect, place a flat tumbled stone or a cabochon in the shoes or gloves.

Rhodochrosite brings heat to the whole body. Its effect is very rapid in cases of sensitivity to cold arising from tiredness and lack of sleep. It mobilises the body's natural energy reserves and produces a freshening effect (though it is best to remember that we are talking of our own energy reserves, and

that they always have to be renewed with sleep and good food).

Amber decreases any sensitivity to cold and helps one to feel comfortably warm, even during the winter (if adequately dressed, of course). It raises the spirits, with an associated warming effect on the body.

Ruby stimulates the circulation and the distribution of energy throughout the whole body. Like Garnet, it helps with mild hypothermia and in changing one's attitude toward frost and cold. As one of the most robust of crystals, it communicates the sensation that one can overcome anything. In this context, that is in not shrinking from the cold.

For all the above, wear as a bracelet, necklace or pendant, while awake. In addition, or as an alternative, take as gem essence (5-7 drops, 3 times daily), or as gem water (100–300 ml taken in small sips over the course of the day).

Throat Pains

Throat pains can be caused by straining the voice, irritation (e.g. cigarette smoke), infections (diseases in the airways, sore throat), and thyroid gland problems. They can also be caused by emotional stress (literally, a result of holding something back and the resulting tenseness of something unspoken and "stuck in our throats"). Dislocated cervical vertebrae, tensed neck muscles, jaw tension and dislocations, abnormal occlusion or the consequences of problems with teeth are other causes not as easily recognised.

There is also a connection with the intestines and the lymphatic system, as the mucous membranes in the airways often take over the job of detoxification that the intestines or the lymph cannot cope with when overloaded. This situation can also arise as the result of allergies, especially food allergies. So, intestinal cleansing (see Detoxification) and a conscientiously followed diet (preferably with no sugar or cows' milk and low intake of animal protein) are helpful with acute throat pains, especially recurrent ones.

In all cases, a professional medical diagnosis should also be made. It is not only colds that have a key role in respect of infectious diseases. In fact, there are others with a greater potential for real danger, such as diphtheria, mumps, flu or glandular fever. Possible complications – including abscesses, laryngitis, catarrh and acute middle ear inflammation, bronchitis or pneumonia – should be prevented at the earliest possible stage.

One general and helpful remedy for throat pains is to rinse the mouth and the teeth with organic, cold-pressed sunflower oil for some 10-20 minutes every day. When you have finished, spit out the oil and rinse out thoroughly with tepid water. Do NOT swallow the oil under any circumstances!

When throat pain occurs with feverish, general symptoms (tiredness and listlessness), the body is signalling its urgent need for rest. However, even when this is not the case, one should always take care of oneself. If need be, stay in bed whenever suffering from a painful throat; there is a real chance that it may become even worse. Finally, relief and recovery can also be obtained by gargling with sage and thyme tea.

Crystals can relieve acute throat symptoms, and also help at a causal level. This is especially the case when the problems occur repeatedly. Then, vertebrae and neck muscles can also be treated with various treatments such as cranio-sacral therapy, osteopathy, the Dorn-Breuss Method and others.

See also: Neck Pain; Tonsillitis

Amazonite helps with painful throats and hoarseness caused by jaw tensions or straining the voice or when we "have a lump in our throat", because of being unable to express grief, suffering, feelings of unhappiness and an inability to unload our troubles.

Apophyllite helps when throat pain is connected with shyness, fears, inner pressure, anxiety and insecurity. In these cases, it can also help prevent infections from developing into bronchitis.

Aquamarine helps with throat pains, dry coughs, hoarseness connected with allergies, thyroid gland problems, excitement and stress. It also helps one to assert oneself verbally.

Chalcedony relieves throat pain, coughs and swallowing difficulties that may be caused by irritation from smoke, alcohol, etc. It also alleviates infections and diseases of the airways, overloading of the lymphatic system, allergies and straining the voice. It can also play a part when something that really should be said up front to another person, is suppressed and "blocks" the throat. According to Hildegard von Bingen, it is also the crystal of "speakers", and so helps with hoarseness, laryngitis and vocal cord problems.

Chrysocolla helps with throat pain, with difficulty in swallowing, and when the throat feels dry, rough and tender. It boosts the healing of swollen tonsils and the cure and regeneration of mucous membranes. As a detoxifying crystal, Chrysocolla also helps relieve the lymphatic system and strengthen the immune system – both of which are vitally important in preventing any recurrent throat pain.

Dumortierite helps with the consequences of jaw tension, abnormal occlusion or problems of the alimentary tract. Further, it helps when grief, fear or dejectedness make the throat contract. It helps one open up and to unload the mind.

Noble Opal helps with throat pain, coughs and problems in swallowing that are caused by excessive irritation, colds, infections and an overworked lymphatic system. Emotionally, it assists with the consequences of worries, grief and a general lack of *joie-de-vivre*.

Fluorite helps with a severely irritated, raw and contracted throat – one which feels as if it is burning – and with stubborn, barking and irritating coughs, problems with swallowing and pains caused by stress, irritation, allergies, strains on the lymphatic system and respiratory illnesses. Any feelings of personal restriction, as well as crises and desperate situations can all indicate a need to apply Fluorite in connection with throat pain.

Heliotrope helps with the early stages of a cold, problems in swallowing, tonsillitis and with suppressed, depressive or aggressive personal feelings or problems.

Lapis lazuli helps with throat pain that is caused by suppressed anger or when something unspoken is "stuck in our throat". Lapis lazuli makes it easier to "swallow" any uncomfortable truths or to express them vigorously. Apart from that, it also helps when a severe strain on the voice leads to hoarseness or even loss of voice.

Larimar helps with chronic throat pain, hoarseness and loss of voice.

Moss Agate helps with throat pain and stubborn coughs that are associated with mucus and severe inflammation of a sore throat, swollen lymph nodes etc.

Ocean Jasper, the green coloured variety containing pure Chalcedony in the form of transparent, colourless spots is especially effective.

Rutile Quartz must be applied when the

throat pain appears to be 'moving downwards', i.e. down into the bronchi (see also Bronchitis).

Sardonyx helps particularly with a lessening of throat pain, but where some middle-ear inflammation and similar complications remain.

Emerald helps with throat pain with inflammation in connection with head colds and common colds. It should, in particular, be applied when the throat pain threatens to rise into the sinuses.

Sodalite helps with problems in the throat, the larynx or the vocal cords, like Lapis Lazuli, when something that has not been expressed has got stuck in the throat. It furthers consciousness about the fact that one should always say what has to be said, so that there will be no further blockages. It also has a fever lowering effect in cases of infection and helps in particular with a very dry throat and continuous hoarseness.

The practical application is the same for all of the above and one should preferably wear a necklace or a pendant on the throat. If rapid relief is required, take either gem essence (5-7 drops, 5 times daily) or gem water (200–300 ml taken in small sips over the course of the day).

Raw crystals (Aquamarine and Emerald) or tumbled stones can also be put into the mouth (for safety reasons NOT while you are lying down!).

Apophyllite is held in place with a scarf around the neck, as it is mostly only available in the form of a crystal or cluster.

See also: Bronchitis; Colds; Coughs; Hoarseness; Thyroid Problems; Loss of Voice.

Thrush

see Fungal Infections

Thyroid Problems

The thyroid is a hormonal gland, which regulates the entire human energy metabolism of protein, carbohydrate and fat, as well as controlling respiration and blood circulation. It does this chiefly by the secretion of two hormones that contain the element iodine. In addition, the thyroid gland regulates body growth, bone generation and overall development throughout childhood, as well as the sexual requirements and the emotional state of adults.

In turn, the thyroid function is regulated by the pituitary gland, which ensures that a suitable amount of hormones are produced. Consequently, any disturbances of the thyroid gland function will have an effect on the whole individual because of the many-sided effect of its hormones.

Thus, an over-active thyroid – which can be caused by high iodine levels, benevolent cysts in the gland, its acute inflammation, impaired regulation by the pituitary gland, or Graves' disease (an autoimmune ailment) – leads to increased irritability, nervousness and inner unrest. This syndrome is accompanied by extreme and debilitating tiredness, as well as by fears, tremors, raised body temperature, heavy perspiration, visual disturbances, tachycardia, sleep disturbances, negative attitudes towards sex, loss of body weight (in spite of a good appetite), diarrhoea and goitre (swellings in the thyroid region of the neck and a bulging of the eyes).

Conversely, an under-active thyroid gland –which can be caused by extreme lack of iodine, disturbances in the pituitary gland, chronic inflammation, malignant cysts, or side-effects from medicines – shows up as general physical weakness, low temperature, puffy appearance of the face, goitre, excess weight and dry, brittle skin, hair and nails. A reduced heart rate, a slowed down metabolism and a lowering of emotional/mental processes also occur.

Overall, then, the consequences of thyroid over- or under-activity show clearly how important it is that a balanced hormonal production occurs in this gland as the central regulator of our energy output, it is, – so to speak – the body's "accelerator pedal". Therefore, all diseases of the thyroid gland should always be investigated and treated by a doctor or an alternative practitioner.

Unfortunately, medical science remains imprecise as to some causes of regulatory disturbances in the pituitary gland – and

hence the thyroid – but a couple of crystals can be beneficial.

Aquamarine is helpful with both high and low thyroid activity. Apparently, it harmonises the regulatory function of the pituitary gland,

Place a tumbled stone or a slice on the forehead, or wear a necklace or a pendant. Just as effective is to take gem essence (4-6 drops, 3 times daily) or gem water (100–200 ml taken in small sips over the course of the day).

Rock Crystal likewise harmonises the function of the thyroid gland. However, this crystal seems to have a more direct effect, as it is most efficient, when it is placed or fixed in form of a tumbled stone on the throat, or when it is worn in the form of a pendant or a necklace.

Amber is especially helpful with an under-active thyroid gland. It furthers the absorption of iodine through the intestine and the iodine digestion within the thyroid. For this reason, it has been applied since ancient times in cases goitre caused by iodine deficiency. Amber necklaces for babies have the advantage in that they encourage and support growth and development and, at the same time, have a pain relieving effect when the baby is teething.

Wear as a necklace or a pendant. As an alternative, take gem essence (5-9 drops, 3 times daily) or gem water (200–300 ml taken in sips over the course of the day).

Blue Chalcedony and Ocean Jasper help primarily with an over-active thyroid gland and have a relieving effect on Graves' disease. They normalise the body temperature, perspiration, visual disturbances, the heart rate, tremors, and help eliminate nervousness and fear.

Wear as a necklace or pendant, for best effect; or, alternatively, take gem essence (5-7 drops, 3 times daily) or gem water (200–300 ml taken in sips over the course of the day).

Lapis lazuli has a harmonising effect on both over and under-active thyroid glands. As with Aquamarine, a harmonization of the pituitary gland is also achieved.

Place a tumbled stone or a section/slice on the forehead, or wear as a necklace for greater effect, or as a pendant at the throat. Alternatively, take gem essence (3-7 drops, 3 times daily) or gem water (100–200 ml taken in sips over the course of the day).

Tick Bites

The tick is a blood-sucking member of the arachnid family but is only about the size of a pin head with a flat, firm body, short legs and a sucker equipped with barbs. There are about 850 species of tick worldwide. Of these, eight species that occur in European and North American latitudes have a very bad reputation as carriers of the viral infections Rocky Mountain Fever, Meningeal encephalitis (sometimes called Central European Brain Disease or CEBD) and Lyme Disease (also called Borrelia or Borellosis) which is caused by a spiral bacteria.

Ticks can attack many different kinds of hosts, including humans and their relatively long average life expectancy of 2 to 4 years makes them ideal carriers of many kinds of disease causing germs.

They can survive for months and years without food, lurking in the small branches of undergrowth, in the shrubbery of a parking lot, or in bracken and tall grass, while they wait for a host. As they need to protect themselves against dehydration, they never live more than about 80 cm (about 30 inches) above ground, i. e. never in trees, as was previously believed. Potential hosts are recognised by their body odours and their body heat. When the ticks receive such signals, they allow themselves to be brushed off the vegetation and then cling to the skin and hair of the host and find a suitable place to bite. This search for a suitable spot may take from a couple of hours to several days. This increases the chances of finding the tick in good time, before it fastens itself to the skin. Only one out of 100 to 500 ticks in the affected areas are carriers of the CEBD – but one in three ticks carries Lyme's Disease.

However, the harmful bacteria are often not carried over when the tick attaches itself to the host. So, providing the tick is removed in good time, using specific tick tweezers, an infection can nearly always be avoided.

Therefore, it is well worth always carrying out a meticulous "tick check", after been out in woodland, tall grass, bracken or in a meadow. Refrain from applying oil or glue to kill the tick, as ticks, which are exposed to such treatment, are known to excrete the contents of their stomach, including disease germs, into the blood of the host! Because of this and as the tick is hard to remove, being attached to the skin, a common method of removal "in the field" used to be to apply the still hot head of an extinguished match to the tick, which will then release its hold without the damage caused by pulling it away with tweezers, etc.

Then, once the tick has been removed, the spot where one has been bitten can be treated with the ointment of the wild plant, dog's mercury (*Mercurialis perennis*), in order to reduce the danger of infection.

Crystals can also help the process.

Heliotrope is probably the number once choice for applying to the bite location

Prase is effective where the tick bite has become reddened

Rhodonite is good for particularly painful bites

Emerald is recommended for use on an infected bite

For all the above, place a flat section/slice or a tumbled stone directly on the bite, holding it in position by sticking

plaster or bandage. The relevant essence (5-9 drops), or gem water (100–200 ml), can be also taken as a supplement.

If there is any suspicion whatsoever that CEBD, Lyme Disease, Rocky Mountain Fever or any other infection has been contracted (e. g. any strong, flu-like symptoms), seek out a doctor immediately for a full and professional investigation.

See also Insect Bites and Stings

Unfortunately, when it comes to using crystals for the direct treatment of theses serious diseases, there is still work to be done before any recommendations can be made.

Crystals listed elsewhere (see Flu) can relieve some of the associated problems, but they cannot cure or help in the real healing of these diseases. Further, the traditional treatment of Lyme Disease with antibiotics is often not very effective either. Successful recovery can just as easily be obtained through individual combinations of natural remedies – although this should always be overseen by a reputable alternative practitioner. Indeed, herbal medicine has recently enjoyed some success using teasel tincture in the treatment of Lyme Disease – though the jury is still out on this particular remedy.

Overall, a careful check remains the best prophylaxis at present! And, if we do not want to give up enjoying walks in woods and meadows, there are still a couple of ways in which we can make ourselves much less "interesting" to ticks.

Because they react to human body odour, it is important to think about this in relation to one's metabolism and diet. For this reason, ticks never bother some people at all, whilst others seemed forever plagued by them. A diet with a reduced consumption of meat, sausage, and dairy products will reduce the odour of our sweat. Thorough cleansing of the skin and tissues (see Detoxification) will further this even more.

The milder body odour may also be more easily covered by perfumes and scents, which make the ticks stay away. Ticks do not like garlic, for example (this applies to all blood-sucking creatures).

The same goes for strong essential oils, such as tea tree, eucalyptus, cedar, mint, lemon balm and cloves. A corresponding scent mixture can thus provide effective protection.

As a further supplement, crystals that change the metabolism have already been tried out on animals with great success.

Amethyst is an important crystal in treating tick bites as it cleanses the skin (see Skin Care) and thereby alters the secretion of sweat and the body odour. As a supplementary aid, carry a raw or a tumbled stone – or wear it as a bracelet, necklace or pendant on the body.

Finally, apply Hildegard von Bingen's Amethyst Water (see page 25), both externally (washing) and internally (10 ml as required).

Heliotrope, with its properties of "warding off unwanted influence" seems to have an effect on ticks as well. It stimulates the immune defences, improves lymph flow, aids detoxification of the metabolism and so alters perspiration rates and associated and body odour.

Carry a raw stone; or wear it as or a bracelet, necklace or pendant. If necessary, also take gem essence (5-9 drops, when required), or gem water (100–200 ml taken in small sips over the course of the day.)

Amber has the same effect, as it regulates the digestion and metabolic processes and is helpful with skin diseases that are a consequence of these problems. Amber has been shown to have good results with animals, used in the same way as Heliotrope.

Serpentine, in particular the variety known as Zebra Serpentine is very helpful for tick bites on both humans and animals. Applied like Heliotrope, it has also regulates the digestion and metabolism.

Black Tourmaline also helps to prevent tick bites in humans and animals and reduces their probability. It also changes body odour by means of improved metabolism, etc. as well as relieving the inner tensions that might cause the body to attract insects and ticks.

Preferably wear it as a bracelet, necklace, pendant or a crystal on the body. Also, take gem essence (3-7 drops, when required), or gem water (100–200 ml).

Tinnitus

see Hearing Problems

Tiredness

Tiredness, a lack of energy or feelings of weakness after a long working day or after a night without sleep require no other specific treatment than adequate rest and sleep. Nevertheless, if one is still tired and drained after a normal night's sleep, the situation merits further investigation.

Physical problems, such as an unrecognised inflammatory state or infection, iron deficiency, disturbed circulation; nervous complaints and so forth can all be a source of or lead to tiredness and weakness. However, these conditions can also be caused by severe emotional upsets, a real or imagined sense of conflict and serious worries. Furthermore, the state of one's liver is another thing to consider in this context – for weakened liver function is often considered by alternative medical thought as "tiredness is the pain of the liver" (see Liver Health).

Nevertheless, any sudden onset of tiredness, weariness and overall lassitude occurring without any apparent reason, should be regarded as being serious and, if necessary, medical or other professional advice sought.

In the long run, of course, only treatment on a truly causal level can help alleviate the above. Nevertheless, it may be necessary to do something restore energy and vitality as quickly as possible. Crystal therapy can help in many ways here, especially during difficult times, when e there seems to be too much work and too little sleep. However, one should never try to "replace" sleep and rest solely by crystal influence for any long period. No crystal can actually supply true physical or mental strength (even if elsewhere in this book this terminology or description is used as a kind of shorthand or for convenience of description) as crystals simply stimulate natural energy reserves – and, in the end, even these can be depleted.

Apatite harnesses our natural energy reserves in times of persistent physical and emotional weakness or apathy. It has a strengthening and enlivening effect, especially when there are phases of extreme activity and lack of energy that seem to alternate in rapid succession. Apart from that, Apatite also enhances a healthy appetite and thus contributes to "stocking up" energy reserves.

Fire Opal has a stimulating and encouraging effect that can be experienced even within a couple of minutes. It makes one feel dynamic and active, especially in "getting started" more quickly in the morning. Not surprisingly, Fire Opal awakens the latent "fires of enthusiasm" and makes it possible to achieve a great deal within a very short time. However, it should only be employed for a short period, so that energy reserves are not depleted too rapidly.

Garnet Pyrope helps stimulate energy reserves in states of tiredness, etc. whilst simultaneously encouraging the body's innate regeneration processes. Thus, it also ensures long-lasting stamina and courage of purpose in trying times. More mundanely, but just as important, it helps in what has to be done every day, even if there seems no hope of an immediate or speedy improvement of a disagreeable situation.

Rhodocrosite has a rapid, encouraging and stimulating effect, helping to overcoming tiredness and the like within a relatively short time. However, it should not be used for too long, as energy reserves are depleted rapidly with its application, resulting in feelings of an even greater lack of energy.

Tiger Iron provides new strength, when one is tired and weak, through stimulation of the iron metabolism. It works slowly; however, it builds up continuously and should only be avoided, if the exhaustion is caused by inflammation. Apart from that, its nickname, "tiger in the tank", is fully justified.

For all of the above, wear as a necklace, or pendant, with body contact. Fire Opal and Rhodocrosite should only be worn for short periods; the others can be worn for longer.

Alternatively, take gem essence (5 drops, 3 times daily) or gem water (200–300 ml taken in small sips during the course of the day).

Tonsillitis

Tonsillitis is much more than a sore throat. It is a disease characterised by inflammation, feverishness and problems in swallowing. Bed rest is necessary to cure the condition and prevent any complications. In addition, I recommend avoiding the drinking of cow's milk, as it has an adverse effect on the production of mucus in the throat tissues (see Detoxification) and slows the process of recovery.

Proven home remedies include the application of hot, moist compresses for the throat, gargling with sage and thyme tea, or with essential sandalwood oil (mix 2-3 drops with a teaspoon of honey in a glass and add hot water; drink once every hour).

As tonsillitis and any severe sore throat are acute illnesses, there may well be emotional causes. In order to get a handle on the problem, it is worth posing questions, such as: "What is stuck in my throat?" or "What makes my throat seems to contract?"

It is important to clarify these causes in order to avoid recurring bouts of infection. The following crystals are also useful for this purpose.

Chalcedony soothes a sore throat fastest of all. It should be applied when you can feel or see heavily swollen lymph nodes, but there is, at most, only a small amount of coating to be seen on the tonsils. Chalcedony is also a good choice if you have communication problems during the course of the illness.

Chrysocolla helps with a throat that feels dry and rough. It stimulates the shrinking of swollen tonsils and the healing and regeneration of the mucous membranes. As a detoxifying crystal, it further helps cure the causes of the disease (e. g. an overworked lymph system or weakened immune system). This is particularly important in recurrent cases.

Heliotrope helps particularly with suppurating and heavily coated tonsils. It is also beneficial with the effects of suppressed anger or conflicts. It has its most obvious effect when applied immediately as soon as throat pain begins.

Moss Agate and **Ocean Jasper** help with a "full-blown" sore throat and tonsillitis, where there is severe inflammation, pain and swollen lymph nodes, etc. Green-coloured crystals that also include pure chalcedony in a transparent and colourless form are particularly effective.

Emerald helps generally in cases of any type of throat infection. However, it should definitely be applied when your upper respiratory passages are affected, in cases of sinusitis, or if you feel you have lost your way in life at the time when you are suffering from a sore throat.

For all of the above, wear as a short necklace or pendant around your neck. At the same time, take gem essence (5-7 drops, 3 times daily), or gem water (200–300 ml taken in sips during the course of the day).

Small crystals (Emerald) or tumbled stones can also be put directly into the mouth. However, **for safety reasons**, NOT whilst lying down.

Toothache

Toothache is the pain we feel when a softening of the tooth, caused by caries (see Tooth Disease) or decay, reaches further into the tooth and is close to the nerve, or when the tooth is affected by an inflammation in the area of the nerve.

The worst type of toothache occurs when the nerve itself is dying. In such cases, small pockets of gas form and then press on the remains of the still-sensitive nerve. The resulting pain can truly be excruciating – although personal pain thresholds can vary greatly. Nevertheless, the purpose of toothache is probably to prompt the sufferer to see a dentist as soon as possible.

In order to alleviate the pain on the way to the dentist or whilst awaiting treatment, there are some home remedies that can be used as painkillers. These include cloves (which have an anaesthetising effect when they are placed in the mouth) or tea tree oil.

Crystal therapy too is applicable, and whilst it is useful before dental work is carried out, it is more effective afterwards, when any lingering pain may have to be relieved quickly.

Kunzite and **Sugilite** are first and foremost when it comes to controlling pain. Kunzite has a more rapid effect, (taking only a couple of minutes to act; but the effect fades just as quickly). Sugilite has a slower effect and can take up to an hour before it is effective. However, the pain relief lasts much longer than is the case with Kunzite.

Place a tumbled stone of either of the above in the mouth, or place it outside, on the cheek, over the aching spot. If the pain is really severe, it is also possible to take gem essence (5-9 drops), or gem water, when required.

Lavender Jade is, however, best used instead if the area around the nerve of the tooth is inflamed. It has both pain killing and inflammation reducing properties and is especially effective when combined with tea tree oil.

Rub the gums or the cheek with tea tree oil and place a section/slice, or a tumbled stone, on the aching spot. In addition, one can also rinse the mouth with gem essence (10 drops into 100 ml of water) or gem water.

Tooth Disease

The most common disease to affect the teeth is dental caries, in which the teeth become soft and brown and eventually decay. Whilst the exact process is not yet fully understood by medical science, what is certain is that there is a connection with bacteria and carbohydrates (particularly sugar) in the mouth.

Consequently, it remains essential and of vital importance to brush one's teeth regularly – and to see the dentist immediately if tooth cavities appear.

However, even people who brush their teeth regularly can sometimes contract caries; while other people, in spite of inadequate tooth care, still manage to have sound and healthy teeth. It seems unfair, but there may also be some internal factor at play here. Emotionally and psychologically, our teeth are affected directly – as in our tendency to clench our teeth in order to endure and overcome problems, when making difficult decisions and to maintain control in trying situations. So, it can be that the condition of one's teeth is often the result of other people's actions, against which it hard to defend oneself. Thus, therapeutic help with any conflict of this kind can indeed have an indirect influence on the teeth.

Apatite supports the solidity and health of our teeth. As fluorine that contains calcium phosphate, its chemical composition

263

is not unlike that of teeth, and so it seems to have a favourable influence on them. Apart from that, Apatite furthers self-motivation and drive, enabling one to regain control of life and live by one's own choices.

Apatite is best to worn in the form of a necklace or pendant around the neck.

Travel Sickness

Travel sickness is a temporary disturbance caused by swaying or turning movements, exposure to centrifugal force (driving around bends), the feeling of not having solid ground under one's feet (sea travel and ferry journeys especially – as seasickness), or in connection with monotonous shaking (bus or train). It is caused by an irritation of the balance organ within the ear and of the autonomous centres of the brain stem. Emotionally, of course, it can also arise via any tension associated with travel nerves, fear of flying, etc.

Typical symptoms are fits of dizziness, sweating, skin pallor, nausea and vomiting. As a precaution, one can take soothing remedies, such as ginger tablets, which also reduce feelings of nausea. Two hours before the trip, take one tablet every hour. An alternative is a homeopathic remedy called coculus, which is made from the seed of a southeast Asian poppy. It can be taken in the form of 7 drops or as 5 small pills of coculus and sucrose/lactose (Coculus C30). The

Bach flower remedy scleranthus is also helpful.

Dumortierite ("the take-it-easy-crystal"), a mineral rich in boron, provides excellent relief from feelings of nausea and from vomiting. It also encourages the necessary emotionally calmness and relaxation during journeys.

Wear as a necklace or pendant the day before the journey (necklaces give the best results). Also, take gem essence as a supplement (5-7 drops) at the beginning of the journey.

Varicose Veins

Varicose veins are caused by expansions of veins located immediately beneath the upper skin layers most typically occurring in the legs; they are a consequence of an accumulation of blood that should be returning via normal circulation to the heart.

This accumulation is caused by a weakening of the surrounding connective tissue or by the venous valves, which normally reflux of the blood. Hormonal changes during pregnancy may also encourage this condition and the occurrence of varicose veins. Otherwise, their development is encouraged by conditions such as being overweight, lacking in physical exercise and from too much standing or sitting over long periods.

There are emotionally linked causes, too, such as frustration, general stress or general feelings of lack of energy.

Physical exercise, like taking walks or riding a bicycle, and weight reduction is generally recommended as major method of prevention. The consumption of, or bathing in, horse chestnut extract is also claimed to further the regeneration of the veins and to prevent further formation of a varicose condition.

However, any physical or surgical treatment ought to be accompanied by holistic cleansing (see Detoxification), which strengthens any weak connective tissues and stabilises the walls of the veins.

On an emotional level, of course, it is also important to determine just what is causing any frustration and stress

Agates with a relevant configuration and composition will support the cleansing and stabilising process. Those with circular, concentric rings – the so-called **Eye-Agates**, which look like the cross section of blood vessels – and **Mexican Lace Agates** with red tracery, which look like varicose veins, are particularly suitable. Inflammations of the veins, which often occur as a complication of varicose veins, can be avoided and cured with **Pink Agates**.

Emotionally, Agates also support protection, safety, stability and perseverance.

Place or fix a crystal directly on the affected spot and/or take water, in which crystals have been placed for two previous days.

Vision Problems
see Ametropia

Voice Problems
see Hoarseness; Loss of Voice

Vomiting

Vomiting, the convulsive emptying of the stomach contents is not an illness in itself, but a symptom with a variety of causes. In most cases, the stomach tries through vomiting to get rid of consumed substances that are either harmful, or when the stomach cannot process them because of other illnesses or disturbance. Vomiting can be also caused by, among other things, the following; congestion and irritation of the stomach (e. g. because of alcohol), general feverish illnesses (particularly in children), stomach/intestinal illnesses, gall bladder colic, metabolic diseases, various types of inflammation, poisoning or migraine. In addition, unpleasant experiences, smells, disgust, shocking images or sights, etc. may also result in vomiting. Mental impressions which cannot be absorbed and digested can also cause vomiting.

As long as vomiting provides relief and helps to eliminate anything that cannot be digested, it should by not be suppressed. However, nausea that continues when no vomiting has been experienced for a long time, and nothing more can be brought up, can be relieved with healing crystals or other remedies. The cause of the vomiting should, however, always be clarified with a doctor or an alternative practitioner especially if there is no obvious cause, such as excessive alcohol consumption or indigestible fast food.

Rock Crystal relieves vomiting that is accompanied by strong nausea and unproductive retching. Either hold a natural crystal in the hand, or hold it on the stomach pointing upwards.

Dumortierite relieves nausea and vomiting and is particularly helpful when there is nothing left to vomit up, yet there is no end to the vomiting reflex.

It is best to hold a tumbled stone or a flat section on the stomach, or to wear a necklace or a pendant on the body. Taking gem essence (8-12 drops in 50–100 ml water) or gem water (50–100 ml) is also helpful.

Malachite stimulates the act of vomiting and can cause nausea. This can actually be useful and particularly helpful when it is really necessary to "get rid of" consumed liquids or food that is causing the sickness.

Place a tumbled Malachite stone in the mouth for a short while, hold it on the stomach, or take gem essence (10 drops in 100 ml water) or gem water (50–100 ml taken in sips during the course of the day).

Warts

Warts are benevolent, virus-based growths that show up in the form of unusual occurrences of hard skin. They can be contagious, if a tendency toward formation of warts is present. Flat warts are soft, round, mall knots, which often occur in rather large numbers, but only cause little discomfort. As with verrucas and corns, they grow within skin r calluses, like an embedded thorn, deep into the tissue and can be very painful if they are exposed to pressure.

Popular and home-based folk remedies for their treatment include moistening the wart with one's own urine (for several weeks!); the use of oil of red thyme and tea tree; fixing a clove of garlic with sticking plaster directly on the wart; rubbing the wart with the juice of half an onion at the time of the waxing moon in Cancer, Scorpio or Pisces. (If you wish to follow this idea through, the onion must, afterwards, be buried deeply in the earth so that it can never germinate, but will merely rot away. Gradually, as the onion rots away, the warts will fall off.)

Amethyst, Heliotrope, Peridot and **Amber** have turned out to be the most suitable minerals for removing warts, with Peridot demonstrating the best results. Amethyst is most effective as Hildegard von Bingen's Amethyst Water.

Place the crystals on the wart in the form of a crystal (Amethyst), a slice/section

(Heliotrope) or a raw stone (Peridot) respectively, or a polished stone (Amber); or in the form of gem essence (for moistening).

Amethyst can also be applied externally in the form of gem essence. An ointment of Peridot essence and tea tree oil (10 drops of each in 10g of ointment base, which consists of 1 part bee's wax and 4-5 parts jojoba oil) has also proved to be very effective.

Weakness

see Tiredness

Weather Sensitivity

Sensitivity to changes in the weather is a heightened response to climatic changes that can provoke distinct symptoms associated with poor circulation, rheumatism, previous brain injuries, scars or emotional upheaval. Changes in the barometric pressure, humidity and temperature; especially associated with certain types of wind, e. g. the Fohn, Mistral, etc. in Europe, Blue Northern and the Hawk in the USA; are all factors that come into play here. In addition, atmospheric electrical charges (before a thunderstorm, or when two weather fronts meet), can also produce similar effects – such as disturbed concentration, mood fluctuation, anxiety, discomfort, tiredness, sleep disturbances, headaches and pain in scars or old wounds.

It seems that our bodies have difficulty in adjusting their natural regulation mechanisms when faced with these types of atmospheric change.

See also: Sunburn; Sunstroke

Agate is helpful, as it stabilises the blood circulation and strengthens the natural ability to cope with emotional strain. Thus it helps counteract disturbances in concentration, discomfort, disrupted sleep, headaches and general anxiety.

Blue Lace Agate and Ocean Jasper are probably even better to apply for sensitivity to changes in the weather. Because these crystals stimulate the flow of body fluids and sooth the nerves, they help to cope with a whole range of external influences that are caused by the weather. In particular, they can relieve pains of any kind, tiredness, and general discomfort.

Petrified Wood has a stabilising effect, physically as well as emotionally, which is similar to that of Agate, and has a soothing effect on the nerves. It helps with concentration and alleviates moodiness, general discomfort; sleep disturbances and feelings of anxiety.

Wear as a bracelet, necklace or pendant with direct body contact.

In severe cases, take as gem essence (5-9 drops when required), or gem water (200–300 ml taken in small sips over the course of the day).

Weight Problems

A tendency towards excess weight is widespread nowadays in our modern, industrialised and urban society. In rare cases, it is caused by glandular disturbances (for example, in the thyroid gland) or brain disease (inflammation). However, the most common cause, obvious as it may seem, is, quite simply over-eating – and this is the aspect addressed here.

The main foods which pile on the extra pounds are those rich in calories – for example, sweets of all types – and so when we talk about nutrition, the main focus should not only be on the main meals, but also on those "snacks" in between, which are often marketed (both cynically and erroneously) as "breaks to boost your energy".

Quite simply, eating less remains the very best way to get rid of that extra weight. So, all those television commercials and advertisements that are trying to sell certain so-called "foods" (with the emphasis very much on "sell"), which supposedly make layers of fat melt away without having to give up that daily cream bun, are a total waste of time and money. Such alleged remedies often have little or no effect and can even be downright harmful to your health. Therefore, we are left with diet as the key to it all.

It is often difficult to change one's diet – not because one may feel hungry under a new one, but because of ingrained eating habits. Apart from simple eating, consumption of food has many other associations and aspects, ranging from an enjoyable social activity, all the way to being a substitute for love. Consequently, in making a diet change, keep in mind all of these extra connotations. It is easier to replace a daily chocolate snack with an apple than with nothing at all. Be creative: change unhealthy eating habits for healthy ones – but make the change step by step. Gradual change is much better (and more effective) than plunging straight into a crash diet for a few weeks. What is the point of adopting the very latest fashionable or fad diet (and one comes along almost monthly, with all the attendant hype) if any benefit, however tediously won, then results in a relapse and a couple of days of "sinning" indulgence, spoiling all the effort.

There is another factor to consider; as well as healthy and unhealthy nutrition, there is the concept of a healthy and unhealthy time to eat. For example, a rich meal is much harder to digest in the evening than in the morning or at noon. Not only is sleep negatively affected by a full stomach, but food can become, quite literally, lodged in the wrong place. There is quite a lot of sense in the old adage: "Breakfast like a king; lunch like a lord; dine like a pauper!" Even the modern nutritional research costing millions has proved unable to add anything significant to these words of wisdom. Yet, dinner in the evening remains a feature of life for many, especially as a social event.

So, if we eat healthy, whole food with a high nutritional value and do so at the right time, and if we replace small indulgences between meals with healthy little snacks, there ought to be little left to prevent low-key weight reduction. It is the very nature of our genes, which dictates that we will not all end up with the shape of a Barbie doll or a truly handsome hunk. Those kinds of genes have quite simply not been "allocated" to 97% of the population. Teddy bears are much more inviting and cuddly than some anorexic fashion model!

Despite strict adherence to the above, there are three other important factors that may, still, create a tendency towards one being overweight.

First, there are the toxins embedded in body fat, which the human organism simply does want to be burdened with. This is where systematic detoxification, through a special diet and elimination process, supervised by a doctor or an alternative practitioner, is required (see Detoxification).

Second, the fat layer might even be acting as an emotional shield, even if only subconsciously. In losing weight, one becomes more "thin-skinned', i.e. more sensitive, easier to attack and more vulnerable. There is a direct connection between the physical and mental meanings of the expression, in fact. In this case, try to determine if there are reasons behind a feeling of needing protection. If one feels safe, secure and stable emotionally, it may well be that the parallel, physical "buffer zone" will often become superfluous (see also Psychic Protection).

Third, any emotional, psychological or mental state of not feeling "grounded" may result in translation to the physical condition and lead to a weight gain. Simply put, an increase in physical weight provides the "mass" required to stand firmly on the ground. It is something worth considering, with a view to bringing thoughts and feelings down to a realistic level. One has to develop a sense of reality and drive in order to feel grounded again. In many cases, if that happens, the inner and outer need for extra weight will also disappear.

As always, crystals can be helpful in this process in many ways as they can help in changing ingrained negative habits.

Fluorite, among others, is very effective. Simply replace that scrumptious cream gateau in the fridge with Fluorite..... But, joking aside, it really can help change one's eating habits.

Other crystals may stimulate the metabolism, so that the tendency to put on "spare tyres" is reduced.

Magnetite is a good choice as it helps with self-acceptance and also an acceptance of change in general – important in taking on a new eating regime, etc. and attaining goals. It also has a relieving and harmonising effect, reducing the feeling of a need for protection, and thus helps dissipate what caused the overweight problem in the first place.

Ultimately, though, anything and everything to do with nutrition always have something to do with self-awareness. Come the evening, it is very important to try and recall exactly what has been eaten during the day.

Sodalite may help in remembering and creating the essential awareness in such a context. It is, after all, a crystal that aids in creating the space and time in which to live life according to one's own wishes. Furthermore, it also reduces the need for any other form of "expansion' – physical or otherwise.

With Fluorite, Magnesite and Sodalite, wear as a bracelet, necklace or pendant for as long as seems necessary to see their effect.

Petrified Wood is another interesting mineral that should be considered in this context. As a form of Chalcedony, it may help with problems of being overweight, especially when there may be some psychological basis, where aspirations and ideas are raised well beyond and above the reality of life. Fossil wood induces a feeling of security and of giving a solid basis, standing firmly, with both feet on the ground – physically and emotionally.

Try placing a slice or section of the fossilised material on a chair and then sit on

it. Alternatively. Wear a piece as a bracelet, necklace or pendant – or place unpolished pieces around the bed.

Wounds

The healing of wounds can be speeded up and improved considerably by crystal therapy. This applies equally to simple cuts, cracks, abrasions and other injuries, all the way to major surgical wounds after an operation. The generation of unsightly scar tissues can either be avoided totally, or at least partly, depending on the specific case? Of course, crystal treatment of large injuries, presupposes that first aid has been administered and the necessary measures (e.g. stitches for major wounds) have been performed professionally by a surgeon or doctor.

The most important factor in connection with wounds and injuries (after the necessary first aid, of course) is ensuring that one is fully aware of the incident or accident. If necessary, repeat the sequence of events– exactly as it took place, on the same spot and as quickly as possible after the incident (without hurting oneself again!). Sometimes, it is necessary to repeat the whole thing several times, until the pain suddenly increases –and then decreases dramatically. This is the point at which to stop. Such consciousness-raising focuses our attention and associated life energy directly upon the affected spot – so, in turn furthering the healing process.

If the above procedure is impractical, try crystal therapy.

Obsidian in the form of a tumbled stone, is held in the hands, or placed it close to the wound, so that the remaining state of shock within the body cells can be dissipated.

Rhodonite and **Mookaite** can then be applied by placing a tumbled stone, or a section/slice directly on the affected spot. Alternatively, wear them as a bracelet, necklace or pendant; or take as gem essence (5-9 drops), or gem water (up to 1 litre a day).

Worry

see Melancholia

Part 3

Home Remedy
Kits

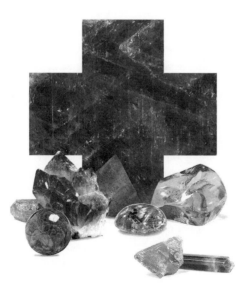

Making Home Remedy Kits

It is important to have to hand all of the remedies when they are needed. This applies especially to the kind of "medicine chest" of healing crystals that you can create for yourself, as the commercial availability of specific minerals and gemstones can subject to considerable fluctuation. It can take days, weeks and sometimes even months, before a specific healing crystal can been supplied – and that's far too long to wait when there is an acute ailment to deal with!

Therefore, maintaining a sensibly thought out home remedy kit is well worth the while. They can prove to be very valuable assets.

However, two things should be kept in mind, when putting together the assortment of healing crystals. Firstly, all of the crystals in the remedy kit should be able to supplement each other, and in such a way that a wide range of properties and applications is possible. Of course, whist any such assortment should be created to suit personal needs, it is worth looking at having three separate kits as follows:

- **The travel kit** (24 healing crystals)
- **The small home kit** (48 healing crystals)
- **The large home kit** (90 healing crystals)

The second point to remember is that in addition to the assortment of individual types of crystals, one should ensure that those selected as the primarily choice ought to be those that can be employed in as many different ways as possible.

Ideally, they are best used in the form of actual crystals, or as raw or tumbled stones with holes, which can be held in the hand, placed on the body or be worn as pendants. This is especially important for the "travel kit", with its limitations of space and weight.

With some specific minerals, however, there are no real options. For example, certain Amethyst-based treatments can only be carried out with the crystals in the form of a druse. This form of Amethyst can be used for cleansing other crystals, so a piece of Amethyst druse is an essential part of all home remedy kits.

The various physical forms that crystals can take are depicted later in this section (see pages 284-288).

There is also a complete "A to Z" of all the crystals mentioned in the book, along with colour photographs showing which forms that are most commonly available.

The Travel Kit

The travelling medicine chest contains 24 crystals that can be applied for the most important illnesses and ailments, etc. These include colds, fevers, headache, circulation problems, menstruation problems, injuries, wound healing, toothache, etc. The selected and listed crystals can, in addition, also be applied for typical travel complaints, such as, for example, travel sickness, nausea, vomiting, diarrhoea, constipation, insect bites, sun burn, tension, etc.

In order to acquire a collection which takes up as little space as possible, it is recommended that you choose crystals that can most easily be placed on the body, fixed there with sticking plaster, be worn on a string, or be used for gem water production. In this way, every single crystal covers a wide range of practical applications.

The Travel Kit

Healing Crystal	Recommended Forms
Amethyst	Druse, (drilled) tumbled stone, gem essence
Amazonite	Bracelet or (drilled) tumbled stone
Apatite	Crystal or (drilled) tumbled stone
Aventurine	(Drilled) tumbled stone
Amber	Necklace or (drilled) tumbled stone
Chalcedony with bands (Blue Lace Agate)	(Drilled) tumbled stone
Chrysoprase	(Drilled) tumbled stone
Dumortierite	(Drilled) tumbled stone, gem essence
Emerald	(Drilled) tumbled stone, gem essence
Garnet Pyrope	(Drilled) tumbled stone
Heliotrope	(Drilled) tumbled stone, gem essence
Kunzite	Crystal or (drilled) tumbled stone
Lavender Jade	(Drilled) tumbled stone
Magnesite	(Drilled) tumbled stone

Healing Crystal	Recommended Forms
Malachite	(Drilled) tumbled stone
Obsidian (Apache's Tear)	Raw stone or (drilled) tumbled stone
Ocean Jasper (Ocean Agate)	Section/slice, (drilled) tumbled stone, gem essence
Prase	(Drilled) tumbled stone
Rhodochrosite	Section/slice, (drilled) tumbled stone
Rhodonite	(Drilled) tumbled stone, gem essence
Sardonyx	(Drilled) tumbled stone
Turquoise	Raw stone or (drilled) tumbled stone
Tourmaline, Blue	Crystal, (drilled) tumbled stone, gem essence
Tourmaline, Black	Four small crystals, (drilled) tumbled stone

To check what each of these looks like, see pages 289-317 under "Healing Crystals A to Z".

In cases of special needs the travel kit contents can be supplemented with the following:

Agate in the form of a section/slice, in connection with digestive problems; Apophyllite in the form of a crystal or a crystal cluster against asthma attacks; Aquamarine in the form of a drilled crystal or drilled tumbled stone; and as gem essence for treating allergies, especially hay fever; Blue or Pink Chalcedony without bands, in the form of a drilled tumbled stone, in order to support milk generation during breastfeeding, which can be particularly important on a journey; Hematite/Tiger Iron in the form of a drilled tumbled stone in cases of iron deficiency; Moonstone especially on honeymoon.

The Small Home Kit

The small medicine chest contains 48 crystals, for treating the most frequently occurring illnesses and conditions. It contains among, other things, crystals for the treatment of acne, allergies, asthma, circulation problems, inflammation, fevers, joint problems, heart problems, coughs, headache, menstrual problems, migraine, nerve problems, rheumatism, back pain, sleep disruption, stress, obesity, tension, warts, etc. It includes everything that is in the travel kit, of course.

The forms recommended in the following table are only suggestions and other alternative forms of the crystal or mineral can be seen below in "Healing Crystals A to Z" (pages 289-317).

The Small Home Kit

Healing Crystal	Recommended Forms
Agate (best with eye signature)	Section/slice, (drilled) tumbled stone, gem essence
Amazonite	Bracelet or (drilled) tumbled stone, gem essence
Amethyst	Druse, (drilled) tumbled stone, gem essence, necklace
Apatite	Crystal, (drilled) tumbled stone, gem essence
Apophyllite	Crystal, crystal cluster
Aquamarine	Crystal, (drilled) tumbled stone, gem essence
Aragonite with bands	Section/slice, (drilled) tumbled stone
Aventurine	Necklace, (drilled) tumbled stone, gem essence
Rock Crystal	Generator crystal, (drilled) tumbled stone
Amber	Raw unpolished stone, necklace, (drilled) tumbled stone, gem essence
Calcite	Raw unpolished stone, (drilled) tumbled stone, gem essence
Carnelian	Raw unpolished stone, (drilled) tumbled stone, gem essence
Chalcedony with bands (Blue Lace Agate)	Section/slice, (drilled) tumbled stone, necklace, gem essence
Chrysocolla	Necklace, (drilled) tumbled stone, gem essence
Chrysoprase	Section/slice, (drilled) tumbled stone, gem essence
Dumortierite	Necklace, (drilled) tumbled stone, gem essence

Healing Crystal	Recommended Forms
Emerald	Crystal, (drilled) tumbled stone, necklace, gem essence
Epidote	Necklace, (drilled) tumbled stone, gem essence
Fluorite	Raw unpolished stone, (drilled) tumbled stone, necklace, cut forms
Garnet Pyrope	Crystal, (drilled) tumbled stone, necklace
Jet	Raw unpolished stone, (drilled) tumbled stone, necklace, gem essence
Hematite	Necklace, (drilled) tumbled stone, gem essence
Heliotrope	Section/slice, (drilled) tumbled stone, necklace, gem essence
Kunzite	Crystal, (drilled) tumbled stone
Lapis lazuli	Raw unpolished stone, (drilled) tumbled stone, necklace, gem essence
Lavender Jade	(Drilled) tumbled stone
Magnesite	Raw unpolished stone, (drilled) tumbled stone, necklace, gem essence
Malachite	Section/slice, (drilled) tumbled stone, necklace
Moon Stone	Necklace, (drilled) tumbled stone
Mookaite	Raw unpolished stone, Section/slice, (drilled) tumbled stone, gem essence
Moss Agate	Necklace, pendant, (drilled) tumbled stone, gem essence
Noble Opal	Raw unpolished stone, (drilled) tumbled stone, gem stone, gem essence
Obsidian (Apache's Tear)	Raw unpolished stone, (drilled) tumbled stone
Obsidian (Snowflake)	Cabochon, (drilled) tumbled stone, necklace, gem essence
Ocean Jasper (Ocean Agate)	Section/slice, (drilled) tumbled stone, gem essence
Peridot	Necklace, (drilled) tumbled stone, gem essence
Prase	Necklace, (drilled) tumbled stone, gem essence
Pyrite Sun	Raw unpolished stone
Rhodochrosite	Section/slice, pendant, (drilled) tumbled stone, necklace, gem essence
Rhodonite	Section/slice, pendant, (drilled) tumbled stone, necklace, gem essence
Sardonyx	Raw unpolished stone, (drilled) tumbled stone, gem essence
Smoky Quartz	Crystal, (drilled) tumbled stone, necklace
Sugilite	Gem stone, (drilled) tumbled stone, gem essence
Topaz Imperial	Crystal, pendant, (drilled) tumbled stone, gem essence
Turquoise	Raw unpolished stone, (drilled) tumbled stone, gem essence
Tourmaline, Blue	Crystal, (drilled) tumbled stone, gem essence
Tourmaline, Black	Four small crystals, (drilled) tumbled stone, necklace, gem essence
Zoisite	Necklace, (drilled) tumbled stone, gem essence

The Large Home Kit

The large medicine chest contains all the 90 crystals, which are mentioned in the book. With these it is possible to treat all the 160 illnesses, complaints and mental problems described in the book. This assortment contains the central range of crystals applied for treatment in crystal healing. Only in special cases do they need to be complemented with further crystals.

The forms of individual crystals mentioned below are chosen as a function of how often they are applied. For other forms of some of the crystals listed below, see pages 289-317 under "Healing Crystals A to Z".

The Large Home Kit

Healing Crystal	Recommended Forms
Agate	Section/slice, pendant, (drilled) tumbled stone, gem essence
Agate (eye signature)	Section/slice, pendant, (drilled) tumbled stone
Agate (bladder signature)	Section/slice, pendant, (drilled) tumbled stone
Agate (intestine signature)	Section/slice, pendant, (drilled) tumbled stone
Agate (inflammation signature)	Section/slice, pendant, (drilled) tumbled stone
Agate (uterus signature)	Section/slice, pendant, (drilled) tumbled stone
Agate (vessel signature, Lace-Agate)	Section/slice, pendant, (drilled) tumbled stone
Agate (skin signature)	Section/slice, pendant, (drilled) tumbled stone
Agate (stomach signature)	Section/slice, pendant, (drilled) tumbled stone
Agate (water agate)	Raw unpolished stone, tumbled stone, partly polished geode
Amazonite	Bracelet, necklace, (drilled) tumbled stone, gem essence
Amethyst	Druse, (drilled) tumbled stone, necklace, gem essence
Antimonite	Crystal, crystal cluster (to be put into water)
Apatite	Crystal, (drilled) tumbled stone, necklace, gem essence
Apophyllite	Crystal, crystal cluster
Aquamarine	Crystal, (drilled) tumbled stone, necklace, gem essence
Aragonite with bands	Section/slice, pendant, (drilled) tumbled stone
Aventurine	Necklace, pendant, (drilled) tumbled stone, gem essence

Healing Crystal	Recommended Forms
Amber	Raw unpolished stone, necklace, (drilled) tumbled stone, gem essence
Biotite-Lens	Raw unpolished stone, drilled, if possible
Bronzite	Pendant, (drilled) tumbled stone, gem essence
Calcite	Raw unpolished stone, (drilled) tumbled stone, pendant, gem essence
Carnelian	Raw unpolished stone, (drilled) tumbled stone, pendant, gem essence
Chalcedony with bands (Blue Lace Agate)	Section/slice, (drilled) tumbled stone, necklace, gem essence
Blue chalcedony (unbanded)	Necklace, pendant, (drilled) tumbled stone
Pink Chalcedony	Raw unpolished stone, pendant, (drilled) tumbled stone, gem essence
Chrysoberyl	Crystal, pendant, gem stone (cabochon etc.), gem essence
Chrysocolla	Necklace, pendant, (drilled) tumbled stone, gem essence
Chrysoprase	Section/slice, pendant, necklace, (drilled) tumbled stone, gem essence
Citrine	Crystal, pendant, (drilled) tumbled stone, gem essence
Diamond	Raw unpolished stone, gem stone, gem essence
Diaspor	Raw unpolished stone, crystal
Dioptase	Crystal, small crystal cluster, gem essence, eye drops
Dumortierite	Necklace, pendant, (drilled) tumbled stone, gem essence
Emerald	Crystal, gem stone, (drilled) tumbled stone, necklace, gem essence
Epidote	Necklace, pendant, (drilled) tumbled stone, gem essence
Fire Opal	Raw unpolished stone, (drilled) tumbled stone, necklace, gem essence
Fluorite	Raw unpolished stone, (drilled) tumbled stone, necklace, ground Forms
Garnet Pyrope	Crystal, (drilled) tumbled stone, pendant, necklace, gem essence
Jet	Raw unpolished stone, (drilled) tumbled stone, necklace, gem essence
Hematite	Raw unpolished stone, pendant, (drilled) tumbled stone, necklace, gem essence
Heliotrope	Section/slice, pendant, (drilled) tumbled stone, necklace, ear-olive, gem essence
Kunzite	Crystal, pendant, (drilled) tumbled stone, necklace, gem essence
Landscape Jasper	Necklace, pendant, (drilled) tumbled stone, gem essence
Lapis lazuli	Raw unpolished stone, Section/slice, pendant, (drilled) tumbled stone, necklace, gem essence
Larimar	Section/slice, pendant, (drilled) tumbled stone, gem essence
Lavender Jade	Pendant, (drilled) tumbled stone, gem essence
Magnesite	Raw unpolished stone, (drilled) tumbled stone, Necklace, gem essence
Malachite	Section/slice, pendant, (drilled) tumbled stone, necklace, gem essence
Moon Stone	Necklace, pendant, (drilled) tumbled stone, gem stone, gem essence
Mookaite	Raw unpolished stone, section/slice, (drilled) tumbled stone, gem essence
Moss Agate	Necklace, pendant, (drilled) tumbled stone, gem essence
Noble Opal	Raw unpolished stone, (drilled) tumbled stone, gem stone, gem essence
Nephrite	Pendant, (drilled) tumbled stone, gem essence
Obsidian (Apache's Tear)	Raw unpolished stone, (drilled) tumbled stone

Healing Crystal	Recommended Forms
Obsidian (Rainbow)	Section/slice, pendant, (drilled) tumbled stone, polished stone
Obsidian (Snowflake)	Cabochon, (drilled) tumbled stone, necklace, gem essence
Obsidian (black)	Mirror (polished section/slice), pendant, (drilled) tumbled stone, gem essence
Ocean Jasper (Ocean Agate)	Section/slice, (drilled) tumbled stone, bracelet, necklace, gem essence
Peridot	Necklace, pendant, (drilled) tumbled stone, gem essence
Petrified wood	Raw unpolished stone, Section/slice, pendant, (drilled) tumbled stone, gem essence
Pink Moss Agate	Pendant, (drilled) tumbled stone
Prase	Necklace, pendant, (drilled) tumbled stone, gem essence
Pyrite Sun	Raw unpolished stone
Rhodochrosite	Section/slice, pendant, (drilled) tumbled stone, necklace, gem essence
Rhodonite	Section/slice, pendant, (drilled) tumbled stone, necklace, gem essence
Rock Crystal	Generator crystal, (drilled) tumbled stone, necklace, gem essence
Rock Crystal (Herkimer Diamonds)	Three small double-ended crystals
Rose Quartz	Raw unpolished stone, pendant, (drilled) tumbled stone, necklace, gem essence
Ruby	Crystal, cross Section, pendant, (drilled) tumbled stone, gem essence
Rutile Quartz	Crystal, pendant, (drilled) tumbled stone, gem essence
Sard	Pendant, (drilled) tumbled stone, gem essence
Sardonyx	Raw unpolished stone, pendant, (drilled) tumbled stone, gem essence
Serpentine	Necklace, pendant, (drilled) tumbled stone, gem essence
Smoky Quartz	Crystal, pendant, (drilled) tumbled stone, necklace, gem essence
Sodalite	Necklace, pendant, (drilled) tumbled stone, gem essence
Sugilite	Gem stone, pendant, (drilled) tumbled stone, gem essence
Thulite	Raw unpolished stone, (drilled) tumbled stone, pendant, gem essence
Tiger's eye	Necklace, pendant, (drilled) tumbled stone
Tiger Iron	Necklace, section/slice, pendant, (drilled) tumbled stone, gem stone (triangle), gem essence
Topaz Imperial	Crystal, pendant, (drilled) tumbled stone, necklace, gem essence
Turquoise	Raw unpolished stone, pendant, (drilled) tumbled stone, gem essence
Tourmaline Dravite	Crystal, section/slice, pendant, (drilled) tumbled stone, gem essence
Tourmaline, Blue	Crystal, section/slice, pendant, (drilled) tumbled stone, gem essence
Tourmaline, Red	Crystal, Section/slice, pendant, (drilled) tumbled stone, gem essence
Tourmaline, Black	Four-six small crystals, section/slice, pendant, (drilled) tumbled stone, necklace, gem essence
Tourmaline, Green	Crystal, pendant, (drilled) tumbled stone, gem essence
Tourmaline, Watermelon	Crystal, section/slice, pendant, (drilled) tumbled stone, gem essence
Zircon	Crystal, gem stone, gem essence
Zoisite	Necklace, pendant, (drilled) tumbled stone, gem essence

Crystal Forms and Signatures

Not all healing crystals are available in all of their natural forms. The forms and signatures listed here are therefore intended as a general overview of the possible forms that might be suitable for one of the home remedy kits

To check other forms of a specific mineral or stone, see pages 289-317 under "Healing Crystals A to Z".

The term 'form' is used to describe the physical appearance of a crystal in the kit. It makes little or no difference whether or not its form can be traced back to its state in natural deposits (a single crystal, druse, raw stone, etc.) or whether it is processed or enhanced in some way (tumbled stone, section/slice, necklace, etc.). In order to make things as simple as possible, gem essences are also included within this terminology.

The term 'signature', on the other hand, describes the affinity between an inclusion, appearance or markings on a crystal with the similar appearance of some part of the human anatomy and is attributed with having an effect on that organ or body part. Only naturally occurring characteristics can be legitimately ascribed in this way as having a category of signatures.

Forms, which are the result of deliberate cutting, polishing and processing (for example, creating a heart-shaped crystal) cannot be said to have a signature.

Signatures play an especially important role in Agates and Ocean Agates (Ocean Jasper), but other crystals too are ascribed with having specific healing properties resulting from their signatures. For example: Amber is sometimes found containing a skin signature, Pink Chalcedony with a mucous membrane signature; Hematite with a kidney and intestine signature; Heliotrope with a pus signature; Magnesite and Malachite with a brain signature; Rhodochrosite with a vessel signature and Rhodonite with a tissue signature.

Overall, one can summarise all of this by saying that whenever the appearance of a crystal makes one think of something specific in or on the body, there is probably a connection between the crystal and the organ or tissue it looks like. It would seem to be the case that it is no coincidence for nature to produces the same form in many situations and locations.

Most healing crystals are used in one or other of the following described **Forms**.

Raw stones are minerals and gems in the form of rough pieces of stone or aggregates. Within this category belong Biotite-lenses, Chalcedony Rosettes, granular Diamond aggregates, Fluorite split-octahedrons, Pyrites, chunks of Rose Quartz, compact Thulite or lumps of Turquoise.

Crystals are naturally occurring minerals, whose form is characterised by even surfaces and edges. For particular therapies and treatments (e. g. lowering a high temperature with generator rock crystals) specific surface combinations are required on the crystal.

Crystal clusters comprise several individual crystals as naturally occurring conglomerates. They are used in this form for specific treatments (e. g. clusters of Apophyllite or Dioptase).

Druses are cavities with in rock formations but which are lined heavily with crystals. Pieces of druses are, in fact, fragments

Fig. 21: Raw Crystals

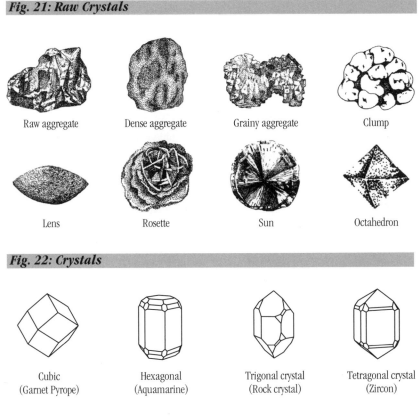

Raw aggregate	Dense aggregate	Grainy aggregate	Clump
Lens	Rosette	Sun	Octahedron

Fig. 22: Crystals

Cubic (Garnet Pyrope)	Hexagonal (Aquamarine)	Trigonal crystal (Rock crystal)	Tetragonal crystal (Zircon)

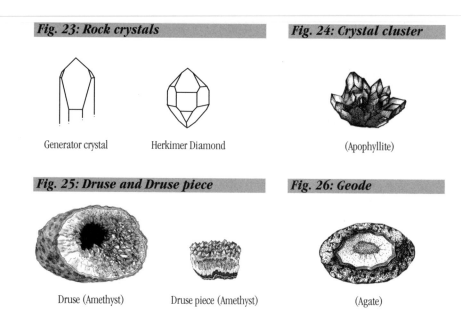

Fig. 23: Rock crystals

Generator crystal   Herkimer Diamond

Fig. 24: Crystal cluster

(Apophyllite)

Fig. 25: Druse and Druse piece

Druse (Amethyst)   Druse piece (Amethyst)

Fig. 26: Geode

(Agate)

from such an "inner lining" of crystals within a cavity. Amethyst, in particular, is usually applied in form of a druse or piece of druse.

Geodes are, in effect, small druses only a few centimetres in size. Agates are sometimes applied in the form of geodes, in particular the unbroken Water Agates

Section/slices are small slabs of crystals, which are cut on both sides and usually highly polished. Agates, especially, are applied in this form, as it clearly brings out the signature of the stone. Mirrors are section/slices, which have been highly polished. For the time being, only mirrors made of Obsidian are applied.

Cross-sections are thin section/slices, cut from crystals, whose external form still

manifests the original profile of the crystal. Tourmalines, especially, are often applied in the form of cross sections.

Tumbled stones are irregularly shaped raw stones, which have been polished into a round shape in tumbling machines and are reminiscent of Quartz pebbles that have been tumbled naturally in rivers. They are the most commonly applied crystals in connection with crystal healing. When they are equipped with a drilled hole to thread them on leather or silk strings, they are called drilled tumbled stones; with a glued metal eye or a hanger [ring; loop] they are called pendants.

Specially polished/ground stones can be made into a wide range of shapes – including the classic ball, egg, and pyramid

Fig. 27: Slice

(Agate)

Fig. 28: Section

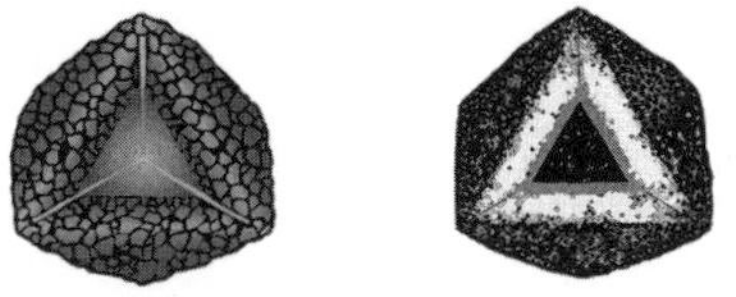

(Tourmaline) (Tourmaline)

Fig. 29: Tumbled crystal

Fig. 30: Polished

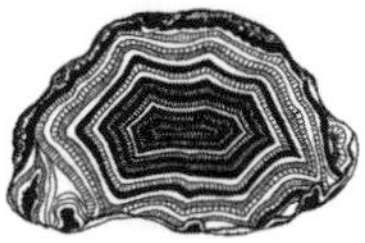

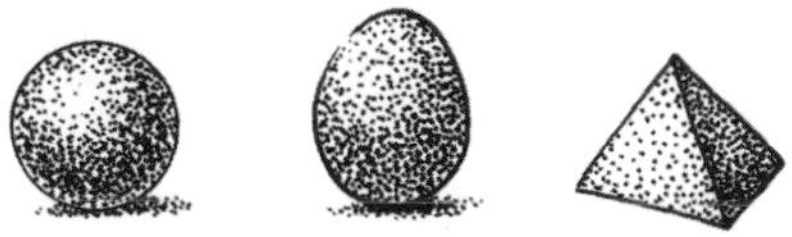

Sphere Egg Pyramid

forms. New shapes are constantly being created, including so-called "free", irregular forms. In principle, any form can be applied, as the inner quality of a crystal (origin, structure, minerals, and colour) will not change substantially, when the outer form is changed.

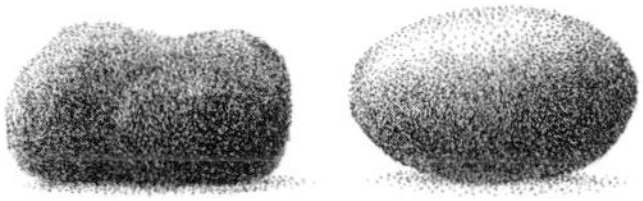

Pendants are raw stones, crystals, tumbled stones or gem stones, which have been mounted, or have a metal eye or a metal hanger, so that they can be carried on a necklace or a string.

Necklaces are raw or polished stones, balls or stones in other forms, which are threaded on a string. In the field of crystal healing, it is necklaces made of small fragments of crystal or round crystal beads that are used most often.

Bracelets are raw or polished stones, which are threaded on elastic, so that they can be worn on the wrist, or the ankle, if required.

Ear olives are small stones, that have been ground and polished in a long oval shape (for example, Heliotrope) and which can be placed in the outer ear. They are equipped with a small metal eyelet, to which a string is attached, so that they can be removed again after use from the ear.

Gemstones have been especially ground, cut and polished to be worn as jewellery. Gem cutting is highly skilled work and follows a wide range of patterns, each with its own style and name. The range of possible forms and working methods has been considerably expanded during the last few of years.

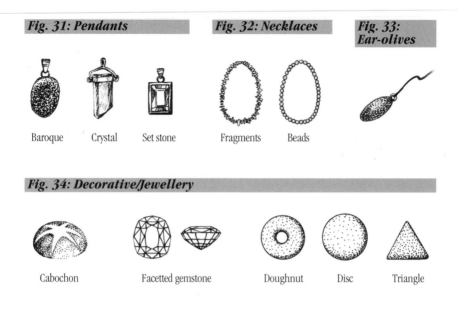

Fig. 31: Pendants

Baroque   Crystal   Set stone

Fig. 32: Necklaces

Fragments   Beads

Fig. 33: Ear-olives

Fig. 34: Decorative/Jewellery

Cabochon   Facetted gemstone   Doughnut   Disc   Triangle

For crystal healing, several forms are generally used: cabochon (hemispherical); facetted (stones polished with many facets) stone; flat torroidal (like horizontal slices from a ring doughnut); discs (round section/slices of stones but which have a slightly convex surface); and, occasionally, triangles.

In the description of treatments in these pages, a gemstone can always be used in place of the same mineral when the wearing of a pendant or tumbled stones is indicated. However, as a rule, raw stones and crystals (and sometimes tumbled stones), are used for the production of gem essences and gem water, as well as for other special preparations in water (Amethyst), wine (carnelian), or oil (Peridot) (see page 25). Gem essences can also be used for preparation of ointments (see page 24).

The above forms are summarised visually in the inside rear cover, which can be left folded out for easier identification of the crystals, etc. mentioned in the treatments comprising Part 2 – or you can double check under "Healing Crystals A to Z" on pages 289-317 – in order to be sure of the appearance of a specific form.

Healing Crystals A to Z

Here are all of the 90 crystals recommended in the treatments described in Part 2 – with descriptions and colour photographs. Each description consists of two main parts as follows.

Forms: these first few lines indicate the range of forms of the respective crystal that are commonly available for crystal healing. This is not necessarily complete, but, nevertheless, it provides essential information on selection of crystal forms for a personal home remedy kit.

Applications: the second section of each description refers the main entries in Part 2, where use of the individual crystal is discussed. However, do not use this section alone when choosing a crystal. Always check the actual entry in Part 2 for the specific application in the treatment of illnesses and complaints. Only in this way can

the best selection be made and the correct application ensured.

For further information, see also *Crystal Power, Crystal Healing*, first published in English by Cassell, London in 1998 and reprinted many times. This book gives comprehensive descriptions of each crystal on the basis of its spiritual, emotional, mental and physical levels of effectiveness. Only Bronzite, Diaspor, Jet, Pink Moss Agate, Sard and Ocean Jasper are absent from the book as their therapeutic effects have only been researched very recently.

To summarise, please use this reference when seeking further detailed information about a specific crystal. The purpose of the following summary is chiefly to assist in finding the specific crystals described in Part 2 and to help in creating your own home remedy kits.

Agate

Forms: Section/slice, bracelet, necklace, pendant, (drilled) tumbled stone, gem stone doughnut, etc., gem essence. Gem essences made from Agates with specific signatures are still not available, though it is worth trying special types of Agate placed in water – e. g. Agates with a vessel signature in cases of haemorrhoids and varicose veins.

Applications: Nightmares, eye complaints (general), stomach pain and problems, leg ulcers, bloatedness, bladder problems, blisters, intestinal problems, ametropia, homesickness, sleep problems, a need for protection, weakened sight, pregnancy, synovitis, growth problems, weather sensitivity and cysts.

Special signatures:

Agate with an eye signature has round, concentric circles or markings, similar in appearance to the human eye. As a result, it is used in connection with the following: tired eyes; eye complaints (general); conjunctivitis; ametropia; varicose veins; enlarged prostate; a need for protection; weak sightedness; pregnancy and cysts.

Agate with a bladder signature has a marking, which corresponds with the hollow section of the bladder. This Agate is used with bladder problems, intestinal problems and cysts.

Agate with an intestine signature (e. g. Mexican Fire Agates) contains curved bands reminiscent in appearance of the intestines.

It is used in connection with stomach ache; bloatedness; intestinal problems; diarrhoea and constipation.

Agate with an inflammation signature has a natural pink colouring, embedded with signatures in shades of grey or brown. It can be used in connection with inflammation, particularly, if it also displays the signature of the affected organ. **Warning**: do not apply so-called "Apricot Agates"! These are artificially heated grey Agates, which tend to have an adverse effect on inflammation.

Agate with a uterus signature has a marking reminiscent of the form and structure of the uterus. It is used in connection with: stomach ache; menstrual problems; as a pregnancy protection crystal; and for normal retraction of the uterus after the birth.

Agate with a blood vessel signature has an appearance similar to the "eye Agates" above, displaying concentric circles reminiscent of sections taken through blood vessels, or with markings looking like the actual course of blood vessels. This Agate is used in connection with ulcerated legs, haemorrhoids and varicose veins – especially during pregnancy.

Agate with a skin signature contains either parallel bands – looking similar to the structure of the skin, with cuticle, sclera, and sub cutis tissues – or markings which correspond to typical skin complaints, such

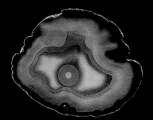
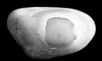

Agate slice, Brazil, and tumbled crystal,
Botswana, with 'eye' signature

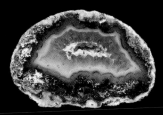
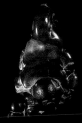

Agate geode, Brazil, with 'bladder'
signature

Agate, partly polished, with 'intestine'
signature (Fire Agate, Mexico)

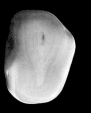
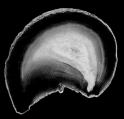

Agate, tumbled crystal, Botswana,
with 'inflammation' signature

Agate slice, Brazil, with
'uterus' signature

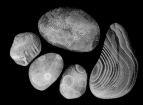
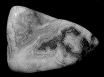

Agate, tumbled crystals, Botswana,
with various 'skin' signatures

Agate, tumbled crystal, with 'organ'
signature (Lace Agate, Mexico)

as rashes, inflammation or scars. It is used in connection with these skin diseases and also with intestinal problems, blisters and fungal infections.

Agate with a stomach signature has a marking, which corresponds to the curved hollow organ of the stomach. Especially suited are the yellow-brown Agates, if possible with a Rock Crystal nucleus. This Agate is used in connection with intestinal and stomach problems.

Water Agates are water-filled Agate geodes, still containing fluid from the time when the Agate was actually formed! This signature is reminiscent of the uterus, which is filled with amniotic fluid during pregnancy. So, it is used as a protective crystal for pregnant women, as well as in connection with bladder problems and cysts.

Amazonite

Forms: Raw stone, section/slice, (drilled) tumbled stone, bracelet, necklace, pendant, gem stone, gem essence, gem water.

Applications: nightmares, fear, slipped disc, bed-wetting, depression, poor memory, painful throat, hoarseness, hyperactivity, carpal tunnel syndrome, improving liver function, learning problems, synovitis, tennis elbow, ganglia and growth problems.

Amber

Forms: Raw stone, section/slice, (drilled) tumbled stone, bracelet, necklace, pendant, gem stone, gem essence and gem water.

Applications: Allergy, stomach ache, intestinal problems, diabetes, gall bladder problems, gout, pains in the extremities, homesickness, itching, carpal tunnel syndrome, headaches, stomach problems, neck tension, nervousness, rheumatism, thyroid gland problems, pregnancy, synovitis, sensitivity to temperature, nausea, constipation, warts, teething, gum disease and tick bites.

Amethyst

Forms: Crystal, piece of a druse, section/slice, (drilled) tumbled stone, bracelet, necklace, pendant, gem stone, gem essence, gem water (as per Hildegard von Bingen).

Applications: Abscesses, acne, tired eyes, eye diseases (general), nystagmus, blisters, high blood pressure, intestinal problems, diarrhoea, ametropia, birth, haemorrhoids, skin care, homesickness, insect bites, itching, headaches, melancholia, migraine, neck tension, dermatitis, bruising, squinting, sleep problems, dandruff, sun burn, sensitivity to temperatures, grief, muscle tension, warts, bedsores and tick bites.

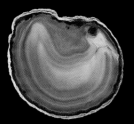

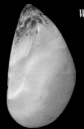

Water Agate,
Brazil

Agate slice, Brazil, with 'stomach'
signature

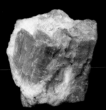

Amazonite, raw crystal,
Namibia

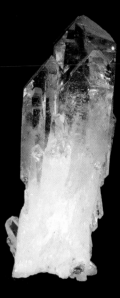

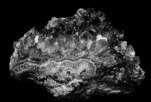

Amethyst, druse piece, Uruguay

Amethyst crystal, Mexico

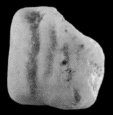

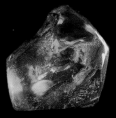

Amber, East Prussia

Amber, East Prussia

Antimonite

Forms: A crystal or a crystal cluster is placed in water.

Applications: stomach ache, dandruff, psoriasis and nausea.

Apatite

Forms: Crystal, (drilled) tumbled stone, bracelet, necklace, pendant, gem essence and gem water.

Applications: joint problems, hyperactivity, knee problems, broken bones, tiredness and weakness, operations, osteoporosis, ganglia, growth problems, teeth and dental diseases.

Apophyllite

Forms: Crystal, crystal cluster.

Applications: asthma, bronchitis and painful throats.

Aquamarine

Forms: Crystal, crystal cluster, (drilled) tumbled stone, bracelet, necklace, pendant, gem stone, gem essence and gem water.

Applications: Allergy, tired eyes, eye diseases (general), nystagmus, stomach ache, bladder problems, ametropia, birth, painful throat, hoarseness, hay fever, coughs, hyperactivity, dermatitis, squinting, thyroid gland problems, sensitivity to temperatures, nausea and growth problems.

Aragonite (with banding)

Forms: section/slice, (drilled) tumbled stone, bracelet, necklace, pendant, gemstone (a mineral with 80% Aragonite is also available in the specialist trade as "Onyx-Marble"), gem essence and gem water.

Applications: Slipped disc, knee and growth problems.

Aventurine

Forms: (drilled) tumbled stone, section/slice, bracelet, necklace, pendant, gemstone, gem essence, gem water.

Applications: arteriosclerosis, heart problems, nervousness, stroke, sleep problems, dandruff, psoriasis, sun burn, sun stroke, stress and temperature sensitivity.

Biotite-lens

Forms: Raw stone (lenses) sometimes drilled or polished.

Applications: stomach ache, intestinal problems, birth, knee problems and menstrual problems.

Bronzite

Forms: (drilled) tumbled stone, bracelet, necklace, pendant, gem essence and gem water.

Applications: exhaustion and stress.

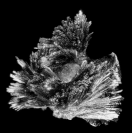

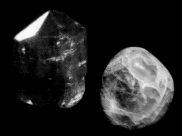

Antimonite crystal cluster, Romania

Apatite crystal and tumbled crystal, Mexico

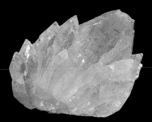

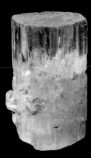

Aquamarine crystal, Pakistan

Apophyllite crystal cluster, India

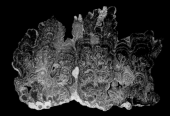

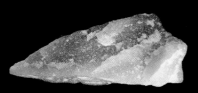

Aragonite slice, Germany

Aventurine, raw crystal, Zimbabwe

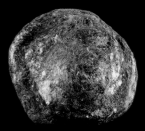

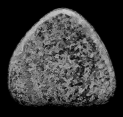

Biotite lens, Portugal

Bronzite, tumbled crystal, Brazil

Calcite

Forms: Raw stone (massive), (drilled) tumbled stone, bracelet, necklace, pendant, ball, gem essence and gem water.

Applications: intestinal problems, birth, broken bones, osteoporosis, constipation and growth problems.

Carnelian

Forms: raw stone (lump), (drilled) tumbled stone, bracelet, necklace, pendant, gem essence, gem water, raw or tumbled stones which have been simmered in wine.

Applications: leg ulcer, bleeding (slight), intestinal problems, colds, fever (rising), birth, nosebleed, temperature sensitivity and bedsores.

Chalcedony, Blue

Forms: Raw stone, section/slice, (drilled) tumbled stone, bracelet, necklace, pendant, gemstone, ground and polished forms, gem essence, raw and tumbled stones that are placed into water

Applications: *Chalcedony with bands / Blue Lace Agate*: eye diseases (general), bladder problems, blisters, high blood pressure, allergy, throat inflammation, conjunctivitis, detoxification, colds, fever (lowering), tired feet, pains in the extremities, influenza, glaucoma, throat pain, hoarseness, coughs, learning problems, stimulation of the lymph system, sinusitis, strengthening of the kidneys, oedemas, thyroid gland problems, weak sightedness, pregnancy, loss of voice, stuttering, sensitivity to temperature, weather sensitivity, and teething.

Unbanded Chalcedony : Eye diseases (general), bladder problems, blisters, high blood pressure, diabetes, fever (lowering), birth, glaucoma, throat pain, learning problems, milk generation, strengthening of the kidneys, thyroid gland problems, weak sightedness, breast-feeding, loss of voice, menopausal problems, sensitivity to temperature and weather sensitivity.

Chalcedony, Pink

Forms: Raw stone, (drilled) tumbled stone, bracelet, necklace, pendant, gem essence, raw and tumbled stones placed in water

Applications: throat inflammation, diabetes, detoxification, colds, birth, influenza, homesickness, hoarseness, heart problems, learning problems, stimulation of the lymph system, milk generation, oedemas, thyroid gland problems, breast-feeding and stuttering.

Chrysoberyl

Forms: Raw stone, crystal, crystal cluster, tumbled stone (rare), bracelet, necklace, pendant, gem stone, gem essence and gem water.

Applications: bad memory, hyperactivity, concentration problems, learning problems, nervousness, weak sightedness, and loss of voice and stuttering.

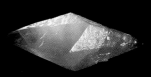

Calcite crystal, Brazil

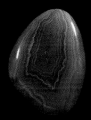

Carnelian, tumbled crystal, Botswana

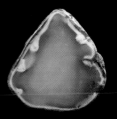

Blue Chalcedony without bands, Turkey

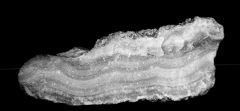

Banded Chalcedony, Brazil

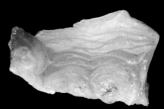

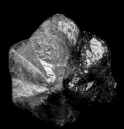

Pink Chalcedony, USA (rosette)

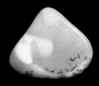

Pink Chalcedony, Turkey (tumbled crystal)

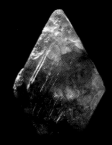

Chrysoberyl crystal, Zimbabwe

Chrysoberyl triplet, Brazil

Chrysocolla

Forms: Raw stone (massive to compact), (drilled) tumbled stone, bracelet, necklace, pendant, gem stone, gem essence and gem water.

Applications: throat inflammation, stomach ache, fever (lowering), gall bladder problems, birth, painful throat, strengthening of the immune system, carpal tunnel syndrome, scars, pregnancy, synovitis, stress, tennis elbow and ganglia.

Chrysoprase

Forms: Section/slice, (drilled) tumbled stone, bracelet, necklace, pendant, gem stone, gem essence and gem water.

Applications: acne, allergy, nightmares, eye diseases (general), stomach ache, bedwetting, intestinal problems, detoxification, fertility, athlete's foot, gall bladder problems, gout, glaucoma, homesickness, herpes, insect bites, cramp, sorrow, strengthening of the liver, dermatitis, strengthening of the kidneys, operations, fungal infections, rheumatism, sleep problems, psoriasis and growth problems.

Citrine

Forms: crystal, (drilled) tumbled stone, bracelet, necklace, pendant, gemstone, gem essence and gem water.

Applications: Stomach ache, bed-wetting, depression, diabetes, birth, sadness and growth problems.

Diamond

Forms: raw stone, crystal, pendant, gemstone and gem essence.

Applications: arteriosclerosis, eye diseases (general), bad memory, gout, cataract, concentration problems, strokes and weakened sight.

Diaspor

Forms: raw stone, crystal.

Applications: stomach ache, stomach problems, heartburn and acidification.

Dioptase

Forms: crystal, crystal cluster, gem essence, gem water and eye drops

Applications: tired eyes, eye diseases (general), slipped disc, knee problems, strengthening of the liver, weak sightedness and growth problems.

Dumortierite

Forms: (drilled) tumbled stone, section/slice, bracelet, necklace, pendant, gemstone, gem essence and gem water.

Applications: fear, stomach ache, intestinal problems, depression, diarrhoea, vomiting, gall bladder problems, painful throat, homesickness, carpal tunnel syndrome, sorrow, nervousness, operations, travel sickness, pregnancy, stress, grief and nausea.

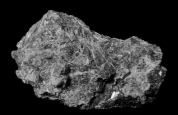

Chrysocolla, raw crystal

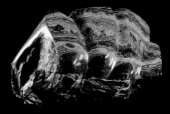

Chrysocolla, partly polished

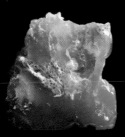

Chrysoprase slice, Australia

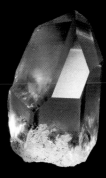

Citrine crystal, Brazil

Diamond crystal, South Africa

Diaspor crystal, Turkey

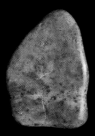

Dumortierite, tumbled crystal, Mozambique

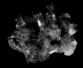

Dioptase crystal, small cluster, Namibia

Emerald

Forms: crystal, cross section, (drilled) tumbled stone, bracelet, necklace, pendant, gem stone, gem essence and gem water.

Applications: throat inflammation, tired eyes, eye diseases (general), stomach ache, conjunctivitis, bloatedness, bronchitis, intestinal problems, inflammation, ametropia, gall bladder problems, birth, influenza, painful throat, carpal tunnel syndrome, head ache, cramp, strengthening of the liver, middle ear inflammation, sinusitis, dermatitis, back pain, squinting, snoring, head cold, weak sightedness, synovitis, growth problems, bedsores and tick bites.

Epidote

Forms: crystal (rarely), (drilled) tumbled stone, section/slice, bracelet, necklace, pendant, gem stone, gem essence and gem water.

Applications: colds, exhaustion, birth, influenza, strengthening of the immune system, strengthening of the liver, regeneration and growth problems.

Fire Opal

Forms: raw stone, (drilled) tumbled stone, bracelet, necklace, pendant, gemstone (cabochon, facetted), gem essence and gem water.

Applications: Low blood pressure, homesickness, tiredness and weakness, potency problems, sexuality and temperature sensitivity.

Fluorite

Forms: raw stone (octahedron), crystal cluster, (drilled) tumbled stone, bracelet, necklace, pendant, polished forms (spheres, pyramids etc.), gem essence, raw or tumbled stones which are placed in water.

Applications: Intestinal problems, painful throat, bad memory, gout, coughs, concentration problems, learning problems, osteoporosis, fungal infection, ganglia, overweight and growth problems.

Garnet Pyrope

Forms: crystal, (drilled) tumbled stone, bracelet, necklace, pendant, gemstone, gem essence, gem water, and ointment.

Applications: bladder problems, circulation problems, exhaustion, cold feet, joint problems, circulation problems, tiredness and weakness, weak muscles, ear problems, pregnancy, sexuality problems, numbness, temperature sensitivity and bedsores.

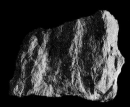

*Epidote, raw crystal
(Unakite), USA*

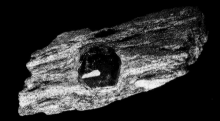

*Garnet Pyrope crystal
in a matrix, Alaska*

*Fire Opal,
raw crystal, Mexico*

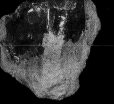

*Emerald crystal,
Brazil*

*Fluorite
octahedrons, USA*

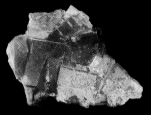

*Fluorite crystal cluster,
Black Forest, Germany*

Haematite

Forms: raw stone, (drilled) tumbled stone, section/slice, bracelet, necklace, pendant, gem stone, gem essence and gem water.

Applications: leg ulcers, low blood pressure, intestinal problems, iron deficiency, circulation problems and pregnancy.

Heliotrope

Forms: section/slice, (drilled) tumbled stone, bracelet, necklace, pendant, ear olive, gemstone, gem essence, gem water and ointment.

Applications: abscesses, throat inflammation, arteriosclerosis, stomach ache, bedwetting, conjunctivitis, bladder problems, intestinal problems, iron deficiency, inflammation, colds, gall bladder problems, birth, influenza, painful throat, haemorrhoids, heart problems, strengthening of the immune system, insect bites, carpal tunnel syndrome, middle ear inflammation, sinusitis, ear problems, stroke, snoring, head cold, synovitis, nausea, warts, tick prophylaxis.

Jet

Forms: raw stone, (drilled) tumbled stone, bracelet, necklace, pendant, gemstone, gem essence and gem water.

Applications: intestinal problems, diarrhoea, mouth problems, grief, teeth grinding and gum disease.

Kunzite

Forms: crystal, (drilled) tumbled stone, bracelet, necklace, pendant, gem stone, gem essence, raw or tumbled stones which have been placed in water.

Applications: slipped disc, birth, bad memory, lumbago, nerve problems, back pain, pain, pregnancy, grinding teeth, toothache.

Landscape Jasper

Forms: (drilled) tumbled stone, bracelet, necklace, pendant, gemstone (doughnut, disc), gem essence and gem water.

Applications: allergy, intestinal problems, and hay fever.

Lapis lazuli

Forms: raw stone (massive to dense), crystal (rarely), (drilled) tumbled stone, section/slice, necklace, pendant, gemstone, polished forms (spheres, pyramids etc.), gem essence and gem water.

Applications: high blood pressure, painful throat, hoarseness, herpes (lips), learning problems, menstrual problems, thyroid gland problems, loss of voice.

Larimar

Forms: section/slice, (drilled) tumbled stone, bracelet, pendant, gem essence and gem water.

Applications: painful throat, nerve problems, nervousness, loss of voice, growth problems.

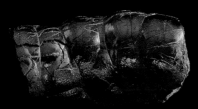

Hematite, raw crystal, England

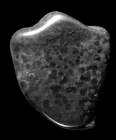

Heliotrope, tumbled crystal, India

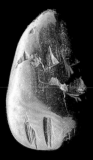

Larimar, Dominican Republic

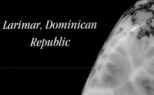

Jet, tumbled crystal, USA

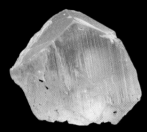

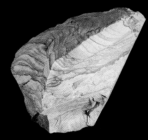

Kunzite crystal, Afghanistan

Landscape Jasper, raw crystal, South Africa

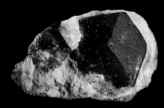

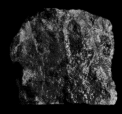

Lapis lazuli, crystal, Afghanistan

Lapis lazuli, raw crystal, Afghanistan

Lavender Jade

Forms: (drilled) tumbled stone, bracelet, necklace, pendant, gem essence and gem water.

Applications: homesickness, carpal tunnel syndrome, nerve problems, strengthening of the kidneys, synovitis and toothache.

Magnesite

Forms: raw stone (lump), (drilled) tumbled stone, bracelet, necklace, pendant, gemstone (doughnut, disc), gem essence and gem water.

Applications: stomach ache, intestinal problems, tired feet, gall bladder problems, birth, pains in the extremities, headache, cramp, stomach problems, migraine, neck tension, nervousness, back pain, heartburn, stress, nausea, overweight, muscle tension, cramp in the calves, grinding teeth, sprains.

Malachite

Forms: section/slice, (drilled) tumbled stone, bracelet, necklace, pendant, gemstone, gem essence and gem water.

Applications: stomach ache, vomiting, gall bladder problems, birth, cramp, strengthening of the liver, menstrual problems, rheumatism, pain and sexual problems.

Mookaite

Forms: raw stone (massive), (drilled) tumbled stone, section/slice, bracelet, necklace, pendant, gem essence and gem water.

Applications: leg ulcers, light bleeding, intestinal problems, birth, homesickness, operations, cuts, abrasions, wound healing and bedsores.

Moon Stone

Forms: (drilled) tumbled stone, bracelet, necklace, pendant, gemstone (cabochon), gem essence and gem water.

Applications: acne, fertility (women), birth, menstrual problems, pregnancy, growth problems and the menopause.

Moss Agate

Forms: (drilled) tumbled stone, section/slice, bracelet, necklace, pendant, gemstone, gem essence and gem water.

Applications: throat inflammation, colds, fever (lowering), tired feet, pains in extremities, influenza, painful throat, coughs, stimulation of the lymph system, sinusitis.

Moss Agate, Pink

Forms: (drilled) tumbled stone, pendant, gem water.

Applications: stomach ache, intestinal problems, nausea, and constipation.

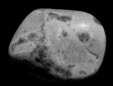

Lavender Jade, Turkey

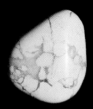

Magnesite, tumbled crystal, Zimbabwe

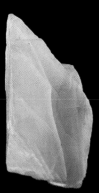

*Moonstone,
raw crystal,
India*

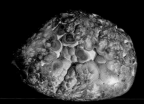

Malachite clump, partly polished, Congo

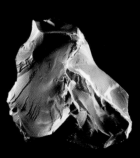

Mookaite, raw crystal, Australia

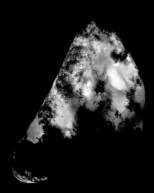

*Moss Agate,
tumbled crystal,
India*

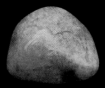

Pink Moss Agate, tumbled crystal, India

Nephrite

Forms: section/slice, (drilled) tumbled stone, necklace, pendant, gemstone, gem essence and gem water.

Applications: bladder problems, strengthening of the kidneys.

Noble Opal

Forms: raw stone, (drilled) tumbled stone, bracelet, necklace, pendant, gemstone (cabochon), gem essence and gem water.

Applications: eye diseases (general), depression, painful throat, homesickness, coughs, cancer, sorrow, improving of the lymphatic system, weak sightedness and grief.

Obsidian

Black Obsidian is regular black obsidian rich in foreign matter.

Snowflake Obsidian has small, grey feldspar aggregates, which are reminiscent of snowflakes or clouds or flowers.

Rainbow Obsidian contains small water blisters that reflect incidental light, and which, in turn, act as a prism and produce the colours of the spectrum.

Apache's Tear has a very high silicic acid content that makes it transparent.

Forms: section/slice (mirror), (drilled) tumbled stone, bracelet, necklace, pendant, gemstone (cabochon, doughnut, disc, etc.), gem essence and gem water.

Applications

(*Black Obsidian*): bruising, bleeding (slight), cataract, operations, cuts, shock, abrasions, need for protection (mirror), sprain, sensitivity to temperature, wound healing, overstretched or torn ligaments.

Snowflake Obsidian: bruising, bleeding (slight), circulation problems, cold feet, operations, cuts, shock, abrasions, sensitivity to temperature, sprains, wound healing, overstretched or torn ligaments.

Rainbow Obsidian: bruising, bleeding (slight), cataract, operations, cuts, shock, abrasions, sensitivity to temperature, sprains, wound healing, overstretched or torn ligaments.

Apache's Tear: bleeding (slight), cataract, operations, back pain, pain, cuts, shock, abrasions, sprains, wound healing, overstretched or torn ligaments.

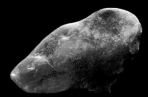

Nephrite, tumbled crystal,
Russia

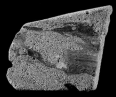

Noble Opal, Boulder Opal,
Australia

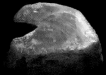

Noble Opal, white Opal,
Australia

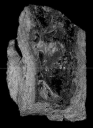

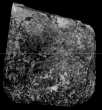

Noble Opal, crystal opal, Australia

Noble Opal, black opal, Australia

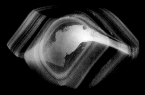

Rainbow Obsidian, Mexico

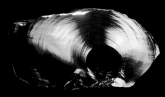

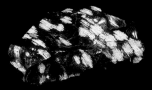

Black Obsidian, Mexico

Snowflake Obsidian, Mexico

Ocean Jasper (Ocean Agate)

Forms: raw stone, section/slice, (drilled) tumbled stone, bracelet, necklace, pendant, gem stone, gem essence and gem water.

Applications: abscesses, allergies, nightmares, throat inflammation, eye diseases (general), stomach ache, leg ulcers, conjunctivitis, bladder problems, blisters, bronchitis, cellulite, intestinal problems, diabetes, detoxification, inflammations, colds, exhaustion, fever (lowering), fertility, tired feet, gall bladder problems, pains in the extremities, influenza, glaucoma, painful throat, hay fever, coughs, strengthening of the immune system, cancer, strengthening of the liver, stimulation of the lymph system, migraine, middle ear inflammation, mouth problems, sinusitis, dermatitis, strengthening of the kidneys, oedemas, ear problems, fungal infections, enlarged prostate, regeneration, thyroid gland problems, sleep problems, snoring, weak sightedness, synovitis, nausea, growth problems, menopause, weather sensitivity, cysts.

Peridot

Forms: raw stone (grainy or massive), (drilled) tumbled stone, bracelet, necklace, pendant, gem stone, gem essence, ointment, raw or tumbled stoned which have been placed in sun flower oil.

Applications: intestinal problems, detoxification, gall bladder problems, birth, strengthening of the kidneys, warts.

Petrified Wood

Forms: raw stone, section/slice, (drilled) tumbled stone, bracelet, necklace, pendant, gem stone, gem essence and gem water.

Applications: homesickness, overweight, weather sensitivity.

Prase

Forms: crystal (rarely), (drilled) tumbled stone, section/slice, bracelet, necklace, pendant, gemstone, gem essence and gem water.

Applications: insect bites, bruising, sunburn, sunstroke and temperature sensitivity.

Pyrites

Forms: raw stone (sun)

Applications: slipped disc, joint problems, lumbago, knee problems, pain, tick prophylaxis.

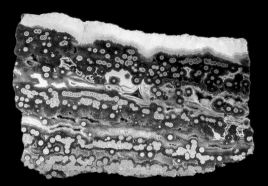

Ocean Agate (Ocean Jasper),
Madagascar

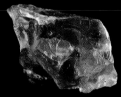

Peridot, raw crystal, (Chrysolith), USA

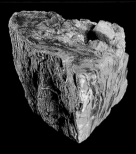

Petrified Wood, raw crystal, Australia

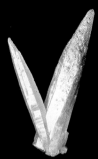

Prase crystals,
Serifos, Greece

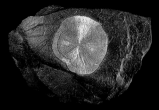

Pyrites in mother lode, USA

Rhodochrosite

Forms: section/slice, (drilled) tumbled stone, bracelet, necklace, pendant, gemstone, gem essence and gem water.

Applications: low blood pressure, circulation problems, exhaustion, migraine, tiredness and weakness, pregnancy, sensitivity to temperature.

Rhodonite

Forms: section/slice, (drilled) tumbled stone, bracelet, necklace, pendant, gemstone (doughnut, disc), gem essence and gem water.

Applications: acne, fear, stomach ache, leg ulcers, blisters, bruising, bleeding (slight), intestinal problems, haemorrhoids, herpes (lips), insect bites, headache, weak muscles, muscle injuries, neck tension, scars, nosebleed, ear problems, operations, pain, cuts, shock, abrasions, grief, burns, sprains, growth problems, wound healing, bedsores, gum disease, overstretched or torn ligaments, tick prophylaxis.

Rock Crystal

Forms: Crystal, crystal cluster, (drilled) tumbled stone, bracelet, necklace, pendant, gem essence and gem water.

Applications: eye diseases (general), vomiting, ametropia, fever (lowering), joint problems, cataract, insect bites, headache, squinting, thyroid gland problems, pain, weak sightedness, stuttering, numbness and temperature sensitivity.

Special Forms:

Generator crystals have an especially large, dominant surface at the point. The latter can "draw off" heat in cases of fever or temperature sensitivity, if the skin is stroked with it.

Herkimer-Diamonds are small, bright and especially clear, double-ended Rock Crystals. Three of them arranged in a triangle on an aching area have a relieving effect.

Rose Quartz

Forms: crystal cluster (rarely), massive raw stone, (drilled) tumbled stone, section/slice, bracelet, necklace, pendant, gem stone, cut corms (spheres), gem essence and gem water.

Applications: circulation problems, fertility (women), heart problems, sexual problems and bedsores.

Ruby

Forms: crystal, cross section, (drilled) tumbled stone, bracelet, necklace, pendant, gem stone, gem essence and gem water.

Applications: low blood pressure, fever (raising), circulation problems, potency problems, back pain, sexual problems and temperature sensitivity.

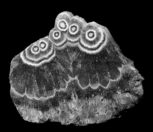

Rhodochrosite slice, Argentina

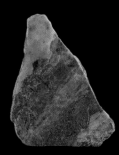

Rhodonite slice, Australia

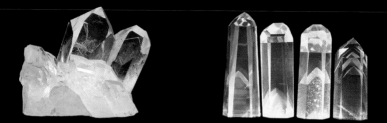

Rock crystal cluster and Phantom Quartz, Brazil

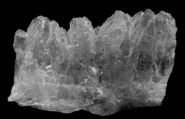

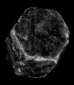

Ruby crystal, India

Rose Quartz crystal cluster, Brazil

Rutile Quartz

Forms: crystal, crystal cluster (rarely), (drilled) tumbled stone, section/slice, bracelet, necklace, pendant, gem stone, gem essence and gem water.

Applications: fear, asthma, bronchitis, depression, athlete's foot, birth, painful throat, heart problems, coughs, regeneration, sexual problems and constipation.

Sard

Forms: (drilled) tumbled stone, bracelet, necklace, pendant, gem essence and gem water.

Applications: Colds, fever (raising), heart problems.

Sardonyx

Forms: raw stone (massive), (drilled) tumbled stone, bracelet, necklace, pendant, gem essence and gem water.

Applications: eye diseases (general), nystagmus, stomach ache, intestinal problems, colds, pains in the extremities, glaucoma, painful throat, middle ear inflammation, ear problems, operations, squinting, weak sightedness.

Serpentine

Forms: section/slice, (drilled) tumbled stone, bracelet, necklace, pendant, gemstone, gem essence and gem water.

Applications: stomach and intestinal problems, diarrhoea, homesickness, strengthening of the kidneys, need for protection, sexual problems, cramp in the calves and tick bites.

Smoky Quartz

Forms: crystal, crystal cluster, (drilled) tumbled stone, bracelet, necklace, pendant, gem essence and gem water.

Applications: Nystagmus, intestinal problems, athlete's foot, headache, neck tension, fungal infection, back pain, sunstroke, stress, muscle tension.

Sodalite

Forms: raw stone (massive), (drilled) tumbled stone, bracelet, necklace, pendant, gem stone, cut forms (spheres, pyramids), gem essence, gem water.

Applications: eye diseases (general), high blood pressure, painful throat, hoarseness, loss of voice, temperature sensitivity to temperature and obesity.

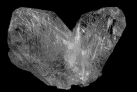

Rutilated Quartz crystals, Brazil

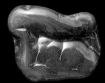

Sard, tumbled crystal, India

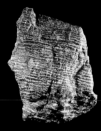

Serpentine, raw crystal (Silver Eye), Australia

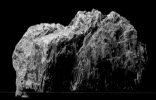

Serpentine, raw crystal, (Tauern green), Austria

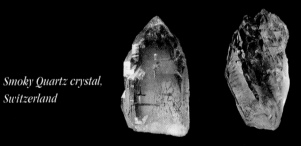

Smoky Quartz crystal, Switzerland

Smoky Quartz, Switzerland

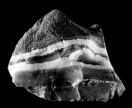

Sardonyx, raw crystal, India

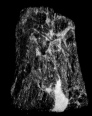

Sodalite, raw crystal, Brazil

Sugilite

Forms: section/slice, (drilled) tumbled stone, bracelet, necklace, pendant, gemstone, gem essence and gem water.

Applications: fear, lumbago, carpal tunnel syndrome, nerve problems, operations, pain, teeth grinding, toothache.

Thulite

Forms: raw stone (grainy), (drilled) tumbled stone, bracelet, necklace, pendant, gemstone, gem essence and gem water.

Applications: fertility (men), potency and sexual problems.

Tiger's Eye (Gold Quartz)

Forms: section/slice, (drilled) tumbled stone, bracelet, necklace, pendant.

Applications: asthma.

Tiger Iron

Forms: section/slice, (drilled) tumbled stone, bracelet, necklace, pendant, gemstone (doughnut, disc, triangle), gem essence and gem water.

Applications: iron deficiency, exhaustion, circulation problems, menstrual problems, tiredness and weakness, pregnancy.

Topaz, Imperial

Forms: crystal, (drilled) tumbled stone, bracelet, necklace, pendant, gemstone, gem essence and gem water.

Applications: stomach ache, intestinal problems, depression, fertility (women), childbirth, nervousness and growth problems.

Tourmaline, Blue (Indigolith)

Forms: crystal, section/slice, cross section, tumbled stone, pendant, bracelet, necklace, gem stone, gem essence and gem water.

Applications: eye diseases (general), blisters, birth, hyperactivity, neck tension, scars, squinting, weak sightedness, numbness, sensitivity to temperature, grief, burns, muscle tension, growth problems.

Tourmaline, Dravite

Forms: crystal, (drilled) tumbled stone, section/slice, cross section, pendant, necklace (rarely), gem essence and gem water.

Applications: cellulite, intestinal problems, neck tension, scars, numbness, muscle tension and, growth problems.

Tourmaline, Black

Forms: crystal (especially thin crystal sticks), crystal cluster, section/slice, cross section, (drilled) tumbled stone, bracelet, necklace, pendant, gem stone, gem essence and gem water.

Applications: stomach ache, bloatedness, intestinal problems, neck tension, scars, ear

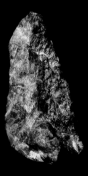

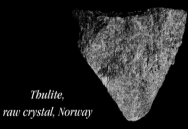

Thulite,
raw crystal, Norway

Sugilite, raw crystal,
South Africa

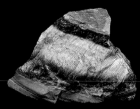

Tiger's Eye, raw crystal, South Africa

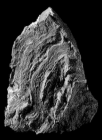

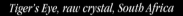

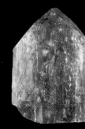

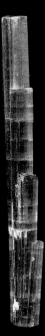

Tiger Iron, raw crystal, Australia

Imperial Topaz crystal, Brazil

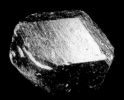

Tourmaline Dravite, Namibia

Tourmaline Indigolith,
Brazil

problems, back pain, sleep problems, pain, need for protection, numbness, muscle tension, constipation, growth problems, tick prophylaxis.

Tourmaline, Green

Forms: crystal, section/slice, cross section, (drilled) tumbled stone, bracelet, necklace, pendant, gem stone, gem essence and gem water.

Applications: eye diseases (general), detoxification, joint problems, hyperactivity, carpal tunnel syndrome, cancer, neck tension, scars, nerve problems, rheumatism, squinting, weak sightedness, synovitis, numbness, tennis elbow, ganglia, muscle tension, growth problems.

Tourmaline, Red

Forms: crystal, section/slice, cross section, (drilled) tumbled stone, bracelet, necklace, pendant, gem stone, gem essence and gem water.

Applications: eye diseases (general), lumbago, hyperactivity, knee problems, neck tension, scars, nerve problems, squinting, weak sightedness, pregnancy, numbness, muscle tension, growth problems.

Tourmaline, Watermelon

Watermelon Tourmalines have a red centre and a green coating.

Forms: crystal, section/slice, cross section, (drilled) tumbled stone, bracelet (rare), necklace, pendant, gem stone, gem essence and gem water.

Applications: eye diseases (general), heart problems, lumbago, neck tension, scars, nerve problems, squinting, weak sightedness, numbness, muscle tension, growth problems.

Turquoise

Forms: raw stone (lump), (drilled) tumbled stone, bracelet, necklace, pendant, gemstone, gem essence and gem water.

Applications: asthma, stomach ache, carpal tunnel syndrome, ear problems, rheumatism, a need for protection, heartburn, nausea and acidification.

Zircon

Forms: crystal (mostly double terminated), pendant, gem stone, gem essence and gem water.

Applications: stomach ache, cramp, strengthening of the liver, menstrual problems, pain.

Zoisite

Forms: (drilled) tumbled stone, bracelet, necklace, pendant, gemstone, gem essence and gem water.

Applications: colds, exhaustion, fertility (men), influenza, enlarged prostate, regeneration, psoriasis and growth problems.

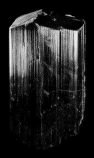

Tourmaline Black, Brazil

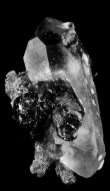

Watermelon Tourmaline, crystal on Quartz, Afghanistan

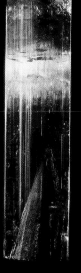

Tourmaline, Rubellite with Verdelith, Brazil

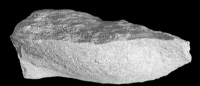

Turquoise, raw crystal, Arizona, USA

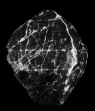

Zircon crystal, Brazil

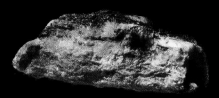

Zoisite with Ruby, Tanzania

Bibliography

Titles selected by the author, along with a brief summary of scope and contents.

Michael Gienger, *Die Heilsteine der Hildegard von Bingen*, Neue Erde Verlag, Saarbrücken, 2004.
Hildegard von Bingen's *Book of the Crystals* from the twelfth century; transcribed and annotated by Michael Gienger. Old wisdom for use with modern knowledge; a beautiful, practical book for the home about the art of crystal healing; lots of unique recipes.

Michael Gienger, *Crystal Power, Crystal Healing*, Cassell Octopus 1998.

Michael Gienger, Healing Crystals – *The A-Z Guide to 430 Gemstones*, Findhorn Press, 2005.
Small practical index and pocket-guide (only 98 pages, in postcard format); includes the important information about the most common healing crystals.

Michael Gienger, *Crystal Massage for Health and Healing*, Findhorn Press, 2006.
Massage with crystals; described by seven contributors as the most agreeable, beautiful and effective applications of crystal healing; includes techniques, methods and experiences with different kinds of crystal massage.

Other References and Research

The information and experience distilled into the pages of this book are based partly on as yet unpublished research by the following groups, societies and persons:

Cairn Elen Lebensschulen u. Steinheilkunde-Netzwerk
Experiences and reworking from this book's suggested treatments, etc.

Forschungsprojekt des Steinheilkunde e.V.
Empirical research on the effectiveness of crystal therapy (address see below)

Walter von Holst, Kornbergstr. 32, 70176, Stuttgart
Healing crystals for treatment of allergies, skin diseases; also some general research

Friedrich Pelz (Kontakt through Michael Gienger/Cairn Elen Lebensschule)
Effects of healing crystals on brain waves' research results of more than 3000 EEG-measurements.

Heilpraktiker Rainer Strebel, Schulstr. 22, 7361,4 Schorndorf
Comparisons of crystal healing, naturopathy and individual therapy

Dr. med Manfred Kuhnle, Heinzlenstr. 1, 72336, Balingen
Comparisons of biophysical medicine, homeopathy and traditional Chinese medicine.

Useful Addresses

Seminars and information
on crystal healing:

Cairn Elen Lebensschulen
Roßgumpenstr. 10
D-72336 Balingen-Zillhausen
Germany
Tel.: +49 7071 / 36 47 19
Fax: +49 7071 / 3 88 68
info@cairn-elen.de
www.cairn-elen.de

Research and consumer
protection:

Steinheilkunde e.V., Sitz Stuttgart
Forschungsprojekt Steinheilkunde
Unterer Kirchberg 23/1
D-88273 Fronreute
Germany
Tel.: +49 7505 / 95 64 51
Fax: +49 7505 / 95 64 52
info@steinheilkunde-ev.de
www.steinheilkunde-ev.de

Authenticity testing of gemstones:

The Gemmological Association
and Gem Testing Laboratory of Great Britain
27 Greville Street, London, EC1N 8TN
UK
Telephone: +44 (0)20 7404 3334
Fax: +44 (0)20 7404 8843
information@gem-a.info

AGTA Gemological Testing Center
18 East 48th Street, Suite 502
New York, NY 10017
USA
Tel: 212-752-1717
Fax: 212-750-0930
info@agta-gtc.org

Institut für Edelstein Prüfung (EPI)
Riesenwaldstr. 6
D-77797 Ohlsbach
Germany
Tel.: +49 7803/600808
Fax: +49 7803/600809
lab@epigem.de
www.epigem.de

General information on crystal healing:
www.steinheilkunde.de

Cairn Elen

After Elen had accomplished her wandering through the world, she placed a Cairn at the end of the Sarn Elen. Her path then led her back to the land between evening and morning. From this Cairn originated all stones that direct the way at crossroads up until today.[1]

(From a Celtic myth)

'Cairn Elen'* is the term used in Gaelic-speaking areas to refer to the ancient slab stones on track ways. They mark the spiritual paths, both the paths of the earth and that of knowledge.

These paths are increasingly falling into oblivion. Just as the old paths of the earth disappear under the modern asphalt streets, so also does certain ancient wisdom disappear under the data flood of modern information. For this reason, the desire and aim of the Edition Cairn Elen is to preserve ancient wisdom and link it with modern knowledge – for a flourishing future!

The Edition Cairn Elen in Neue Erde Verlag is published by Michael Gienger. The objective of the Edition is to present knowledge from research and tradition that has remained unpublished up until now. Areas of focus are nature, naturopathy and health as well as consciousness and spiritual freedom.

Apart from current specialised literature, stories, fairytales, novels, lyric and artistic publications will also be published within the scope of Edition Cairn Elen. The knowledge thus transmitted reaches out not only to the intellect but also to the heart.

Contact: Edition Cairn Elen, Michael Gienger, Stäudach 58/1, D-72074 Tübingen
Tel: +49 (0)70 71 - 364 719, Fax: +49 (0)70 71 - 388 68
buecher@michael-gienger.de, www.michael-gienger.de

[1]Celtic 'cairn' [pronounced: carn] = 'Stone' (usually placed as an intentional shaped heap of stones), 'sarn' = 'Path', 'Elen, Helen' = 'Goddess of the Roads'
*Cairn Elen: in British ancient and contemporary Celtic culture, cairns are generally intentionally heaped piles of stones, rather than an individual stone such as a boulder or standing stone.

For further information and book catalogue contact:
Findhorn Press, 305a The Park, Forres IV36 3TE, Scottland.
Earthdancer Books is an Imprint of Findhorn Press.

tel +44 (0)1309-690582   fax +44 (0)1309-690036
info@findhornpress.com   www.earthdancer.co.uk   www.findhornpress.com

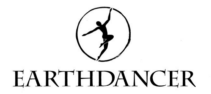

EARTHDANCER

A FINDHORN PRESS IMPRINT

The Healing Crystal First Aid Manual